D1413669

# How to Get Pregnant

# How to Get Pregnant

Sherman J. Silber, M.D.

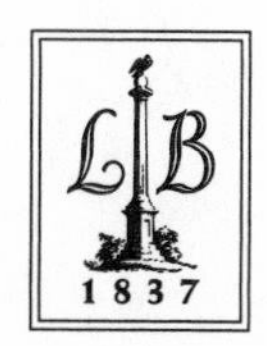


Little, Brown and Company
New York • Boston

Little, Brown and Company
Time Warner Book Group
1271 Avenue of the Americas, New York, NY 10020
Visit our Web site at www.twbookmark.com

Revised Edition: September 2005

The information herein is not intended to replace the services of a trained health care professional. You are advised to consult with a health care professional with regard to matters relating to your health, and in particular regarding matters that may require diagnosis or medical attention.

Library of Congress Cataloging-in-Publication Data
Silber, Sherman J.
How to get pregnant / Sherman J. Silber. — Rev. ed.
p. cm.
Includes bibliographical references and index.
ISBN 0-316-01136-3
1. Infertility — Popular works. 2. Human reproductive technology — Popular works. I. Title.

RC889.S52 2005
616.6'92 — dc22 2005002585

10 9 8 7 6 5 4 3 2 1

Q-MART
Book design by Fearn Cutler deVicq
Printed in the United States of America

To the faithful, hardworking staff at my office and at St. Luke's Hospital in St. Louis, Missouri. For three decades they have acted as tireless workers, organized scientific and medical personnel, and concerned, warm counselors to my patients. The many advances we have made would not have been possible without their exceptional dedication.

I would also like to thank basic research scientists all over the world, with whom I have worked closely, who helped to make much of this clinical progress possible. Some of those who have been especially helpful include: Dr. Frank Barnes, Dr. Keith Campbell, Dr. Jacques Cohen, Dr. Jan DeVries, Dr. Paul Devroey, Dr. Robert Edwards, Dr. Kevin Eggan, Dr. Malcolm Faddy, Dr. Bart Fauser, Dr. David Gardner, Dr. Roger Gosden, Dr. Jamie Grifo, Dr. Alan Handyside, Dr. Marc Hughes, Dr. Rob Jansen, Dr. Hubert Joris, Dr. William Keye, Dr. Jacob Levron, Dr. Willy Lissens, Dr. Jaeon Liu, Dr. Shlomo Mashiach, Dr. Colin Mathews, Dr. David Miller, Dr. Santiago Munne, Dr. Peter Nagy, Dr. David Page, Dr. Rusty Pool, Dr. Sjoerd Repping, Dr. Steve Rozen, Dr. Gerald Schatten, Dr. Karen Sermon, Dr. Roger Short, Dr. Cal Simerly, Dr. Helen Skaletsky, Dr. Andre Speirs, Dr. Catherine Staessen, Dr. Andrew Van Steirteghem, Dr. Yuri Verlinsky, Dr. Leandra Wilton, Dr. Robert Winston, and Dr. John Zhang.

I would also like to thank Michael Pietsch, Jack Galaska, and Susan Richman for starting me on my writing career; Bill Sarnoff, Larry Kirshbaum, and Susan Suffes for nurturing my writing over several decades; Liz Nagle for guiding me through this book; and copyeditor Shannon Langone. Finally, I wish to thank Julie Heintzelman for helping with the manuscript preparation, and Bill Andrea and Jen McCurdy for the illustrations.

— Dr. Sherman Silber
Infertility Center of St. Louis
St. Louis, Missouri
USA
www.infertile.com
314-576-1400

# Contents

PREFACE

# The Infertility Epidemic

We are in the midst of a worldwide epidemic of infertility. Ironically, even in countries with severe overpopulation, one of the most common reasons for a visit to the doctor is the inability to have children. Twenty-five percent of modern couples in their midthirties are infertile. From our teen years (when the last thing we really want is a child) to our midthirties (when we finally feel emotionally and financially secure enough to start a family), there is a twenty-five-fold decline in our ability to get pregnant. Let me explain.

Infertility is defined as the inability to conceive despite one year of regular intercourse (without birth control). The incidence of infertility in teenagers is rare. For women in their early twenties, only 1 to 2 percent are infertile. In their late twenties, 16 percent of women are infertile, and in their mid- to late thirties, 25 percent are infertile. By age forty, more than half of women are infertile, and pregnancy beyond age forty-three is very uncommon. If you are in your thirties, have been working hard to establish yourself, and are now just casually thumbing through this chapter at a local bookstore because you're thinking maybe in a few years you might like to start a family, you should realize that there is a 25 percent chance you will not be able to do so without medical intervention.

These startling figures originally came from the National Center for Health Statistics and were presented to the United States Congress through a panel assembled by the Congressional Office of Technology Assessment in 1988. I was one of five physicians on that Congressional Advisory Panel. We had witnessed an explosive increase since the 1970s in the number of couples desperately struggling to have a child, but it wasn't until these statistics were formally assembled that we were stunned to find out just how staggering the problem was. What accounts for this dramatic increase in infertility over the last forty years? It is apparent that a woman's biological clock is the major reason for this huge increase, because couples are delaying the age at which they try to conceive from their early twenties until their mid- to late thirties.

We could speculate about other causes: the increase in sexually transmitted diseases, environmental pollution, declining sperm count from absorption of toxic substances, and even the increased tension and anxiety of modern life. These may be modestly contributing factors, but the major reason is simply that by the time the modern couple decides to have children, usually in their thirties, the human animal is just not as fertile as it was fifteen years earlier.

I have spent some time studying aboriginal societies, most recently the Hadzi bushmen, a forty-thousand-year-old hunter-gatherer culture in a remote region of western Tanzania. These people own nothing, sleep outside without any hut or tent, and lead a tenuous existence. They marry at age thirteen or fourteen, have children, and usually die in their thirties. I asked them about infertility, and they had never heard of such a thing. Some women might stop bearing children in their mid- to late twenties, but every woman was apparently able to have children. The biology of fertility in humans has not changed in the last forty thousand years. What has changed in the last few centuries is our life span and the age at which we first try to conceive.

One of the views of the Congressional Advisory Panel (which consisted of lawyers, psychologists, sociologists, and religious leaders as well as doctors) was that society clearly benefited from people putting off childbearing until their thirties. Both men and women are now able to obtain fuller educations, develop themselves in their careers, and contribute dramatically to the intellectual and economic prosperity of the modern world. This would not occur so readily if we were saddled with children as teenagers or in our early twenties. So if society is collectively making a decision to delay childbearing, it should be no one's position to advise couples patronizingly just to "hurry up" and have children when they're young.

With dramatic new technology, virtually any couple (with a few exceptions) can have a child. But you must understand the myriad complexities of your reproductive system in order to get the right help instead of the wrong help, and to deal with the emotional and financial costs the process might cause if you are not savvy. Most important, you need to understand your biological clock and how to manage it. My intention in this book is (1) to teach you how to manage your biological clock so that you won't need technology to get pregnant, and (2) to explain how you can use technology safely to get pregnant if that is currently your only option.

## The Importance of Understanding Your Biological Clock

In the *New York Times Magazine* in December of 1989, a forty-one-year-old writer named Paulette conveyed her sense of loss at trying to have a child in her late thirties, not succeeding, and now finding herself a successful forty-one-year-old writer who, sadly, "will probably never have a baby." It wasn't until she reached age thirty-eight that she decided to stop using birth control pills and try to get pregnant. She had read an ill-conceived book and hoped she could get pregnant naturally after learning more about the timing of her cycle and the quality of her cervical mucus. She did not understand her biological clock. It wasn't until she reached forty that she saw a local doctor who began fertility testing, including mucus testing, hormone testing, and two endometrial biopsies (a tiny piece of the uterine lining is tested to see if it is capable of sustaining a pregnancy). None of this plodding got her any closer to getting pregnant.

She was then given a final diagnosis of "luteal phase defect." This was a very popular diagnosis twenty years ago, and many women were treated with progesterone supplementation in the second half of their cycle in an effort to "overcome" this problem. That is worthless treatment. Later she was given a mild ovulatory stimulant pill, Clomid, because of the view that luteal phase defect "might be" caused by a subtle ovulation defect. But she had no way of knowing that her biological clock was too far along for Clomid to be of any use. She then went through a procedure called intrauterine insemination, in which her husband's sperm was placed directly inside her uterus even though previous testing had shown that her cervical mucus was quite able to allow his sperm to penetrate on its own. These are simple, old methods of treatment that sometimes work and might possibly make sense in a young woman trying to have a baby. But not for Paulette.

In fact, what Paulette went through is the conventional approach of trying to make a diagnosis and then using simple, noninvasive treatment appropriate to that diagnosis. The problem with this conventional view is that (1) many of these "diagnoses" are just normal variants that have nothing to do with why the woman is not getting pregnant, and (2) if a woman's time has almost run out, fiddling around for too long with the old-fashioned approaches may waste the few precious years she has left. We now have simple testing that could have told her (when she was younger) just when her particular clock would expire and let her decide (while there was still time left) when to stop procrastinating.

Physicians simply have to admit that we often really don't know why a couple isn't getting pregnant except that the wife is nearing the edge of her biological clock. Of course, a low sperm count in the husband, tubal obstruction, lesions in the uterine lining, and poor ovulation can all contribute to infertility, and all of those problems can be solved. But the biggest problem for a thirty-eight-year-old woman is simply her age. Some women lose their fertility in their twenties and others not until their forties. This book will explain how you can gauge your own biological clock, and if you are too late for that, how you can nonetheless still get pregnant with the proper treatment. But the forty-one-year-old writer of that sad *New York Times* article, in 1989, did not have the availability of this knowledge.

Years ago I celebrated New Year's with our son's high school biology teacher and his thirty-nine-year-old wife, Pam, and their six-week-old baby, who never would have existed without IVF. Pam told me to make sure to tell everyone in this book how awful it is to go through the conventional series of "diagnostic" tests and ineffective treatments for years and years with one contradictory diagnosis after another. She had gone through seven years of this at the previous clinic she had used. She had two laparoscopic operations to remove tiny little spots of "endometriosis" and never got a satisfactory answer to her question of how her mother could have had five children despite much worse "endometriosis." When surgery for endometriosis didn't help, Pam was placed on progesterone because her doctors suddenly discovered luteal phase defect. Later she was given Clomid as well. She had been through literally hundreds of pills, shots, doctors' visits, and tests, not to mention worthless and potentially damaging surgery.

Pam and her husband finally came to me, and after a twenty-minute interview with them, I told her that I really didn't know why she wasn't getting pregnant. But she was in her late thirties and that was enough reason for them to be infertile; I recommended *no more tests.* She was thrilled when I suggested we proceed right to what was then the "new" technology of IVF. She was fed up with trying to figure out why she was infertile and getting nowhere.

Pam conceived with the IVF procedure, and she and her husband had a healthy baby, who is now a healthy teenager. She has no idea why she was infertile and neither do her original doctors, who spent so much of her money on wild-goose chases. For Pam it was not too late. She had the common, "undiagnosable" age-related decline in fertility of women in their thirties. But at least she had an adequate supply of remaining eggs for IVF to work.

## Misleading Diagnoses of the Cause of Your Infertility

### *The Simple, Unexplainable Effect of Age*

Even in the best-conditioned athletes, age has a way of slowing us down, sometimes imperceptibly year by year, and it doesn't mean that there is any particular physical ailment or diagnosis to explain that slowdown. This is usually (though, of course, not always) the case in a couple who tries unsuccessfully to have babies in their midthirties.

In 1982, the French reported in the *New England Journal of Medicine* a large study of 2,193 "normal" women (whose husbands had no sperm whatsoever in their ejaculate) undergoing artificial insemination with fertile donor sperm. These were "normal" women and they were being inseminated with completely normal sperm. There is no logical reason why they shouldn't all have gotten pregnant. Yet it was very clear that the "normal" women under thirty had a high pregnancy rate, and the "normal" women over thirty showed decreasing pregnancy rates as they got older. A study from Ontario published seven years later in the *Journal of Fertility and Sterility* looked at more than two thousand couples with "unexplained" infertility. The chances of getting pregnant with simple, conventional methods of treatment were directly related to how young the woman was. No other factor studied was significant except for the age of the woman.

The decline in fertility as women get older is related to the aging of their eggs. You are born with all the eggs you will ever have, about two hundred thousand to four hundred thousand by the time of puberty, and every month about a thousand of them die. Thus as you get older, your eggs will decrease in both number and quality. Yet some women remain fertile into their forties, and others lose their fertility in their twenties. Chapter 3 of this book shows you how to determine at what particular age you will lose your fertility, so that you can plan to avoid Paulette's dilemma.

A woman I first saw in 1990 is typical of many I see every week. Tammy got pregnant very easily as a young teenager after her first sexual experience and gave the child up for adoption. Five years later, again she got pregnant quite easily and kept this baby as a single mother. She continued to have completely regular, normal periods for six more years, got married, and then used condoms for birth control for three years until she and her husband were certain that their marriage was a stable one. By the time they finally decided to try to have children, she was thirty-three years old, and her menstrual cycles had become irregular, varying from twenty-five to thirty-two days. All of her tests were normal, but now she couldn't get pregnant.

What happened to her subsequently is a terrifying story that exemplifies the pitfalls I am hoping to help you avoid with this book. She saw a doctor who diagnosed her as having "endometriosis" and "adhesions," despite the fact that her organs were quite normal. He performed major surgery to remove the endometriosis and release the adhesions. This completely unnecessary and painful surgery only served to reduce her remaining supply of eggs even further, making it even harder for her to get pregnant.

As long as insurance companies require a "pathological diagnosis" in order to pay for treatment, and as long as major surgery results in no difficulty in getting insurance payment (whereas in vitro fertilization usually is not covered), women like Tammy run a good chance of being mistreated in this fashion.

### *The Endometriosis Myth*

The most commonly overused "diagnosis" for infertility is endometriosis. Endometriosis is a condition whereby some of the lining of the uterus has leaked back into the abdominal cavity and has implanted in tiny nodules either in the abdominal wall, on the outside of the fallopian tube, or possibly in the ovary. When doctors perform a laparoscopy as part of an infertility investigation to see if the woman has a normal uterus, tubes, and ovaries, most of the time the examination is normal. Nonetheless the diagnosis of "endometriosis" is frequently inserted in the operative note simply because the insurance company is much happier to pay for laparoscopy when they see a "pathological" diagnosis, and doctors feel more comfortable that way. The euphemism that avoids outright deception is to call it "minimal lesion" endometriosis. Doctors are often so eager to find a diagnosis to determine the "cause" of infertility (not to mention the desire for patients to get insurance reimbursement) that many couples walk out of their long series of expensive infertility tests thinking incorrectly that they now know why they haven't gotten pregnant. This might be harmless if it weren't for the fact that it may lead to unnecessary or improper treatment, and could delay further the proper treatment. With infertility in older women, any delay caused by foolish treatments is devastating.

### *The Male Factor and Varicocele Myth*

There are many other popular "diagnoses" that may lead to inappropriate treatment. The doctor may obtain a sperm count on the husband and find that it is "low." The husband may then be put on all kinds of totally ineffective drug treatments such as Clomid, Pergonal, human chorionic gonadotropin, or testosterone. But worst of all, he may be given that all too common diagnosis of "varicocele." Very few men escape seeing a urologist for infertility without suffering through this diagnosis.

A varicocele is a varicose vein of the testicle (usually on the left side) that is present in 15 percent of all males on the planet. It is just a common, normal anatomic variant, but it has been argued that 40 percent of infertile men have varicoceles, and it is implied, therefore, that varicocele is the cause of the infertility. But most of these so-called minimal lesion varicoceles are not really varicoceles at all, and are no different from what is found in a normal, fertile male population.

The varicocele has little to do with male infertility. A careful study from Australia of 651 infertile men with varicocele was published in the *British Medical Journal* in 1985 demonstrating absolutely no difference in pregnancy rate among couples in which the husband had the varicocele operated on versus those who did not have the varicocele operated on. Similar studies have been repeated in Belgium, Sweden, and Germany. Furthermore, 15 percent of men who request a vasectomy (because they already have had all the children they want) are found on physical examination to have an obvious varicocele, and in my experience, that is the same as the incidence of varicocele in infertile males.

What happens to infertile couples once the diagnosis of varicocele is made in the man? Typically, the men get operated on, sometimes on one side, sometimes on both sides, and then they wait six months to see if the sperm count improves. Since sperm counts, like the weather, vary from month to month around a mean average value, it only makes sense that if you get one or two sperm counts before this unnecessary surgery, and one or two sperm counts after this unnecessary surgery, at least half of the men will appear to have some improvement. But this is just an illusion created by the variability of sperm counts, and the failure to make equal note of those whose sperm counts seem to have actually gone down after varicocelectomy. Because of the intrinsic variability of sperm counts, half of the patients will appear to have reduced counts after treatment, and half will appear to have improved counts.

Furthermore, many couples can conceive naturally in spite of the husband's very low sperm count. Manuel and Flora were a couple from South America who were married twenty-two years earlier, when she was only seventeen years old. Four years later she became pregnant and had a wonderful little baby boy, but she was never able to become pregnant again. A sperm count performed in their local city was zero. It wasn't until eighteen years later, when Flora was thirty-nine years old and Manuel was forty-five, that they came to see me in St. Louis, and the enigma was solved. Manuel had zero sperm on the first semen analysis; however, after performing many semen analyses over a period of time, we finally found a few rare motile sperm on just one of those occasions. Testicle biopsy revealed that almost the entire testicle was nonfunctioning, except for a tiny island of normal sperm-producing tubules. Obviously, when Flora was very young, at age twenty-one, after four years of regular intercourse, a single sperm from Manuel was finally able to fertilize one of her eggs, resulting in a baby boy. As she became older, however, Manuel's extremely severe infertility, compounded by the naturally decreasing quality of her eggs, made this couple infertile.

## IVF and ICSI Bypass Everything That Can Go Wrong No Matter What the So-called Diagnosis Is

In vitro fertilization (IVF) and intracytoplasmic sperm injection (ICSI) solve the quandary presented by our frequent ignorance of why couples are not getting pregnant. Whatever the diagnosis, the wife's biological clock is the only thing that matters. If the cause of infertility really is low sperm count, the sperm can be microinjected directly into the egg. If the cause of the problem is poor ovulation, the hormonal stimulation and aspiration of eggs from the ovaries removes the need for ovulation. If the issue is poor cervical mucus blocking the entrance of sperm into the womb, these new technologies can bypass that problem as well. If the problem is endometriosis (a highly questionable but very popular diagnosis), again IVF overcomes the unfavorable environment for fertilization that endometriosis supposedly creates in the woman's pelvis. If the problem is poor pickup of the egg by the fallopian tube from the surface of the ovary (a tricky feat in which the fallopian tube has to "reach over" and grab the egg by twisting back on itself), IVF, as well as gamete intrafallopian transfer (GIFT), once again bypasses this event.

Almost anything that can go wrong during the arduous process that sperm and eggs normally have to go through can be bypassed with IVF and ICSI. If the couple is committed to several treatment cycles, and the woman is not too far along on her biological clock, most will get pregnant no matter what the diagnosis and no matter how severe the problem.

### *Change in Thinking Since the Early 1980s*

Much has changed since I wrote the first edition of *How to Get Pregnant* more than twenty-five years ago. We know now that it is a complete waste of time and money for the man to have surgery for varicocele or for the woman to endure a year of Lupron therapy to shrink her endometriosis. We know that treatment of the husband with Clomid or Pergonal and various other drugs will do nothing to increase his sperm count. We understand now more fully just how people do and don't get pregnant, and what is the best strategy for overcoming infertility.

Paulette does not have to waste her few valuable remaining years of potential fertility testing her mucus and wondering whether she's having sex at the right time. Tammy, who got pregnant easily as a teenager and now in her late thirties is happily married and wants a child, does not have to go through unnecessary surgery for endometriosis. We can avoid the emotional drain of literally years of fruitless testing and slingshot-style therapy.

Very often, by the time a couple has gone through years and years of wasted, inappropriate infertility treatments, they're worn out, their funds are absolutely exhausted, and they can't even consider IVF, which would have been so much more likely to have helped them. Cynthia is a thirty-two-year-old woman whose husband underwent two varicocelectomies and who herself was treated for infertility for ten years with Clomid, artificial insemination, several laparoscopies, and several operations to "lyse her adhesions," despite the fact that the cause of her infertility all these years had been completely idiopathic (that means we just don't know the cause). Although she would have a 50 percent chance for pregnancy with each treatment attempt with IVF, she is just too tired, frustrated, and emotionally depressed to go any further. My hope is that this book will give couples the understanding and confidence to know when they can safely temporize, or whether technology like IVF is more appropriate for them to utilize now, before they have exhausted their emotions, time, and resources.

## Progress in Male Infertility

In the early 1990s, the major stumbling block to treatment of infertile couples was the severely infertile male. In about 50 percent of infertile couples, there is a somewhat low sperm count, and in 10 percent the count is extremely low. In such cases, even IVF had routinely failed in the past. There was simply no effective treatment available for the infertile male. That all changed dramatically after 1993, thanks to the pioneering work on sperm retrieval and ICSI performed by Dr. Andre Van Steirteghem, Dr. Paul Devroey, and me, shuttling back and forth between Brussels, Belgium, and St. Luke's Hospital in St. Louis. The work of this team has revolutionized the treatment of male infertility throughout the world and represents the single greatest advance in fertility treatment since the first IVF baby in 1978. Now it is possible to search for just a few sperm in the male ejaculate, and if there is no sperm in the ejaculate, often a few can be found in the testicle. We can then inject a single sperm into each of the female's eggs (ICSI). With this delicate technique, we achieve pregnancy rates for virtually sterile men that are no different from that of men with normal sperm counts. There are now very few cases of severe male infertility that cannot thus be successfully treated.

ICSI (sperm injection) is explained in detail in chapter 11, but essentially this is how the technique works: With ultramicromanipulative instruments attached to special microscopes, the woman's otherwise invisible egg can actually be held secure with a microscope "holding" pipette, and an even tinier micropipette can be used to inject a sperm through the hard outer shell of the egg so that this one sperm is literally forced to fertilize the egg. Can you imagine the delicacy of this type of manipulation? The sperm head is no more than 4 to 6 microns in diameter (that's approximately 1/4,000 of an inch), and an egg is approximately 100 microns in diameter (1/200 of an inch). It took years of painstaking research in Brussels and in St. Louis to perfect it.

One of the biggest fears of those of us who were working on microinjection of sperm was that if the sperm couldn't get into the egg because of poor numbers or poor motility, abnormal shape, or poor maturation, then perhaps they weren't meant to get in. Perhaps it was naive to think that if such a poor sperm were injected into the egg, the chromosomes would be normal, and that a healthy baby could be obtained from such a procedure. Those fears proved to be completely wrong.

Even poor sperm have normal DNA sufficient for making a normal baby, and the only thing wrong with poor sperm (with an occasional exception) is simply that they cannot get into the egg. The incredible complexity of sperm physiology, which will be discussed later in this book, appears to serve no purpose other than to mechanically get the package of DNA that the sperm contains into the egg. Once that package of DNA is inserted into the egg, all the processes of fertilization and embryo formation leading to a baby can take care of themselves.

### *Even Men Who Don't Make Sperm Can Have Children*

In 1985, a young couple, both twenty-two years of age, from New York, came to see me in St. Louis because he had azoospermia (no sperm in the ejaculate) and needed a testicle biopsy to see whether he had an obstruction that could be corrected with microsurgery. In those days, we always prayed that the biopsy would show normal sperm production, because our success rate with microsurgery to correct obstruction in male infertility was over 95 percent. But we could do nothing at that time for couples if the men weren't making sperm at all.

His biopsy revealed what we call "maturation arrest." This means that the early precursors for sperm production were present in the testicle, but there was no continuation of sperm production beyond these early stages. This man was by all definitions 100 percent sterile, and it was my unfortunate job to explain to this otherwise wide-eyed, cheerful young couple (who were looking forward so much to having a family) that they couldn't have children.

But this couple never gave up hope. Ten years later, they came back after they had heard about ICSI. By now we were having exciting success in using ICSI for men with extremely poor sperm counts, and in men with irreparable obstruction requiring retrieval of testicular sperm from a blocked but otherwise normally functioning testicle. But could it possibly work for men who were apparently not making any sperm at all? This determined couple helped us embark upon a new theory with startling consequences.

When I had looked back to my research from the early 1980s on quantitative testicle biopsy, I discovered a phenomenon that had previously eluded my attention. Even in men with zero sperm in the ejaculate, and apparently no sperm production, if one looked carefully throughout the testicular specimens, an occasional sperm precursor could be found that had the same number of chromosomes and the same basic appearance as a normal sperm. Based on this finding, this couple was our first case of a man who appeared to be making no sperm but in whom we were able to find just a few sperm "hiding" in his testicles. We injected these hidden sperm into his wife's eggs, and normal fertilization occurred. They now have a happy baby girl.

Another patient treated around the same time had, as a child, undescended testicles that were brought down surgically into the scrotum very late in his childhood. As is often the case with such men, he was clearly producing no sperm. When we operated on his testes to see if any sperm could be found (under the same theory, that any man with a testicle may have some sperm somewhere), indeed we were again able to find just a few sperm. We injected his wife's eggs with those testicular sperm and again obtained normal fertilization and pregnancy. This young man had been known to be sterile ever since he was a teenager. Yet during extensive exploration of his testicles, we found sufficient sperm to perform ICSI, and he could have a normal family.

The question that might occur to every such couple is, will my baby be normal? The fear might arise that abnormal sperm in men with low sperm counts will cause a higher risk of producing abnormal babies. We have now studied this in over seven thousand such children born through the ICSI procedure as we performed it, and the news is great.

The children are normal, and there is no greater incidence of chromosomal or congenital abnormalities than in the children of normally fertile couples conceiving without any kind of reproductive treatment. There may be occasional exceptions, but they are related to the age of the wife, not the IVF or ICSI treatment. The offspring are more likely to be infertile (like their parents) but are otherwise normal, healthy children.

Poor sperm production represents up to half of the infertility cases in the world, and in the past it prompted couples to undergo billions of dollars's worth of ineffective, unscientific, and frankly stupid surgical and hormonal treatment. ICSI now solves that problem in most couples, but a genetic cure would still be preferable. Our research, in conjunction with the human genome project, the Howard Hughes Institute at MIT, and the University of Amsterdam, thus far indicates that sperm production in men is controlled genetically by many different genes on the Y chromosome and elsewhere in the genome. We have now completely sequenced the Y chromosome and have located the areas on the Y chromosome where sperm production in these men is regulated, and we have identified many of the genes that control spermatogenesis. This discovery means that in the future we may have a genetic cure for male infertility, i.e., replacing the missing gene or genes so that men will be able to resume normal spermatogenesis, thereby eliminating the need for ICSI.

## Egg Donation

With the advent of ICSI, there is now only an occasional need for donor sperm, but there is still a strong need for donor eggs. It is my hope that women who read this book and learn how to plot their own biological clock will be able to avoid having to resort to egg donation by planning their life more knowledgeably. However, an older woman who has already run out of her own supply of fertile eggs can still get pregnant (using her husband's sperm, of course) with embryos derived from the eggs of a younger woman. Egg donation is much more readily accepted emotionally by couples than sperm donation, because the woman still gets to carry and deliver the baby. Because the woman carries the baby, emotional bonding is rarely adversely affected by its being a donor egg. Follow-up on the children who have resulted from egg donation, and on their parents, is wonderful. These are really happy families.

The question, whose baby is it? creeps into every aspect of egg donation, gestational surrogacy, and adoption controversies. Adopting eggs, i.e., using donated eggs, is much more secure for the infertile couple than struggling beyond struggle and traveling around the world to try to find a baby to adopt (a baby that could possibly be taken away in the future) at enormous cost. With donor eggs, which are legally recognized in every state, there is no risk (as with adoption) that the egg donor could ever interfere or lay claim to the child or to the embryos. I will discuss the issue of bonding and the question of whose child it is in chapters 16 and 17.

Even a woman without a uterus can have a child. It is possible for her mother, a very close friend, or a sister to carry her biological child for her and then give that child back to her after the delivery. This is called gestational surrogacy. It is possible to arrange legal adoption from the surrogate even before the delivery. These procedures are medically and legally extremely safe and reliable.

In the mid-1980s, I saw a lovely woman who had undergone surgery by a well-meaning gynecologist for severe pelvic adhesions (scarring) caused by previous infections. If I were to see a woman with such severe adhesions in the pelvis, I wouldn't even think about doing surgery — we would go straight to IVF. However, the surgeon who explored her decided to try to release the adhesions on her fallopian tubes and ovaries. Unfortunately, the doctor performing the surgery got into some problems with bleeding that were beyond his ability to handle, and the only way he could solve the dilemma was by removing the woman's uterus (she was only twenty-five years of age). The doctor who removed her uterus did not feel the sense of tragedy he should have, because he was not aware that this woman could have gotten pregnant easily with IVF without ever attempting that hopeless operation to open her completely cemented-down tubes and ovaries. If this woman had only known that all she needed in order to get pregnant with IVF was a uterus, she might have avoided this foolhardy operation, gone to a proper IVF program, and had her baby.

Miraculously, four years later, I called this woman back to tell her what, at the time, seemed absolutely incredible: that she could have a baby after all, even without her uterus. We could use her eggs and her husband's sperm and put the fertilized embryo into her own mother's uterus. Then, nine months later, her mother would give her newly delivered baby back to her. We have helped many women who have no uterus, or for whom pregnancy would be dangerous, have their babies this way. In many cases, their mother carried their baby, and in other cases, a sister, an aunt, or a close friend. Thus, a mother can give birth to her own grandchildren, and a sister can give birth to her own nieces and nephews.

## Can You Save Your Eggs for Later?

Although human embryos can be successfully frozen and thawed, and can result in happy, healthy babies, unfertilized eggs, until very recently, could not be very successfully frozen and thawed. The success rate in freezing eggs had always been very low, but this is changing. For young female cancer patients, whose ovaries would surely be destroyed by heavy chemotherapy and radiation, we can now remove an ovary, freeze it, and save it to be grafted back to the woman after she has been cured of the cancer. Both egg and ovary freezing might also help women who feel a need to delay childbearing until their late thirties and forties, by which time their egg supply will very likely have been depleted. These are options for the woman who wants her own genetic child but does not anticipate starting a family for many years.

For many years we have been able to use cryogenic technology to freeze and store embryos derived from IVF in order that women not have to risk having a dangerous multiple pregnancy. The embryos can be thawed safety at a later date, and the pregnancy rate with these frozen embryos is still very high. That is nothing new. We have been able to do this since 1983, and long-term follow-up shows no deleterious effect on subsequent offspring. In fact, young couples who are happily married, but want to put off childbearing until later, can readily have their embryos (derived from the husband's sperm and the wife's eggs) frozen and saved for later so that they do not sacrifice their chances for later parenthood.

However, freezing embryos for a future date does *not* solve the problem for unmarried women who want to have children in the future but have not yet met the right man. For these women, freezing their unfertilized eggs, or even an entire ovary, would be the ideal solution. Until very recently, this holy grail of IVF was unattainable. The reason is that in order for fertilizable eggs to be retrieved, they must be in a mature state of development, with a complex alignment of chromosomes, and this makes them susceptible to even the slightest ice-crystal damage. However, with a fairly simple new technique called vitrification, recently refined in Japan, ice-crystal formation is avoided completely, and early results indicate that high pregnancy rates may be achieved with frozen eggs. Thus, a woman who knows that she is nearing a time when she will lose her fertility because of her biologic clock can freeze her eggs, or an ovary, and have her babies later.

In St. Louis, we have now demonstrated for the first time that an entire ovary can be removed and then grafted back after freezing and thawing so that even a menopausal woman can gain back her youthful fertility many years later. This new capability will be especially important to women undergoing treatment for cancer, because all the eggs that might have been lost to chemotherapy can be preserved by first removing and freezing the ovary.

If you are considering freezing your unfertilized eggs, or one of your ovaries, the best approach is to first determine just where you are on your biological clock so that you can know when it's time to worry. You can now monitor your own biological clock from your early twenties on, so you can decide when you ought to try to have a baby naturally. I will show you exactly how you can do this in chapter 3 of this book. If you find out that your biological clock is more advanced than you feel comfortable with, you now have the additional alternative of freezing an ovary or eggs and saving them until you are ready.

## How Can I Be Sure My Baby Will Be Normal?

Why is the egg of an aging female less likely to result in a pregnancy and more likely to result in miscarriage or an abnormal baby than that of a younger woman? Why is it that a young egg placed in an older woman results in a high pregnancy rate, while an egg from an older woman results in an extremely low pregnancy rate? How can we now prevent Down syndrome, or other genetic diseases, without the need for amniocentesis and pregnancy terminations? It's all in the DNA.

In this book, I will explain, in terms you can fully understand, the emergence of DNA technology, and how it can ensure that you have a healthy baby. Otherwise fertile couples who are carriers of genetic diseases such as Tay-Sachs, cystic fibrosis, retinitis pigmentosa, hemophilia, and so on, can now use this technology to be assured that they will have normal children. We can easily screen couples for such genetic risks before they ever decide to have children, and if they have such a risk, preimplantation evaluation of the embryos can save them from having a child who would otherwise die or be handicapped with severe defects.

Several years ago, a twenty-seven-year-old woman with Marfan's disease (inherited from her father) came to my office with her fiancé. She was told quite correctly by her doctors that a pregnancy could easily be fatal to her because of her condition (which results in a weakened main blood vessel in the chest and leaky heart valves). She was about to be married the following year, and she came in with her mother and father, proposing that her mother be a surrogate and carry her baby via IVF. She was surprised when we told her that not only could her mother be a surrogate and carry her baby, but that as long as we were doing IVF anyway, we could test her embryos (derived from her eggs and her husband's sperm) before placing them in her mother, and transfer only the healthy ones. Thus, not only could we allow this woman to have a child via IVF, but also we could assure her of having a baby that would not carry her disease.

Most patients who had previously delivered a child with Down syndrome or had elected to have such a pregnancy terminated simply would not ever try again to get pregnant and undergo the risk of enduring this agony once more. Even patients with cystic fibrosis, who are managing to survive with modern medical treatment, tell us that they don't want their baby to have cystic fibrosis. Using IVF, we can test their embryos and put back only the healthy ones, thereby avoiding these heart-wrenching problems. For obvious ethical reasons, the unhealthy but viable embryos can be frozen and saved for a future date when gene therapy would be able to correct the genetic defect.

There are many couples in their twenties and early thirties who are married and committed to each other, but just don't want children yet. But they are afraid to put off having children into their late thirties or early forties for two reasons: (1) They are afraid that with their biological clock ticking, they will not be able to have children if they wait another ten years, and (2) they are afraid that if they do get pregnant later they will be in an age category where this poses a high risk of abnormal embryos and chromosomal defects in their children, for reasons I will explain in chapter 12. These couples can undergo IVF while they are still young and have their embryos successfully frozen and stored. At a later date, the embryos can be thawed, and the wife can get pregnant even when she is older, with no increased risk of Down syndrome. Alternatively, they can have the wife's ovarian reserve tested (see chapter 3) and can then make a more informed decision about when they should actually begin to try to have children naturally.

## Achieving Pregnancy Without the New Technology

Do not misinterpret the focus of what I am saying. It is better to avoid the need for infertility treatment, and in this book, I will give you tools for doing just that.

In one couple who had been infertile for many years, the wife ovulated perfectly on day fourteen of every twenty-eight-day cycle like clockwork. In fact, because her ovulatory cycle was so perfect and so regular, she always ovulated on Tuesday or Wednesday. Her husband, who was a traveling workaholic businessman, was only in town on the weekends, so for years they never got pregnant simply because they were having sex only on the weekends. A simple rescheduling of their intercourse resulted in her getting pregnant rather quickly without any high technology. But simple approaches like this only work if you have not yet reached the descending point in your biological clock.

One lady begged me to review her case even though she and her husband could not travel to our clinic in St. Louis. At that time, we were estimating the quality and time of ovulation from basal body temperature (BBT) charts (rather than ultrasound and simple leutinizing hormone [LH] urine testing). Her BBT charts clearly showed poor ovulation, but her doctor had insisted on not treating her because he felt the husband's low sperm count was the problem. In fact, the local urologist had put the husband on the male hormone testosterone, which would make his muscles bigger but would certainly lower rather than raise his sperm count. After her husband discontinued these steroids and she went on Clomid, she promptly became pregnant. I still receive a Christmas card every year from her despite the fact that we never met. There are countless similar stories in which very simple approaches work, but only if you learn about your own particular fertility clock.

The problem of infertility in our modern society is getting worse, and the simpler methods do not work well for older would-be parents. These simpler methods should be discontinued after they have been shown to be ineffective for a couple, and the newer technology should be used before too much time, energy, emotion, and money have been wasted on old-fashioned approaches. However, it is my hope that by knowing where you are on your own biological clock, you will be able to have your family naturally, without having to resort to the high technology.

## Where Do We Go for Help?

How do you decide where to go for help with infertility? When our U.S. Congressional Advisory Panel met back in 1988, we amassed figures that showed that of 150 IVF clinics in the United States, half of them had never achieved a pregnancy at all. Furthermore, of those that achieved pregnancies, the success rate varied from extremely low (less than 5 percent) to reasonably high (greater than 30 percent). Evaluating the quality of the clinics was an extremely muddled mess at that time. In 1984, it was reported at the World Congress in Helsinki, Finland, that of more than ten thousand women entering IVF cycles, there were only six hundred live births, for a success rate of only 6 percent. In the United States in 1987, out of a total of twelve thousand women undergoing IVF cycles, there were a little more than one thousand live births, for an overall success rate of about 9 percent. Such a low success rate would hardly be encouraging to a couple.

It was for this reason that the congressional bureaucrats who reported on the discussions of our advisory panel promulgated the claim that the success rate with this new technology was too low and the cost too high to consider it anything other than a last resort and that more resources should be spent on "conventional" therapy for infertility. The bureaucrats also refused to accept the recommendation of the advisory panel that infertility is a medical condition, which would have given strong weight to forcing insurance companies to pay for infertility treatment. The politicians were actually afraid that the female vote would be "offended" by referring to infertility as a medical condition and mandating insurance coverage. If they had not been so erroneously afraid of losing the female vote, IVF today might be affordable to more couples.

Today, your odds are very good that you'll eventually get pregnant with IVF. But you must choose the right doctor and the right program. The Wyden bill, passed by Congress in the early 1990s, is not of much help. It requires that all IVF clinics report their pregnancy rates to the Centers for Disease Control (CDC). But this information doesn't help infertile couples decide where to go for help. Some excellent clinics might have a lower pregnancy rate simply because they direct their attention to the most difficult cases with the longest duration of prior infertility, the greatest amount of scarring, the oldest women, the poorest sperm quality, or the lowest ovarian reserve. If the clinic had the kind of expertise that suited these difficult cases, it could easily have a lower pregnancy rate than a clinic that takes on more simple, routine cases.

In fact, since the Wyden bill became enforced by the Society for Assisted Reproductive Technology (SART) and by the CDC (the U.S. government's main epidemiology arm), many clinics have simply "canceled" cases with low numbers of eggs because they don't want inclusion of such cases to lower their pregnancy rate. Pregnancy rates can easily be manipulated upward by selecting only those patients who have a large number of eggs, or by not recommending continued IVF to those who do not get pregnant in the first or second cycle. By law, these statistics are not supposed to be used for comparison shopping or marketing because they can be so misleading. But they always are.

We have seen many patients in St. Louis who were refused IVF treatment in their own communities because they appeared to have a dismal prognosis. I remember a forty-two-year-old woman from Canada who had gone through multiple IVF cycles when she was younger and failed to get pregnant. No credible IVF program in the United States would accept her because they were concerned about what that would do to their statistics. We warned her that her chance of pregnancy was extremely low, approximately 9 percent, because of her age and her very low ovarian reserve. Her first IVF cycle with us yielded only three eggs, and she failed to get pregnant. However, she insisted on coming back for a second cycle several months later, at which time we retrieved four eggs. This time she became pregnant and delivered a healthy little baby that has grown up to be a very fine young man. Similarly, we took care of a basketball executive and his wife who were both forty-two years old and had gone through many failed IVF cycles elsewhere in good programs. When we put her through IVF, we obtained relatively poor-quality embryos with a great deal of fragmentation, and we felt quite sure she would not get pregnant. Nonetheless, she did get pregnant with healthy twins.

These examples are not meant to imply that our program was any better than the previous IVF programs that these couples went to. The pregnancy rate in forty-two-year-old women with less than five eggs, even in the best IVF programs, including ours, is less than 20 percent, and the delivery rate is only about 10 percent. The only reason for citing these examples is to emphasize that even couples who are in a poor prognostic category can get pregnant but often don't get the chance to undergo IVF because accepting such patients would lower the IVF program's statistics and impede their marketing efforts.

Some clinics have become so commercialized that they publish misleading advertisements in local newspapers and magazines, and even in the *New York Times* and the *Wall Street Journal.* These advertisements promise high pregnancy rates based on carefully selecting only the youngest, most fertile cases and offer money-back guarantees after overcharging for every cycle to cover the cost of rebates. Indeed, many unnecessary and expensive tests, which can cost as much as ten thousand dollars or more, are sometimes insisted upon before the first IVF, thus guaranteeing hefty revenue exclusive of any potential rebate. This commercialized Kentucky-fried IVF franchising has become a cause of great distress and confusion for patients trying to figure out what to do. This is not meant to disparage honest clinics that offer insurance programs referred to as "shared risk." With such a program, if you are in a high prognostic category (e.g., you are under thirty-five, have lots of eggs, and have had no previous IVF failures), you can pay a lump sum for three cycles, and if you do not get pregnant, you'll get 70 percent of your fees returned. This is more or less an insurance plan, but most couples in a high prognostic category do not care for it because it is likely to cost them more than if they just pay separately for each cycle.

Because many clinics make false claims of exaggerated pregnancy rates by selecting younger patients (with a short duration of infertility and large ovarian reserve), published rates are simply an unreliable measure. Therefore, the patients' only resource in deciding where to go for treatment is to understand fully how their reproductive system works, and to learn in a detailed way how IVF and ICSI work. You will need in-depth understanding in order to go through the many steps that are part of every IVF cycle. Furthermore, only with this detailed understanding will you be able to decide where to go for help. You need to learn how to pick the right place by interviewing the doctors and the nurses who are directly involved so you can evaluate their results in a sophisticated manner.

A list of specialists or clinics is never going to be reliable. I can assure you that anyone and everyone who says that he or she is a "fertility specialist" gets on such a list. In an effort to maintain neutrality and avoid libel suits, organizations such as the American Society of Reproductive Medicine (ASRM), the American Medical Association (AMA), RESOLVE (a lay organization of infertile couples), and county medical societies, as well as various books and manuals, are unable to recommend which clinic is right for you or is most likely to give a successful result. For the energy, the time, and the money that must be put into the effort to conceive, you must make a good choice for yourself, based on your own understanding of your reproductive system.

With the information provided in this book, you can now monitor your own biological clock from your early twenties on so that you can decide when you ought to try to have a baby naturally and avoid the need for infertility treatment altogether. If infertility treatment becomes necessary, this book explains what you should expect every step of the way. Understanding how this technology works will give you the best chances for a successful pregnancy.

Sherman Silber, MD
Infertility Center of St. Louis
St. Luke's Hospital
St. Louis, Missouri 63017
314-576-1400
silber@infertile.com
2005

CHAPTER 1

# Getting Pregnant Naturally

Getting pregnant is not an easy task, but understanding the essential physiology of the process is the best place to start. In this chapter I will describe the arduous journey that sperm must make through the female genitals to reach the egg, as well as the simultaneous adventure of the egg during which it matures to become genetically ready for fertilization, erupts from the ovary, and gets grabbed by the fallopian tube, fertilized, and then hustled along into the womb at exactly the right moment to implant. Failure of the sperm or egg to make an important connection anywhere along this complicated itinerary will prevent pregnancy from occurring.

## A Brief Review of Female Anatomy

The vagina is an elastic canal, about four to five inches long. At the end of this canal, in the deepest recess of the vagina, is a structure called the cervix, which is the entrance to the womb, or uterus. The uterus is a hard, muscular, pear-shaped structure with a narrow, triangular cavity inside, so small that it would barely hold a teaspoonful of fluid (see figs. 1.1 and 1.2). Yet this is where the fertilized egg must implant itself and grow during the next nine months into a full-size baby. The uterus has a remarkable capacity to expand to allow room for the developing baby, pushing aside and squashing all the other organs of the mother's abdomen. When the baby is ready to be born, the muscles of the uterus contract during labor to squeeze the baby out into the world.

Far back in the corners of the uterus, on each side, are microscopic canals through which the sperm must squeeze in order to reach the fallopian tube, where it may encounter an unfertilized egg. Once the egg has been fertilized, it will pass through the canal in the opposite direc-

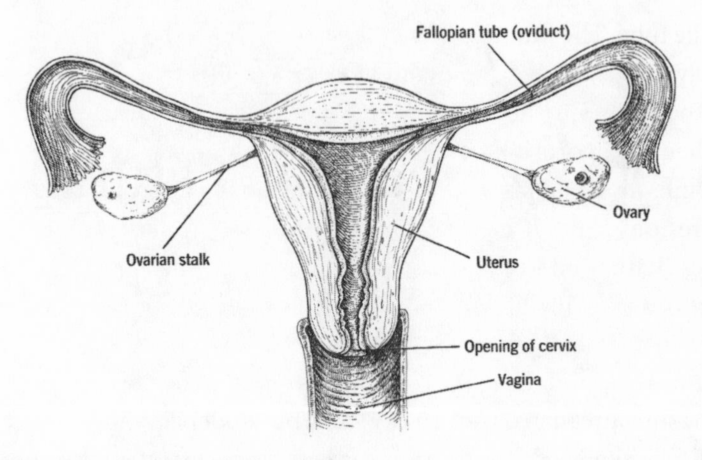


**FIGURE 1.1.** The female reproductive organs.

tion to reach the uterus. These microscopic canals leading from the uterus into the fallopian tubes are only about one-seventieth of an inch in diameter (the size of a pinpoint). The fallopian tubes are four inches long and hang freely in the abdomen. They widen at the ends into large, flowerlike openings called fimbriae.

The ovaries are the organs that make the female's eggs and sex hormones. They lie outside of the uterus and fallopian tubes. When an egg is extruded every month from the surface of one of the ovaries (ovulation), it is released freely into the abdominal cavity rather than directly

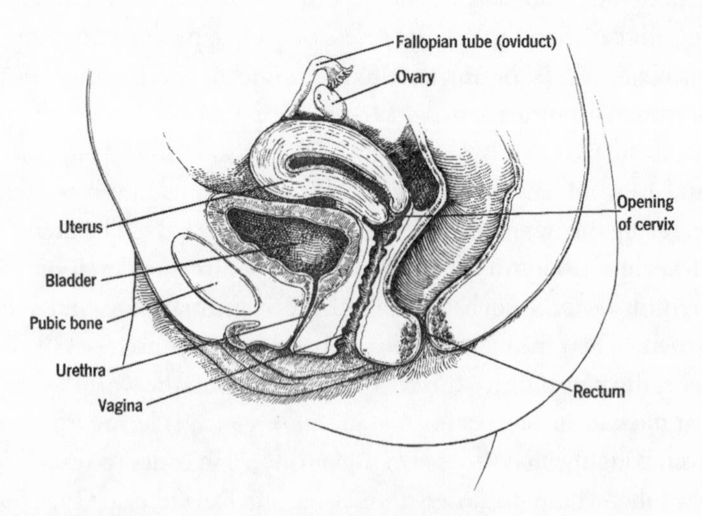


**FIGURE 1.2.** The female reproductive organs (side view).

into the tube. The fimbria then comes to life like an octopus tentacle and actively grasps the egg, pulling it into the fallopian tube. The tube swallows the egg, nourishes it before and during fertilization for three days, and then transports it into the uterus (see fig. 1.3).

While the male produces billions of sperm every week, the female matures only one of her existing eggs for ovulation each month. The ovaries mature and release about four hundred such eggs during the course of a woman's lifetime. Generally, the most fertile eggs are released earlier in life, and of her limited supply of four hundred thousand, about one thousand eggs will die inexorably every month. Thus with advancing years, though a woman may still be able to get pregnant, she is much less fertile than she was in her youth.

### *How Do the Egg and the Sperm Reach the Fallopian Tube?*

The journey of the egg, or ovum, through the fallopian tube and finally into the uterus after fertilization is extraordinarily hazardous. The woman's tube is not simply a passive channel through which the egg is transferred; many events must work in precise synchrony for successful pregnancy to occur.

There are, on the surface of the fimbria, microscopic hairs called cilia, which constantly beat in the direction of the uterus at a fantastically rapid speed and create a kind of conveyor-belt effect for moving the egg into the tube and toward the uterus. The cilia work this magic by digging into the sticky gel, called the cumulus oophorus, that surrounds the egg, and they transport this whole sticky, gooey mass. The egg itself is invisible to the naked eye, but the gel that envelops it is easily visible. If this sticky substance were not present, and the egg were placed bare upon the surface of the fimbria, the beating of the cilia would never move the egg along. The cilia are only able to dig in and transport the egg with this sticky, gooey material encasing it.

The process of grasping the egg and moving it into the interior of the tube requires only about fifteen to twenty seconds. Once the egg is safely within the tube, it is transported quickly toward the narrower region of the tube, the ampullary-isthmic junction, located two-thirds of the way toward the uterus. Here, the egg must wait for a successful sperm coming from the opposite direction to fight its way into the egg's tough outer membrane, the zona pellucida, score a direct hit, and thereby establish pregnancy. While the egg is held in this location by the tight resistance of

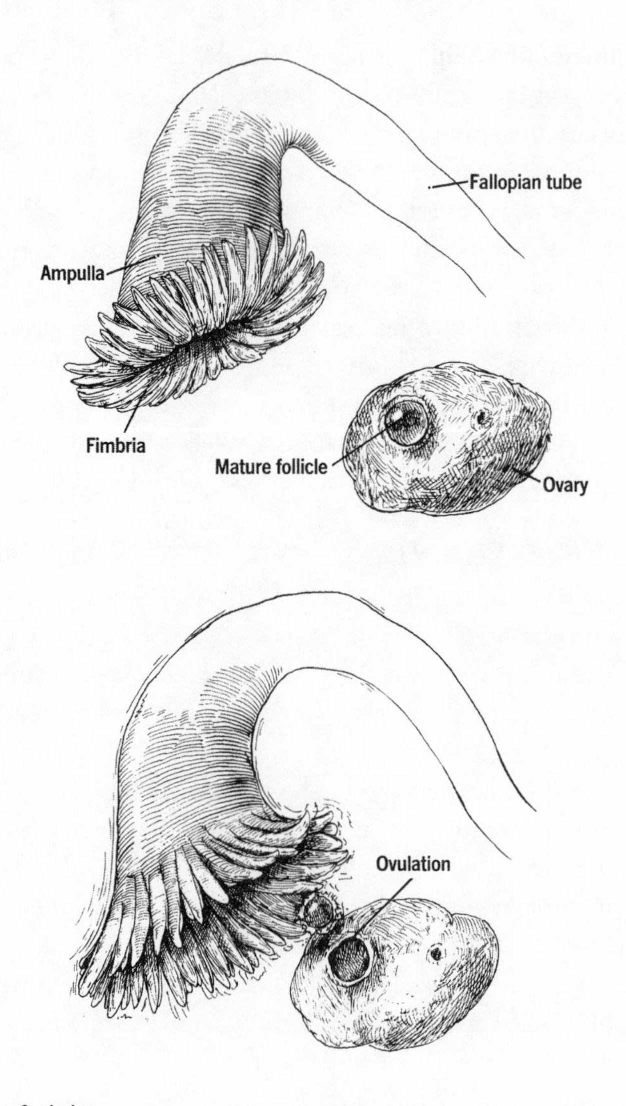


**FIGURE 1.3.** Ovulation.

the narrow region of the tube, the much tinier sperm nonetheless must struggle through this area of resistance to arrive from the opposite direction. Once it is fertilized, the egg must be nourished for several days in the ampulla of the tube before it can be allowed to pass into the uterus. If it is transferred into the uterus too soon, it will not be ready to implant, and it will die. If the transfer of the egg into the uterus is delayed too long, a tubal, or ectopic, pregnancy will occur (the fertilized egg will implant in the tube rather than the womb). Once the egg has been allowed to develop in the tube for three or more days, the isthmus suddenly opens up and the early embryo passes quickly into the uterus. Because the journey of the egg from the ovary to the site of fertilization, its nourishment in the tube, and the precise synchrony of the continuation of its journey into the womb are so intricate, problems with this egg and embryo transport process are frequently responsible for female infertility.

If the egg is not penetrated by sperm soon after ovulation, it becomes overripe and dies. After the egg is released from the ovary, it is only capable of fertilization for about twelve, or possibly at most twenty-four, hours. The likelihood of intercourse taking place during such a specific interval in any month is rather slight. So nature must provide some mechanism for providing a continuous flow of healthy sperm to the site of fertilization. That way, if intercourse is perhaps one or two days off schedule, some sperm can still arrive at the site of fertilization at the right time. For this reason, complicated barriers to sperm transport are necessary.

The success of IVF demonstrates that if eggs can be recovered at precisely the right time, they can be fertilized in the laboratory with only a small number of sperm. Then the complicated barrier mechanisms provided by nature to allow a slow, continuing flow of a small number of sperm at any moment is not necessary and the large numbers of sperm normally required for fertilization through intercourse are not needed.

### *Ejaculation into the Vagina*

Most of the spermatozoa in the ejaculate are contained in the very first portion of fluid that squirts out of the penis and enters the vagina. The remaining squirts usually contain very little sperm. Thus, at the first moment of ejaculation the female's cervix (the opening leading into her uterus) is bathed by a high concentration of sperm. Within just a few minutes after ejaculation, sperm begin to invade a very thick fluid (called cervical mucus) that is pouring out of the cervix. The sperm must be able to invade the cervix via the cervical mucus by virtue of their own swimming ability. Nothing about the sexual act will help those sperm get into the cervix. They simply have to swim into the mucus on their own, and this requires a great deal of coordinated, cooperative activity on their part.

Ejaculation is a challenging moment for the sperm, as the vagina presents a very harsh, acidic environment, which would normally immobilize them quickly. The alkalinity of the semen (the fluid that contains the sperm), as well as the alkalinity of the cervical mucus, allows the sperm to survive in this difficult vaginal milieu. Any acidity at all quickly kills sperm.

Yet even the semen is a potentially dangerous milieu for the sperm; any sperm that remain in the semen for more than two hours are likely to deteriorate. In order to survive long enough to get to the egg and fertilize it, the sperm must gain rapid access to the cervical mucus. Any sperm that have not penetrated the cervical mucus within a half hour after orgasm will not be able to do so later on, because by then they will have lost their ability to swim into the more friendly environment of the cervix.

### *Sperm Invasion*

Spermatozoa can be seen invading the cervical mucus within seconds after ejaculation, but most will not make it (see fig. 1.4). Of some 200 million sperm deposited into the vagina near the cervix in a typical ejaculation, only 100,000 ever get into the womb. Thus, over 99.9 percent of the sperm never have a chance of getting beyond the vagina.

Once the sperm enter the canal of the cervix, they are capable of fertilizing the egg for as long as forty-eight to seventy-two hours, though they may actually live for up to six days. Remember, since the egg is only fertilizable for about twelve hours after ovulation, it is important to have a continuing flow of sperm across the tube so that whenever the egg appears, there will be sperm available. In this sense, the canal of the cervix can be looked upon as a receptacle through which platoons of spermatozoa migrate and in which some are detained in order to ensure a continuous supply of smaller numbers, over a prolonged period of time, to the deeper recesses of the female where fertilization takes place. Of course, these delaying mechanisms can do more harm than good in infertile couples if events do not allow the invasion of sperm to be mounted successfully.

To understand how this invasion of sperm gets launched effectively, we must first understand the remarkable liquid that covers the opening of the womb — the cervical mucus. The cervical mucus presents a very effective barrier to bacteria and thus protects the womb against infec-

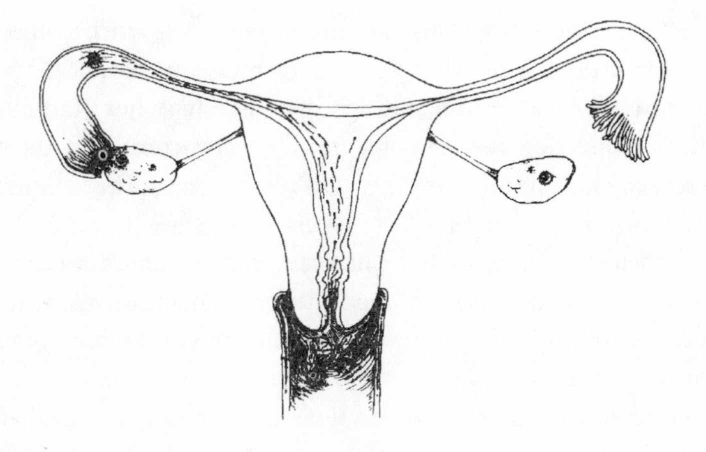

**FIGURE 1.4.** Sperm invading cervical mucus from vagina.

tion. It is a selective filter, which favors normally active sperm and excludes other objects (including poor-quality sperm) from access. But it doesn't even permit access to normal sperm except during a specific period at midcycle when ovulation is imminent and fertilization is possible. Cervical mucus resembles a thick, clear liquid that can be poured from one container into another. However, in a technical sense, it is not a liquid. As it is being poured, it can actually be cut with scissors; therefore, although it seems to behave as a thick liquid, it also has the characteristics of a very pliable, transparent plastic.

Cervical mucus is absent or very scanty during most of the monthly cycle, gradually becoming more abundant around the middle of the cycle, under the influence of increasing estrogen levels, when ovulation is about to occur. Just prior to ovulation it becomes almost optically clear, although it is translucent at other times. At the moment when fertilization is possible, near the time of ovulation, the mucus can be stretched out into a very thin strand; at other times in the cycle it is more sticky, and if stretched it will break. All of these changes in the cervical mucus, which occur around the time prior to ovulation, are designed to help sperm gain access to the uterus. The more liquidlike character, the greater transparency, and the greater stretchability (called *Spinnbarkheit*) are all characteristics that favor the successful invasion of an army of sperm. When the mucus is sticky and thick, not as abundant, and translucent rather than transparent, it is difficult if not impossible for any sperm to gain access.

Microscopically, the cervical mucus consists of a dense mesh that, during most of the monthly cycle, represents a solid barrier to invasion. Just prior to ovulation, under the effect of the female hormone estrogen, mucus production rises tenfold, and the water content of the mucus increases. The otherwise impenetrable mesh opens up and allows a successful invasion of sperm. When semen first reaches the cervical mucus after ejaculation, a clear barrier line can be seen separating the two different fluids. Semen does not "mix" with cervical mucus. Soon, however, phalanges of sperm begin to penetrate the mucus, forming branching structures that invade it.

Observing the sperm's penetration of the cervical mucus under the microscope is an exciting event. Sperm at first seem to bounce against the cervical mucus without any evidence that they will ever be able to gain access. Their movements while in the ejaculate are haphazard and not specifically aimed toward the mucus. However, within a matter of minutes, one or two spermatozoa begin to make an indentation in the line separating the cervical mucus from the ejaculate. Once one sperm has been able to initiate the penetration of the mucus, other sperm then quickly follow at that same point of entry. Sperm then continue to invade the cervical mucus at that point much like a single-file line of army ants. Only one or two spermatozoa at a time can pass through this entrance.

The sperm swim in a straightforward direction along parallel rows of the invisible microscopic molecular structure of the mucus. Once this invasion of the cervical mucus has been established, sperm can reach the fallopian tubes in about thirty minutes.

Pregnancy would not be likely if all the sperm got into the fallopian tubes at one time, because they would soon pass on into the abdominal cavity, and not be available to fertilize the egg except during a very brief, lucky interval. If they were not lucky enough to pass through the fallopian tube at exactly the moment of ovulation (or within twelve hours of ovulation), they would be long gone by the time the egg arrived. Thus, nature had to invent some mechanism for allowing a continuous entry to the site of fertilization by a smaller number of sperm. To accomplish this, the cervix and the cervical mucus act as a reservoir from which spermatozoa are slowly released into the uterus and up to the fallopian tubes over a period of several days.

### *Capacitation of Sperm*

During the course of their odyssey toward the site of fertilization, the sperm undergo capacitation, a process that was not fully understood before the advent of IVF. It used to be thought that unless sperm resided for a certain period of time outside the male reproductive tract and in the specific fluids of the female reproductive tract, they would not be capable of fertilization, even though in every other respect they looked normal. It was thought that this process of capacitation could occur only in the fluids of the female reproductive tract while the sperm migrated toward the egg. However, in vitro fertilization has demonstrated that capacitation of sperm (once considered one of the greatest problems in successfully achieving test-tube babies) can occur in relatively simple, nonspecific fluids available in any laboratory.

All that is necessary to start the capacitation process going is to remove the sperm from the semen by "washing" it. Removing the sperm from semen and placing them in any laboratory "culture media" fluid results in a dramatic tripling of their swimming velocity, so that even though they are mere human sperm, they begin to swim more like the sperm of horses or bulls. Thus, sperm seem to have a natural tendency toward developing capacitation for fertilization on their own and simply require a period of several hours outside the semen. In nature this happens when they leave the semen and enter the cervical mucus. In the IVF laboratory it happens when sperm are separated from the semen by virtually any washing technique (see chapter 8).

## Ovulation

Before egg and sperm can ever meet up in the fallopian tube, the egg must be matured and extruded from the ovary in a process called ovulation. Since many women who seem unable to have children owe their problems to a disturbance in ovulation, and since part of the IVF procedure involves stimulating the ovaries to prepare many eggs for fertilization, we should understand how the repeatable, monthly series of changes leading to ovulation occurs naturally in the ovary. Later we will unravel the hormonal events of the menstrual cycle, which regulate the clocklike orderliness of ovulation.

All of the hormonal events taking place during the month between menstrual periods are directed at preparing the egg to be genetically ready for fertilization, and preparing the uterus (womb) and the cervix for the moment of ovulation, so that the sperm and the egg have the best opportunity for joining up to form an embryo, which can then implant in a properly prepared uterus and result in successful pregnancy.

### *Formation of the Follicle*

Each month, from the time of sexual maturity on, about one thousand undeveloped eggs, or oocytes, leave their prolonged resting phase and start to mature. This initiation of development is a continuous process, in marked contrast to ovulation, which occurs only once a month. Once the egg starts to develop, it proceeds inexorably and no longer has the choice of returning to being quiescent. It either wins the race to ovulate or must degenerate and die.

The most striking feature of the egg's development is the growth of its surrounding fluid-filled compartment, called the follicle (see fig. 1.5). The growth of this follicle is stimulated by the hormone FSH (follicle-stimulating hormone), which is produced by the pituitary gland in the early phase of the monthly cycle. The time required for the egg to develop the proper follicle necessary for ovulation is about fourteen days. Although the FSH stimulates all of the developing eggs during the month to form follicles, one of the eggs always gets a head start over the others, and once it obtains that lead it never relinquishes it. The other eggs developing that month then degenerate. However, if large

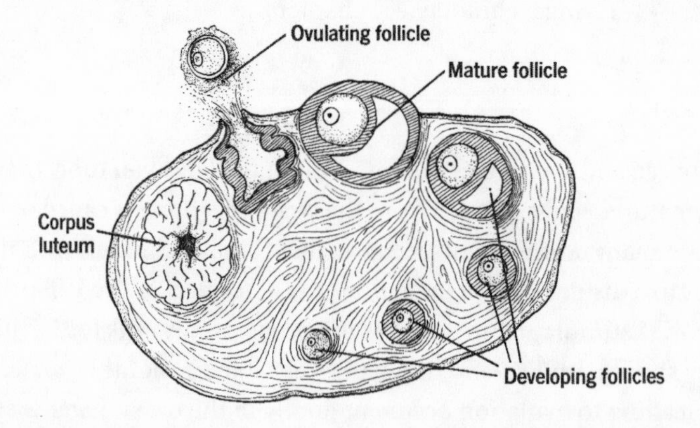


**FIGURE 1.5**

Formation of the follicle, and ovulation and transformation of the ovulated follicle into the corpus luteum.

doses of FSH were to be given to a woman at the beginning of the cycle, far in excess of what her pituitary would normally secrete, she would develop many follicles instead of just one.

The mature follicle is a spherical, bubblelike structure that bulges up from the surface of the ovary, and contains the egg. The egg (which is only 1/200 of an inch in diameter) is surrounded and protected by a mass of sticky, gelatinous fluid called the cumulus oophorus and hangs on a stalk attached to the inside of the follicle wall. The rest of the fluid in the follicle is clear yellow, and the follicle itself is fairly large (four-fifths of an inch in diameter). Occasionally two follicles successfully reach maturity and are both ovulated. In that circumstance the woman may have fraternal, or nonidentical, twins. Indeed, the drugs used to stimulate ovulation in women who would not otherwise ovulate usually cause the development of more than one follicle. Therefore, multiple births are common in women who require medical treatment to help them ovulate.

Two or three days prior to midcycle, when the follicle has reached its maximum size (usually two centimeters, or four-fifths of an inch), it produces an enormous amount of the hormone estrogen. This increased level of estrogen before ovulation stimulates the cervix to make more (and clearer) cervical mucus in order to allow sperm invasion. This dramatic increase in estrogen production by the follicle then stimulates the pituitary gland to release another hormone, different from FSH, called LH (luteinizing hormone). The sudden release of LH is what triggers ovulation (see fig. 1.6). The increase in estrogen indicates to the pituitary that the follicle is ripe, and this beautifully times the release of the LH hormone. Ovulation then occurs normally thirty-eight to forty-eight hours after the beginning of this LH surge.

### *Release of the Egg*

Under the influence of the midcycle LH surge, the wall of the follicle weakens and deteriorates, and a specific site on its surface ruptures. The contents of the bulging follicle are then extruded from the surface of the ovary through this ruptured area (see fig. 1.5). Observed under a microscope, ovulation appears similar to the eruption of a volcano. Occasionally women actually feel several hours of discomfort in their lower abdomen during ovulation; this discomfort is called *Mittelschmerz.* In women who require hormone treatment to stimulate ovulation, so many follicles may grow so large that when ovulation occurs it causes strong cramps, and a woman may even become sick enough to require several days of rest in the hospital. However, this sort of complication is not very likely with modern dosage monitoring. It is mentioned only to underscore what a dramatic intra-abdominal event ovulation is.

### *Production of Progesterone*

The ruptured, empty follicle then undergoes another dramatic change, called luteinization. Luteinization is the process by which the follicle becomes able to make progesterone in addition to estrogen. Prior to ovulation, the follicle could produce only estrogen; after ovulation it can produce the other female hormone, progesterone, as well. Because it is impossible for the follicle to make progesterone before ovulation, the production of progesterone implies that ovulation has occurred. In the past, the presence of progesterone used to be the basis for all clinical methods of evaluating ovulation. The production of progesterone by the transformed follicle after ovulation is necessary for the successful implantation of the embryo in the womb during the second two weeks of the cycle.

The cystlike structure that forms monthly from the ruptured follicle is called the corpus luteum. This is Latin for "yellow body" and simply signifies that the follicle turns yellow as it changes its identity. As soon as the ruptured follicle begins to produce progesterone, the cervical mucus (which had become maximally receptive to sperm invasion just prior to ovulation) is suddenly caused to become sticky and totally impermeable to the invasion of sperm. In addition, progesterone causes the entrance of the cervix to close dramatically, even though just prior to ovulation it had been gaping in readiness for the entry of sperm. In the first half of the cycle, before ovulation, estrogen stimulates the buildup of a thick, hard layer of tissue called the endometrium to line the uterus, but this lining does not become receptive to the fertilized egg until after ovulation, when the secretion of progesterone causes it to soften. If the uterine lining is not softened by progesterone after ovulation (i.e., transformed from proliferative to secretory), implantation of the embryo cannot occur.

The corpus luteum manufactures this progesterone over a very limited time. If no pregnancy develops, the corpus luteum ceases to produce progesterone by ten to fourteen days after ovulation, and subsequently disappears. With this cessation of progesterone production by the ovary, the soft lining that was built up in the womb to prepare for the nourishment of the fertilized egg is shed and the woman menstruates. The decrease in progesterone (and estrogen) levels during menstruation then stimulates a renewed increase in FSH. A new follicle then develops, estrogen production resumes, and the cycle begins again (see fig. 1.6).

## A Review of the Hormones That Control Ovulation and the Menstrual Cycle

The reproductive cycle that animals go through is called the estrous cycle. Only humans and the apes have menstrual cycles. In a menstrual cycle the buildup of the lining of the womb is so lush, and the drop in hormone level supporting that lining so abrupt, that at the end of the cycle the lining actually sheds and the woman bleeds for four to five days in what is commonly known as her period. In all other animals, however, this shedding does not occur, and the thick lining of the womb merely returns to the thinned-out condition, marking the beginning of the next cycle. Furthermore, when animals are about to ovulate in their estrous cycle, they go into heat, or "estrus," and know it is time to copulate.

Since most woman are unaware of when they ovulate, they must try to understand the events of their menstrual cycle more fully, because unlike other animals, we do not automatically copulate at the right time. We will arbitrarily call the first day of the menstrual cycle "day one," which is the day that bleeding commences. Bleeding usually ceases by day four or five and in most cases resumes after day twenty-eight of the cycle. Although the first day of menstruation represents a shedding of the lining of the uterus (womb) from the previous month's cycle, it is actually the beginning (day one) of the next cycle.

On the first day of menstruation the pituitary hormone FSH is already stimulating development of a follicle that will take precedence over all other follicles that month (see fig. 1.6). Interestingly, FSH, which in females causes the follicle to develop, is the exact same hormone that in males helps to stimulate sperm production. Estrogen from the developing ovarian follicle then inhibits further pituitary production of FSH. This is a "negative feedback" mechanism whereby the very estrogen that FSH causes to be produced by the ovary inhibits the pituitary from making more FSH.

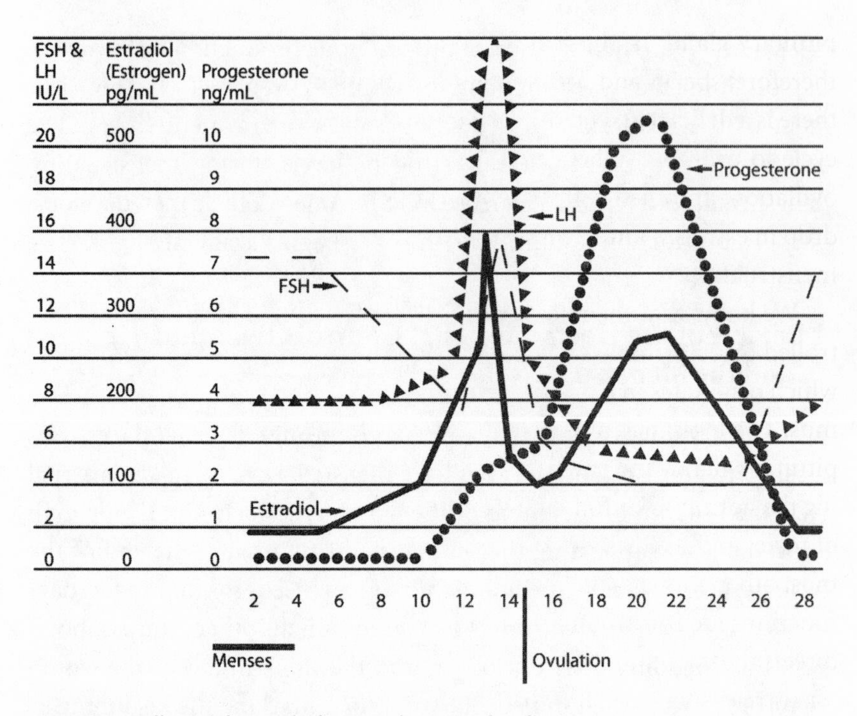


**FIGURE 1.6.** Hormonal control of a normal menstrual cycle.

By day twelve to fourteen of the menstrual cycle, the follicle appears on the surface of the ovary as a fluid-filled bubble ready to burst. In the meantime, the estrogen that has been produced by the follicle during this first half of the cycle has stimulated the uterus to prepare a thick "proliferative" lining. This thick, proliferative uterine lining is not ready to receive the egg until it is "softened" by progesterone in the second half of the cycle.

The final effect of estrogen (in high quantities at midcycle) is to trigger the release of a different pituitary hormone, LH. This enormous surge of LH from the pituitary (see fig. 1.6) is what causes the follicle to burst and then ovulate. But LH does more than simply cause ovulation (release of the egg from the ovary). LH triggers the chromosomes of the egg to separate and thereby prepares the egg genetically for fertilization.

### *How a Primitive Region of the Brain Called the Hypothalamus Controls the Menstrual Cycle*

The entire cycle of follicle development, ovulation, and menstruation depends upon the precisely timed release of FSH and LH from the pituitary gland. In the male, FSH and LH production is constant, and therefore, sperm and hormone production are constant. In the female, there is a delicately synchronized increase in FSH at the beginning of the cycle to promote follicle growth, an LH surge at midcycle to promote ovulation, and then a gradual drop in pituitary hormones that causes a drop in estrogen and progesterone production by the ovary, resulting in menstruation.

We know that the release of FSH and LH from the pituitary is controlled by a hormone called GnRH (gonadotropin-releasing hormone), which originates in a primitive region of the brain called the hypothalamus. The hypothalamus sits right at the base of the brain and above the pituitary gland, and causes the pituitary to release FSH and LH by sending the hormone GnRH directly to it. It used to be thought that the brains of males and females were different in this regard (and indeed they are in most other animals). We now know that this area of the brain in humans functions identically in the male and female, and that it is the ovary that directs the cyclical production of FSH and LH in the female pituitary.

By releasing GnRH, the hypothalamus is simply permissive in allowing the pituitary to stimulate the ovary in the female and the testicle in the male. The brain secretes small pulses (lasting only a minute or so) of the hormone GnRH about every ninety minutes in both men and women. It is the periodic, never-ending release of GnRH from the brain that causes the pituitary gland to start secreting FSH and LH, bringing on puberty, including menstruation in girls.

In men with deficient sperm or testosterone production, the FSH and LH levels are higher because the pituitary is overworking in an effort to compensate. The same phenomenon occurs in women. We know that when the ovary runs out of eggs, and women can no longer produce estrogen (thereby going into menopause), the FSH and LH levels from the woman's pituitary go sky-high in an effort to stimulate what little ovarian reserve may still exist.

To understand estrogen's role in controlling the pituitary hormones, we must look at what happens at midcycle in the woman. The surge in estrogen at midcycle causes the pituitary to suddenly release a high amount of LH (along with some extra FSH), and this stimulates ovulation. The cyclic pattern of hormone production in the female, which is quite different from the constant pattern of hormone production in the male, is not caused by any difference in the female brain's release of

GnRH. If the hypothalamus of any human being were destroyed (male or female), there would be no further GnRH secretion, the pituitary would cease to make FSH and LH, and the ovaries or testicles would shrivel up and completely stop functioning.

### *Clinical Importance of GnRH Release from the Brain for IVF*

Why is the fascinating relationship of a primitive region of the brain to the pituitary, the ovaries, and the testicles so important? It bears very heavily on how we can obtain the best-quality eggs from the female for IVF. When the ovaries are stimulated to make more eggs by administering FSH (a necessary step in the in vitro fertilization process), the tremendous increase in estrogen production over a normal level can cause an early increase in LH secretion. This may result in premature ovulation with complete loss of the eggs or, at best, may hurt the subsequent pregnancy rate resulting from those eggs. In order to prevent this premature LH increase, we need to have a better understanding of GnRH, the hormone from the brain that allows the pituitary to release FSH and LH.

If GnRH were released constantly rather than at pulsatile intervals of ninety minutes, a peculiar reverse phenomenon would take place. The pituitary, rather than being stimulated to release FSH and LH, would become completely paralyzed after two to five days and would no longer secrete any FSH or LH until the constant release of GnRH was stopped and regular pulsatile ninety-minute secretion was resumed. Thus, we can completely turn off the pituitary whenever we want to by simply giving a constant rather than intermittent dose of GnRH. It's as though the pituitary needs a ninety-minute rest before each new GnRH stimulus in order to function properly. If the pituitary doesn't get this ninety-minute rest, it behaves just as though there were no GnRH at all. This process is called down regulation.

GnRH is chemically a very simple hormone called a polypeptide, which can be easily synthesized by drug companies. When a small modification is made in the structure of the GnRH, we have what is known as a GnRH agonist, which, if injected just one time a day, stays around in the bloodstream at a constant level rather than being immediately destroyed within minutes, as the brain's normal GnRH would be. Thus, giving an injection of GnRH agonist once a day creates the same effect as infusing a constant level of GnRH all day long and giving the pituitary no rest. When you give the pituitary no rest, at first it pours out a

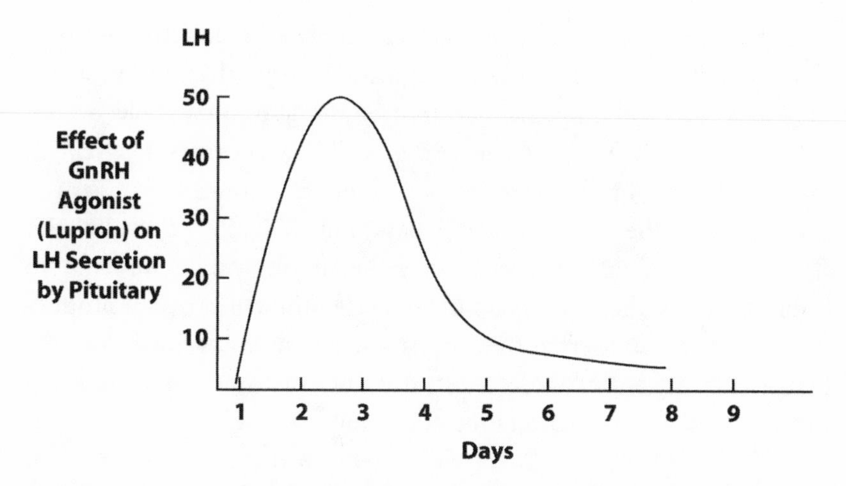


**FIGURE 1.7**

Initial increase in pituitary secretion of LH during the first four days of Lupron (leuprolide) treatment and the subsequent decline to near zero secretion level.

lot of FSH and LH, but then several days later, the depleted pituitary can no longer release LH or FSH (see fig. 1.7).

There are several GnRH agonists on the market, Lupron (leuprolide) being popular in the United States, and Suprefact (buserelin) being a popular one in Europe. Using Lupron along with a stimulation cycle completely turns off the pituitary and prevents a premature LH surge that would interfere with the proper development of the large number of eggs necessary for IVF.

A different variation of GnRH analogue is the GnRH antagonist, e.g., Cetrotide or Antagon. Instead of depleting the pituitary of FSH and LH, as Lupron does, GnRH antagonists work by directly and immediately blocking the pituitary's release of FSH and LH by preventing GnRH from having any stimulating effect on the pituitary.

## How Do Hormones Genetically Prepare the Egg for Fertilization?

Incredible genetic cellular changes take place in a woman's developing eggs each month, beginning with the elevation of FSH at the start of menstruation. Very complex events are taking place in the egg during this monthly development and growth of the follicle. Furthermore, the release of LH stimulated by the estrogen surge at midcycle does much more than just cause ovulation. It finalizes the critical genetic preparation of the egg, without which fertilization would be impossible.

Thus far, only a superficial description of what happens during a menstrual cycle has been given: (1) follicular growth and estrogen production in the first half, (2) ovulation at midcycle, hopefully with fertilization, and (3) preparation of the uterine lining for embryo implantation in the second half of the cycle, stimulated by the production of progesterone from the corpus luteum (newly formed from the ovulated follicle). But these events are only the outward signs of an intricate genetic preparation for fertilization.

### *Reduction Division (Meiosis) of the Egg's Chromosomes*

Every cell in the body has forty-six chromosomes consisting of twenty-three pairs, which carry all of our genes. However, the sperm and the egg at the moment of fertilization must each have only twenty-three single chromosomes, not forty-six, so that when the sperm and the egg unite, the fertilized egg has the normal number of chromosomes.

Like every other cell in the body, sperm precursors in the testicle have forty-six chromosomes. But in the process of sperm production, the chromosomes are reduced to half the normal number by a process called meiosis. So when sperm leave the testicle, they have only twenty-three chromosomes. The eggs also have forty-six chromosomes until the very moment the sperm penetrates an egg and initiates fertilization. Fertilization cannot possibly occur unless the egg's forty-six chromosomes can be reduced to twenty-three. The moment the sperm penetrates the egg, half of the egg's chromosomes must be extruded. Then two half sets of chromosomes, one from the male, and one from the female, merge into a new individual with the normal number of forty-six chromosomes. Without the hormonal stimulation of FSH causing follicle development, followed by the release of LH at midcycle, the eggs would not be genetically prepared for this complex event of meiosis to occur.

The miracle of this separation of chromosomes is the most complicated event in the whole reproductive process; it determines the genetic makeup of the child and results in the genetic variability of the offspring.

### *Development of the Egg During Growth of the Follicle*

At the time of a woman's birth, all of her eggs are fixed in the beginning phase of the first meiotic division. The remaining stages of the meiotic division will not begin until years later, when her egg has finally matured in a developing follicle and the LH surge at midcycle causes the egg to resume meiosis. This resumption of meiosis, triggered by LH, would not occur without the prior preparation by FSH (meiotic competence) during the first two weeks of the cycle.

At the beginning of the cycle, from day one of menstruation, increased FSH production from the pituitary stimulates rapid growth in the egg. The egg will grow during this early follicular phase from a tiny 30 microns to its normal mature size of 140 microns (from 1/1,000 of an inch to approximately 1/200 of an inch in diameter). At this time, the very tough outer membrane, the zona pellucida, forms around the enlarging egg. Next, the follicle expands to form a fluid-filled cavity around the egg. The tiny forming follicle is visible on ultrasound at this point.

When the follicle forms, many compact layers of granulosa cells begin to surround the now enlarged egg, and the outer sheath of these granulosa cells produces the hormone estrogen. Even a brief deprivation of estrogen to the maturing egg during this stage will result in the egg's immediate death. If FSH stimulation were to suddenly cease or be reduced dramatically, estrogen production by the granulosa cells would decline and the egg would die.

The egg remains embedded on one side of the follicle in a mound called the cumulus oophorus. The cells around the egg remain compact until the egg is ready for fertilization. When LH triggers the important genetic events that will allow fertilization after ovulation, these cells spread out in a radial pattern, giving a sunburstlike appearance referred to as corona radiata (see fig. 1.8). If this widely dispersed appearance of cumulus cells surrounding the zona pellucida of the egg is present, physicians performing in vitro fertilization know that the egg is adequately mature for fertilization to occur. It is the most easily observable sign that the egg has gone through enough FSH stimulation to be ready for the genetic events of meiosis, which will ultimately lead to the possibility of fertilization.

It is quite astounding that there is little difference in the maximum

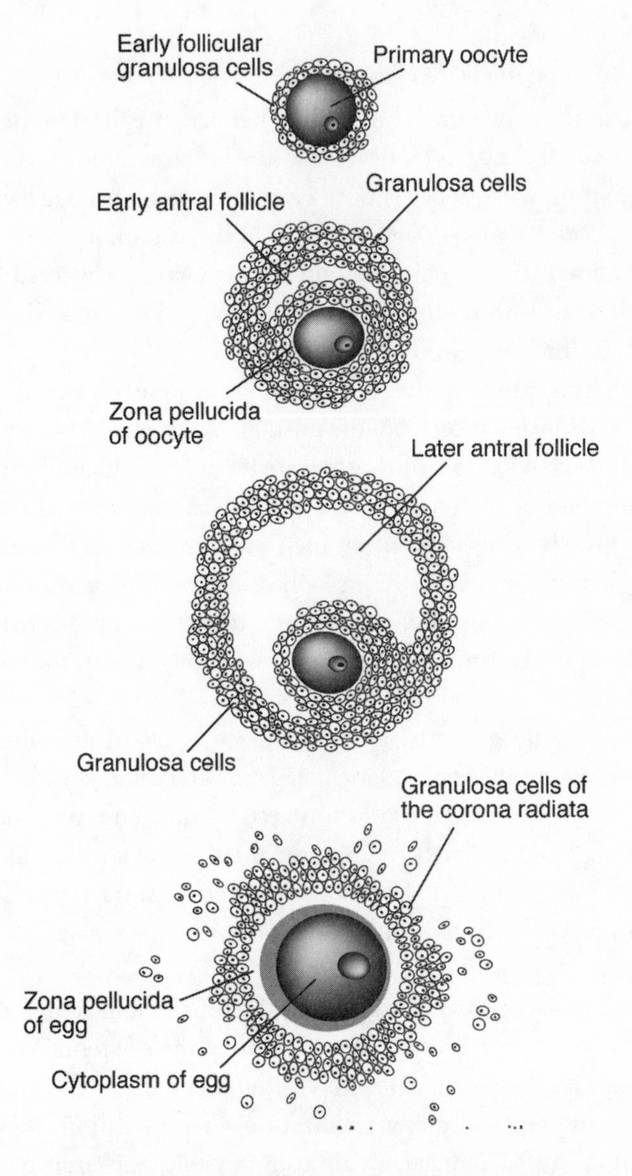


**FIGURE 1.8.** Maturation of egg with full expansion of the corona radiata.

diameter of the egg of almost any species, even though the size of the follicle containing the egg is generally related to the size of the animal. Thus, eggs of a whale could easily pass through the oviduct of the smallest mammal, like a rat, even though the whale's follicle containing that small egg could easily be as large as a whole rabbit. The increasing size of the follicle has nothing to do with any increase in the size of the egg but is merely an indication that the egg is being properly prepared for what it has to do when it receives the surge of LH at midcycle.

### *Resumption of Meiosis After the LH Surge*

LH begins the resumption of meiosis, but the penetration of the egg by a sperm is what causes the completion of that process. After the LH surge, the first meiotic division occurs, but this division does not reduce the number of chromosomes. This is an equal division in which forty-six chromosomes are still left within the egg nucleus. Actually, it is more complex than this, and I will explain it in detail in chapter 12.

The "first polar body" is a small, divided nucleus that is pinched off from the main body of the egg prior to ovulation, about thirty hours after the LH surge. The extrusion of the first polar body from the egg shows that the first meiotic division has occurred under the influence of LH, meaning that the egg is now prepared to undergo the all-important second meiotic division. Many college biology students get confused by these two stages of meiosis. In the first division, all the chromosomes partly divide but do not split completely. In the second division, they actually complete the split. The egg is thus prepared during meiosis for the entrance of a sperm.

### *Penetration of the Egg by a Sperm*

For a sperm to enter and fertilize the egg, it must dig its way through several layers of protective shields surrounding the egg. These outer walls safeguarding the inner confines of the egg represent an impressive barrier to sperm penetration, and a sperm cannot dig its way through these membranes without the aid of chemicals released from its warhead, the acrosome (see fig. 1.9). The acrosome surrounds the front portion of the sperm and acts much like a battering ram. Chemicals released by the acrosome first dissolve the jellylike cumulus oophorus, enabling the sperm to pass through it and reach the tough zona pellucida. This very tough membrane, like the shell of a chicken egg, represents perhaps the most formidable obstacle to sperm. To penetrate this barrier, the sperm cannot just haphazardly liberate chemicals, or the egg might be damaged. The attacking chemicals must remain closely bound to the surface of the sperm and thereby cut an extraordinarily narrow slit into the membrane.

In order for the sperm to make its way through the sturdy zona pel-

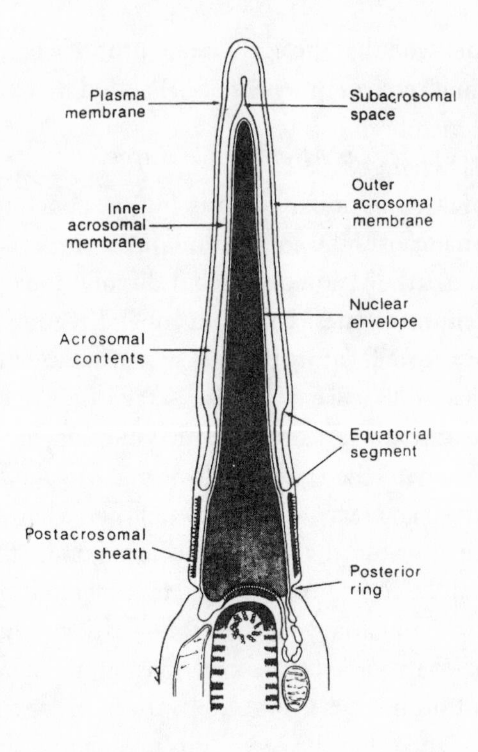


**FIGURE 1.9**

**Diagram of the sperm head and its outer acrosome battering ram before releasing its contents.**

lucida, a process called the acrosome reaction is necessary. The acrosome is attached around the front two-thirds of the sperm head, where it is positioned much like an arrowhead. Its contents are tightly contained because premature leakage of acrosin (the dissolving chemical) would make it impossible for the sperm head to drill its way through the zona pellucida when it finally makes contact. Contact with the zona pellucida stimulates the acrosome to undergo its reaction, during which holes form in the inner and outer acrosomal membranes and acrosin is released, helping the sperm break through the zona pellucida.

Once a lucky sperm makes contact with the zona pellucida (which is purely a random event), it takes a minimum of fifteen minutes before penetration can begin. Some sperm can be seen struggling for as long as an hour before they make their initial penetration. If penetration hasn't occurred within an hour, however, something is wrong and the egg probably won't be fertilized. Sperm enter the zona pellucida at an angle almost exactly perpendicular to the surface of the egg and appear to develop a channel within the zona as they move forward. Despite the important "drilling" effect achieved by the release of acrosin from the outer acrosomal membrane of the sperm head, it is very clear that without the vigorous, hyperactive beating of the sperm tail providing strong mechanical propulsive force, the sperm still would not be able to get in.

Once penetration of the zona has begun, it requires an average of twenty minutes for the sperm to get completely through; once the sperm has broken through, it plunges directly into the egg membrane itself in less than a second. At that moment, the sperm tail immediately becomes paralyzed. Otherwise the thrashing of the sperm within the egg itself would kill the egg. Very soon after the sperm head becomes embedded in the egg, its tightly packed DNA begins to decondense (spread out a little), and the genetic material of the male becomes the male pronucleus.

### *Completion of Meiosis and Union of the Male and Female Genes*

Once the first sperm has successfully invaded the zona pellucida of the egg, a remarkable event takes place. The membrane that surrounds the egg within the zona fuses with the membrane of the sperm, and the sperm and the egg become one. The egg literally swallows the sperm as these two microscopic entities initiate the development of a new human being. Also at this moment the outer zona pellucida becomes transformed into a rigid barrier so impenetrable that other sperm, despite all the chemicals in their acrosomes, cannot possibly enter. Many sperm can be seen attempting to enter the egg in competition with the one that made it first, but their efforts are in vain. Once the egg has been successfully penetrated by a single sperm it shuts its walls so tightly that none of the followers can get through. This protects the fertilized egg from the entrance of extra chromosomes (called polyploidy), which would cause a genetically impossible fetus, and a miscarriage.

Penetration of the egg membrane by the sperm head also sets in motion the second meiotic division of the egg with the release of the second polar body. It is this second meiotic division that reduces the number of the egg's chromosomes to half so that sperm and egg genes can unite. When the sperm head enters the egg, its chromosomes are tightly and densely packed. After fertilization, the sperm head, with its twenty-three chromosomes, expands (decondenses) into what is called the male pronucleus. At the same time, the female nucleus (which is sit-

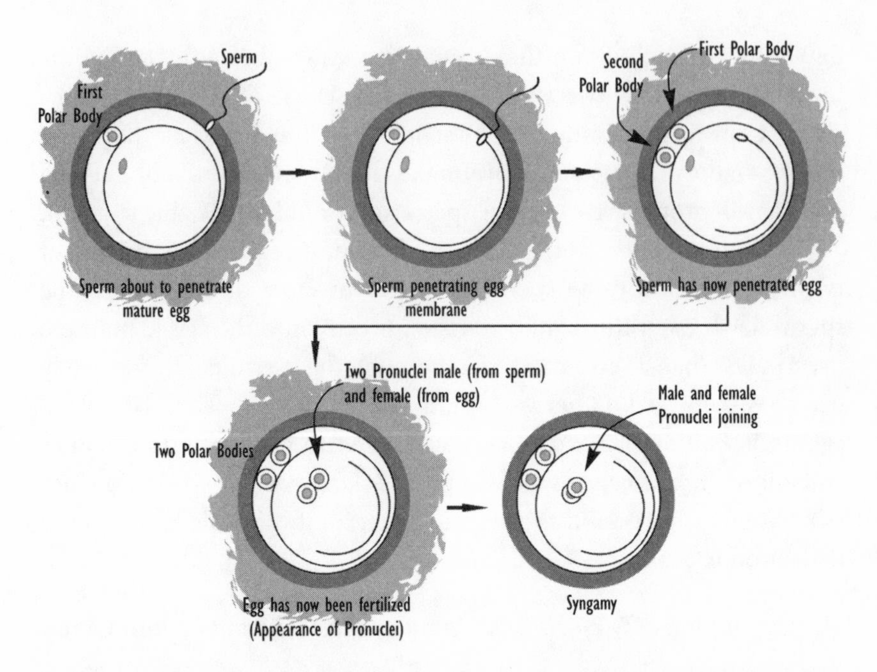


**FIGURE 1.10.** The events of fertilization triggered by the entrance of the first sperm.

ting on the opposite side of the egg) is triggered to undergo its second meiotic division shortly after sperm penetration and become the female pronucleus. This second meiotic division causes extrusion of half the egg's chromosomes to the second polar body, leaving the female pronucleus with twenty-three, just like the sperm. Within eleven to eighteen hours the male and female pronuclei sitting on opposite sides of the egg appear extremely prominent and get ready to converge (see fig. 1.10).

This is truly an amazing event. The two pronuclei (each with twenty-three chromosomes) slowly and majestically move toward the center of the egg and join into one nucleus, which now has forty-six chromosomes and represents an entirely new human being. This merging of the male and female pronuclei is called syngamy. After syngamy, the fertilized egg is ready to divide. Division of the fertilized egg is called cleavage.

## Early Development of the Fertilized Egg

Over the next three days the fertilized egg first divides (cleaves) into two, then four, then eight cells. The first cleavage into two cells occurs sometime before thirty-eight hours after penetration by the sperm. The second cleavage (four cells) begins sometime between thirty-eight and forty-six hours after fertilization. The third cleavage (eight cells) begins between fifty-one and sixty-two hours after fertilization. If any one of those cells were to be removed, the remaining ones would still continue to develop into a normal baby. That is, each cell is still totipotent, and the remaining cells could develop into a completely normal human being. Each one of these early cells formed by the first three or four divisions of the fertilized egg is called a blastomere.

Finally, by the fourth day, the embryo has 64 to 160 cells and is called a morula. These cells have now "compacted" and are no longer totipotent. It's at this stage that the embryo is passed from the fallopian tube into the uterus. By the fifth or sixth day after fertilization, there are so many cells still packed into the same hard, tough zona pellucida that individual cells can no longer be recognized. At this stage the embryo is called a blastocyst. On the sixth or seventh day after fertilization this blastocyst thins out a spot in the otherwise hardened shell of the zona pellucida and actually "hatches," just like a chicken hatches from its shell in an incubator. The blastocyst pushes its way out of this thinned-out crack in the zona pellucida and prepares for implantation (by the seventh day) into the wall of the uterus, or womb. Up until now the zona has protected the embryo. But as a blastocyst, the embryo is now ready for its most treacherous moment when it has to attach to the endometrial lining of the womb. When the blastocyst attaches successfully to the endometrium, that initiates pregnancy.

## Pregnancy Testing

If a pregnancy has been achieved, seven days after fertilization, the embryo begins to secrete the hormone HCG (human chorionic gonadotropin), and this HCG stimulates the ovary to continue to produce progesterone and estrogen, which are necessary for the maintenance of the lining of the womb. Without continued production of progesterone, the pregnancy could not survive. The embryo begins to make HCG when the pregnancy is first established in the uterus, about seven days after ovulation. After three months the fetus, or rather the fetal placenta, actually makes its own progesterone, and the ovaries are no longer needed for production of hormones. After nine months, the baby is ready to be pushed out of the uterus by the mother during labor.

The presence of HCG only signifies that the embryo has implanted and is the basis for almost all of the routine pregnancy tests. Blood tests for pregnancy really just check for the presence of HCG. If it is present, then the pregnancy test is positive. Pregnancy can even be diagnosed with a simple urine test that the woman can perform herself within fourteen days of egg fertilization. However, the laboratory blood test is more reliable. If it is positive, i.e., there is more than twenty-five units of HCG, it should be repeated two days later to see if the HCG level has increased. Normally the HCG doubles every two days for the first month of pregnancy and reaches astronomic levels. If the HCG does not increase, a miscarriage is very likely, and the pregnancy is referred to as a chemical pregnancy.

If the HCG level goes up as it should, then an ultrasound five weeks after fertilization (defined as a seven-week gestational-age pregnancy) should show a normal fetal heartbeat. If there is no fetal heartbeat by seven weeks' gestation, the pregnancy is not viable and miscarriage will follow. Thus, a positive pregnancy test alone does not ensure that the pregnancy is viable. For that you must have an ultrasound exam.

When you have a positive pregnancy test (which just means an elevated HCG level), the chances are 85 percent that you will have a favorable ultrasound at seven weeks and deliver a healthy baby. But miscarriage occurs commonly in early pregnancy despite an elevated HCG level. Because of the biological clock, miscarriage is more common in older women than in younger women, as I will explain in chapter 14.

CHAPTER 2

# Why Are Humans So Infertile?

As you have seen from chapter 1, getting pregnant naturally is a complicated process that requires precise timing. If couples were to have regular intercourse two or three times per week, timing would not be an issue. There would always be sufficient sperm available to the egg whenever ovulation occurred. However, the busy, cluttered lives of modern couples may preclude that. Being aware of the timing of your cycle may thus increase your chances of conception. We can learn some lessons here from a fascinating look at the animal world.

## Humans Don't Know When to Have Sex

In all animals except for humans, the desire for sex is timed to correspond to the female's ovulation. Our inclination to have sex at any time during the month or year is peculiarly human; it separates us from the rest of the animal kingdom and is, reproductively, extremely inefficient. There is only a very brief period of time, just a matter of days during each month, in which intercourse is likely to lead to pregnancy. The timing of sex is thus very important if a species is to have a very high fertility rate. If intercourse doesn't take place around the time of ovulation, it is less likely to lead to a pregnancy. In most animals other than humans, intercourse only occurs at this precise time, when it is likely to result in pregnancy.

Animals go through what is called an estrous cycle, or heat, whereas humans go through a menstrual cycle. In the normal cycle of any animal, as the follicle (or follicles) destined to ovulate begins to grow and prepares the egg for maturation and ultimately fertilization, it produces tremendous quantities of the female hormone estrogen from its granulosa cells. (This high production of estrogen from the developing follicle begins in the human on the first day of menstruation.) In all animals except for humans, this increasing estrogen level chemically triggers the female to desire sex. When this happens, any farmer or animal trainer knows the animal is "going into heat." Whether it's a cow, moose, pig, or rat, the female assumes a peculiarly hunched body position, indicating she is ready for sex. Only at that time in the cycle will she allow a male to get near her. Thus, most animals have sex only when it is likely to result in fertilization and a baby.

Humans, who go through a menstrual cycle, have the same increase in estrogen prior to ovulation. The difference between humans and all other animals is that in humans, the female is just as apt to accept the male in a sexual act at any time during the month. Most of the time, the human female has no idea whether she is having sex at a time of the month that is likely to lead to pregnancy.

Sexual desire in the human is much more complex and is not driven by the female hormone estrogen. In fact, in the human female, sexual drive comes from the male hormone testosterone, the same hormone that is constantly turning on the sexual drive in the male. This is unique in the animal kingdom. Of course, the female level of male hormone is about one-tenth the male level, explaining the lower chemical sexual drive in the female than in the male. The small amount of testosterone that the female makes, however, is quite adequate for her to become willing and interested in being a sexual partner. The amount of testosterone produced by the male is fairly constant from day to day and from year to year. This is true in the female also, although there is a slight increase just around the time of ovulation. Thus, we are similar to our animal friends in that human female-initiated sex is more common around the time of ovulation. But this phenomenon can only be noticed in a small way in large population studies. Usually husbands and wives have sex fairly randomly throughout the month, whereas animals only have sex on a few very specific days, when the female's estrogen level triggers her interest just prior to ovulation.

## Why Is Sex in the Human So Reproductively Inefficient?

Many sociological studies have demonstrated that for the average happily married couple with no psychological problems, and a life not too cluttered by excessive workaholic pressures, sex occurs an average of two to three times per week. Under this circumstance, sex is likely to occur at any time, unrelated to whether it will lead to pregnancy. But what if you have a very busy schedule and a hectic, crowded life, with both partners working, a tremendous amount of stress, and a sexual frequency that is more erratic than a steady two to three times per week? If that is the case and you don't know when you are ovulating, you might be having sex at the wrong time.

Why are human beings so different from animals, and what is the benefit of having this totally random interest in sex? It may be related to our family system.

We know that the human mind today is no different physically than it was forty thousand years ago with the emergence of Cro-Magnon man. But forty thousand years ago, humans were busy learning more efficient methods of hunting and producing primitive art on the walls of caves. Now that same brain is being used to send astronauts into space and to probe the very mysteries of DNA and the genes that create life. How can that same primitive brain be responsible for our incredible civilization? The reason for this is the immense flexibility and capacity for learning that is unique to humans. Other animals are simply born with all the instincts necessary for survival and successful behavior. Humans, however, are born with an enormously educable brain. This requires a family system and a relatively small number of offspring per parent so that the lessons learned in each generation can be passed on from parent to child. If sex in humans were triggered by increased estrogen or testosterone levels timed specifically to when sex is likely to lead to pregnancy, permanent male-female pair-bonding would have been less likely to develop.

It is also worth noting that humans are the only animals that have intercourse facing each other. Throughout the animal kingdom, the female squats in her position of heat and the male mounts her facing her rear end. Only humans face each other during sex, indicating that some kind of communication is occurring other than just a chemically triggered desire for orgasm.

As we will see by the end of this chapter, this reproductive pattern (which is less driven in the human by unthinking, occasional chemical response) promotes the development of permanent mating and a family system. Yet it is partly because of this pattern that human beings are so infertile when compared to the rest of the animal kingdom.

## Seasonal Timing of Sex

For most animals sex is precisely timed by hormones to occur only when it can result in pregnancy, while humans have sex at any time of the week, month, or year. In addition, most animals breed only at a particular time of the year in which getting pregnant is likely to lead to the birth of a baby in the spring months (when the baby is most likely to survive through a warm summer while growing and preparing for its first winter). For example, during midwinter and spring the moose (or any other antlered deer species) has tiny testicles, no horns, and certainly no interest in sex. After June, when the days are getting shorter, the decreasing daylight stimulates a little gland in the moose's brain called the pineal to release a hormone called melatonin, which in the human has very little effect, but in most other animals regulates when breeding will occur. As the days get shorter, the moose's testicles gradually get bigger, and he begins to produce sperm and testosterone, just as the female begins to prepare for ovulation. He goes into rut and she goes into heat at exactly the same time once per year. Sexual desire in the moose is purely mediated by chemicals and in no way relates to any evaluation of each other's personality. When the mating season is over, the male's testicles once again begin to shrink, he stops making testosterone and sperm, and he leaves the female moose to go back on his private wanderings.

Bears have a similar mating pattern except that the mating season is reversed. Whereas the moose's testicles get bigger beginning in late summer and early autumn as the days get shorter, the bear's testicles begin to increase in size in late winter as the days get longer. In fact, it is the increase in the growth of the bear's testicles and the increased production of testosterone that wake him up out of hibernation. He mates after leaving his den in spring, purely because of chemical urges that he does not understand, and shortly after mating leaves the female, who carries on the job of rearing the young completely on her own. With meticulously designed, efficient reproductive systems, most animals have no problem with fertility, but a pair-bonding family environment is not needed for the rearing of their young.

## Reproductive Inadequacy of the Human Male

It is not just the erratic timing of human intercourse that leads to our relative infertility compared to other animals. The fact is that human sperm production is very low compared to sperm production in any other animal. Most male animals produce about 25 million sperm per day per gram of testicular tissue. Humans produce only 4 million sperm per day per gram of testicular tissue. In other words, on a per weight basis, humans produce one-sixth the amount of sperm of any other animal (with a few exceptions such as the gorilla, the cheetah, and the gander).

The average bull ejaculate contains about 10 billion sperm, whereas the average fertile man's ejaculate would contain no more than 100 million sperm. The average bull produces in a single ejaculate one hundred times more sperm than the average human, despite the fact that the actual volume of ejaculate coming from the bull is no more than that of the human. In addition, the bull's sperm are moving at literally three times the speed of the human sperm, in a perfectly straight line, and there are virtually none that are abnormal, weak, or deformed-looking. The human ejaculate is lucky to have 60 percent of the sperm moving at all, most of them move rather slowly compared to those of the bull, and easily 40 percent of the sperm have abnormal structures with atypical head shapes and unpurposeful circular motion instead of linear progression. The average fertile man's sperm looks terribly sick when you compare it to that of most other animals.

Another example of superior animal fertility is the male pig, which ejaculates an entire pint of sperm when he has sex with the sow; the completion of the orgasm requires a full half hour. In addition, the male pig has little screwlike grooves on the end of its penis, which correspond to similar grooves in the female pig's cervix. Thus, the male pig literally screws his penis into the cervix of the female so that there is no leakage or waste during ejaculation, allowing the entire pint of sperm to be delivered directly into the uterus. The amount of sperm in a single pig ejaculate is about four hundred times the amount of sperm in a single human ejaculate, and none of it is lost.

If you were to look at the microarchitecture (histology) of the human testes compared to that of any other animal, you would see a striking difference. The testicular microarchitecture of most animals is perfectly structured, with an orderly wave of sperm production beginning from the earliest immature forms (called spermatogonia) proceeding in a sequential wave through many steps toward the final product — mature sperm. At any given point along the seminiferous tubule of the testicle of most animals, you see a neatly organized progression of sperm production. However, the arrangement seen in human testicle biopsy is a chaotic mess. I will discuss this in greater detail in chapter 7.

Thus, even the normal fertile man has very low sperm production, a high percentage of abnormal sperm in the ejaculate, and a disorganized testicular architecture compared to the rest of the animal kingdom.

### *Is the Environment Causing the Human Sperm Count to Go Down?*

Many people worry that the human sperm count is declining, and numerous popular newspaper articles have suggested that industrial pollution and chemical toxins are the cause. But a cold analysis of available data does not substantiate this fear. Mean sperm counts of American men from fifty years ago were not significantly different than they are today. It is true that 10 percent of fertile men who are actually coming in for a vasectomy have sperm counts in a "very low range," i.e., below 10 million per cubic centimeter (cc). But there is no recent diminution in average sperm count. Sperm count has been declining only in a long-term evolutionary sense. It has been declining not over the last fifty years, but rather over the last several hundreds of thousands of years because of our monogamous mating pattern and family system. Before explaining how our family system has caused this gradual erosion of male fertility, we should discuss the concerns of environmentally conscious researchers who fear, quite justifiably, that modern life can have a negative impact on reproduction.

Let's look at what happened to the Chinese between the 1920s and the early 1930s in the small village of Wang Cun, in the Jiangsu Province, when, for a period of ten years, not a single child was born. The village was panic-stricken and threatened with extinction. They tried praying to Buddha and moved their ancestors' tombs to "luckier" sites. Some of the villagers married previously fertile widows from other villages (who had given birth to children in other places), but they all became strangely barren when they moved to Wang Cun. Then, suddenly, in the mid-1930s, "the curse was lifted," and women began to get pregnant again. It was not understood until many years later that the cause of this sudden sterility of an entire village was a change in the method of cooking — the switch from soybean oil to a cheaper, crude cottonseed oil. When the price of soybean oil went down again in the mid-1930s, the villagers switched back and fertility returned. We now know that cottonseed oil does not necessarily cause sterility if it has been prepared first by heating. But if it has been prepared using a cold press process, without preheating, a chemical in the cottonseed oil, now called gossypol, suddenly and dramatically stops men from producing sperm.

People are often surprised by the little things that can interfere with fertility. Years ago, we scheduled IVF for a forty-year-old couple who had put off trying to get pregnant until the wife was thirty-eight. His sperm count was extremely high, more than 160 million per cc with 90 percent motility, and so they had hoped that she could get pregnant naturally — but they were not tuned in to her biological clock. He was obviously quite fertile, but he began bodybuilding six months prior to the scheduled IVF cycle "to try to build up and be in the best possible shape." He assiduously avoided any hormones or steroids and just worked out physically and took "nutritional supplements." Yet, when the time came for his wife's IVF, his sperm count had dropped to almost zero. He thought the nutritional supplements were harmless. They weren't.

Since 1994 nutritional supplements have been protected from any FDA supervision by a congressional law, so it's impossible to know what companies put into them. This man's sperm count gradually went down from 160 million per cc to only an occasional nonmotile sperm in his ejaculate while he was taking what was thought to be completely safe, protein-only nutritional supplements. We never were able to get the FDA to investigate this case, but when he stopped taking the supplements, his sperm count came back to normal over the next six months.

Although it is clear from large-scale population studies that overall the human sperm count has not suddenly declined in the last fifty years (but rather over hundreds of thousands of years), nonetheless we should be aware that there may be environmental and even emotional factors that can cause fluctuation in sperm count in ways that we don't completely understand.

### *Monogamy and Lack of Sperm Competition*

The major reason that the human male is so reproductively disadvantaged compared to other animals lies in our monogamous mating system and family life, and the inherent lack of "sperm competition." This is a fascinating dilemma that we are forever locked into, and it explains why medical treatments to raise sperm count generally do not work. It also explains why we have to resort to IVF technology to get a woman pregnant when her husband's sperm counts are inadequate, rather than waste time with futile hormonal stimulation approaches that have no impact on sperm production. The infertile male's poor sperm production is genetically determined by hundreds of thousands of years of mating history.

Oligospermia, or low sperm count, is simply part of being human. In family system and mating patterns humans are closest to the gorilla; we are quite different from chimps or smaller monkeys. The ferocious-looking gorilla, who weighs five hundred pounds, has a very tiny penis and very small testicles. On the other hand, the chimpanzee, which weighs only one hundred pounds, has an enormous pair of grapefruit-size testicles — huge compared to those of a human. Why should chimps, who are also great apes and intelligent like the gorilla, have such a tremendous sperm count and be so extremely fertile, when gorillas are probably one of the only other animals on the planet whose sperm production is as poor as that of humans?

Chimps are very promiscuous. They travel in troops of thirty to forty, and all of the males copulate with any female who goes into heat. There is not a single male who does not copulate with any female who has reached her time of ovulation. Gorillas, on the other hand, are virtually monogamous (one male has sex with one female, or sometimes with two females, to whom he remains emotionally attached). When the gorilla's female mate goes into heat, he can be certain there is no other male gorilla who will go near her or have sex with her. They truly have a faithful family system.

If only one male copulates with a given female, there will be no competition from the sperm of any other male, and if she does get pregnant, she will have done so from whatever few sperm that male happens to have. On the other hand, if several males were to copulate with a given female, she is most likely to get pregnant from the male who had the best and highest sperm count. Therefore, in a promiscuous mating pattern, like the chimpanzee's, the male offspring will most likely inherit the genes that result in a higher sperm count. In a monogamous mating system, like the gorilla's or the human's, since there is no competition among sperm from different males for fertilizing the egg, the genes for high sperm count confer little competitive advantage and will not be favored in the population over time.

Human populations with a strictly monogamous lifestyle are much more likely to have low sperm counts and small testicles than those with a more promiscuous lifestyle. One famous study, performed on autopsied men in Hong Kong in the 1980s, compared the testicular size of Chinese males from Hong Kong to that of Caucasian males from the same city. Chinese males had testicle sizes averaging one half that of Caucasian males, showing that many thousands of years of completely monogamous lifestyle resulted in lower sperm counts than in populations where there has been a break from strict monogamy.

## Our Worldwide Infertility Epidemic

Infertility is a global problem. It is not just something that has recently cropped up in the United States. In Russia, China, the Near East, and certainly in Europe and South America, the story is the same. No ethnic, religious, or racial group is spared. In China, where one quarter of the world's entire population resides (1.2 billion people), infertility is the most vexing problem of "upwardly mobile" couples who put off childbearing (as the government has told them to) and then find they can't have children. There is no shortage of patients for IVF in the world's most populous nation. In India, a country with one of the world's most difficult overpopulation problems threatening its economy and way of life, a major family disaster in almost 20 percent of households is the inability to have children. In the new millennium, with westernization and modern development, the problem is growing, and the busiest medical care facilities in India, China, and the Middle East are the fertility clinics. The major cause of this worldwide infertility epidemic is the putting off of childbearing from teen years to a person's thirties and forties. I will explain in the next chapter how you can solve this problem and delay childbearing until you are older, but still not endanger your chances to eventually have a baby.

## Human Destiny and Infertility

If we look at the most remote areas of the world, where humans live today the same as they did tens of thousands of years ago, we can begin to understand better why infertility is not really a curse, but rather an intrinsic part of being human — in fact, it has ensured our survival. The !Kung tribesmen (commonly referred to as the African Bushmen) live in the Kalahari Desert much the same way they did forty thousand years ago. The !Kung have an average of only four children per family and get pregnant only about once every five years; it is the only human tribe whose birth pattern is the same as that of the gorilla. Yet they use no modern birth control and live the most basic, primitive existence on the face of the earth. They have no agriculture, and so the food supply is at best unpredictable. They live strictly by hunting and gathering. They own virtually nothing, and they are chronically undernourished. If they had more children, they surely could not feed them.

The !Kung breast-feed their children exclusively for four or five years (indeed this is necessary because there is so little food available). The child has to derive his or her nutrition strictly from the mother's breast. This constant suckling, without any relief bottles or heaping teaspoonfuls of baby food, completely suppresses ovulation in the female until the child is about four years old, when he or she is truly able to get around and eat the same food as the adults. The family system is secure, and the !Kungs' immense intelligence is unquestioned by anthropologists who have studied them. In a sense, they represent the beginning of our human ascent, which would not have been possible if our ancestors were turning out litters of children.

So when gorillas developed family mating systems and reduced fertility, it was a step toward humanity. Trillions and trillions of ants and bees are born every year, but their mating patterns are governed completely by instinct. There is not a lot that a baby ant or bee has to learn. Human babies are born with a mind that is an open book. It is their early experience and the education afforded by their family in a society that can devote its resources to the education of limited numbers that has resulted in the fullest expression of our humanity.

## Infectious Diseases

About 5 percent of human infertility is caused by tubal obstruction, and that is usually, although not always, caused by sexually transmitted diseases. One-third of African men are sterile because of epididymal obstruction caused by sexually transmitted disease. Gonorrhea and syphilis, which are the most popularly known sexually transmitted diseases (aside from HIV), actually arose in the Renaissance, around the

1400s. The French, of course, blamed it on the English and called it the "English pox," and the English, naturally, blamed it on the French, calling it the "French pox." In reality, gonorrhea and syphilis were rampant everywhere in Renaissance Europe, and these diseases were strictly a result of the increasing promiscuity associated with the liberalization of values during that time. The same phenomenon occurred in the United States and Europe in the 1960s. The increase in infertility after 1960 among women between the ages of twenty and twenty-four (who usually would not yet be undergoing a dramatic age-related decline in fertility) was caused by this increase in sexually transmitted diseases. Because of the current emphasis on "safe sex," brought about by the AIDS epidemic, this problem is declining.

But that, in fact, is why AIDS eventually had to develop. Anyone who has studied the medical history of the Renaissance could have predicted in the 1960s that some terrible disease would develop, most likely generated by a very "weak" organism, which would only be capable of spreading through intimate contact. If the organism (or germ) were strong enough to be transmitted through casual contact, it would be rampant in the population. Chicken pox, for example, is one of the most contagious of all diseases, and few grow up without getting it. But sexually transmitted diseases are usually relatively uncontagious organisms that would never get anywhere if it weren't for the variety of intimate contacts allowed by an increasing promiscuity in the mating pattern of the society.

It is not that a promiscuous sexual pattern will always lead to sexually transmitted disease in a particular culture. For example, well before the arrival of the white man, Eskimos had a very promiscuous-style sex life. A husband would offer his wife to a guest for a night, and he would be terribly insulted by a refusal. In the original Eskimo culture, if a young girl were to get pregnant prior to a marriage being arranged, it would be no problem because she would just give the child to someone else in the community who wanted it. The extended family would take care of the child; the promiscuous sex life was perfectly well accepted. It was with the arrival of white explorers, and the germs that they carried, that they began to contract sexually transmitted diseases.

Not all infectious diseases that cause infertility are sexually transmitted. Smallpox, which is unheard of today, was a scourge of India and the Middle East fifty years ago. Every male child who survived it wound up with epididymal obstruction, i.e., blockage of the sperm ducts, which could only be treated with very sophisticated, modern microsurgery. Twenty years ago, whenever infertile patients from the Middle East or India came to my office and the husband had a few scars on his nose, I knew he had had smallpox as a child, and I knew why they were seeing me.

## What Can I Do?

Infertility is a normal human phenomenon, and if you understand how to manage your biological clock sooner rather than later, it will not prevent you from having a baby whenever the time is right for you.

However, for many women reading this book, IVF technology will be necessary. If you feel a little strange about having your baby through this technology, perhaps you might like to entertain just a page of my "philosophy."

There are those who would reject IVF as being unnatural, and therefore, unethical. These people are afraid of the future. I believe there is a "human destiny" that wants us to continue to develop. Every advance has its potential danger. As Charles Lindbergh flew his little windowless airplane across the Atlantic Ocean to Paris, he probably never dreamed of 747s. The greatest aviator in history could not foresee the future that he was unlocking with that solo flight. Four hundred thousand years ago, humans discovered fire, and 100,000 years ago we began to bury our dead (a custom that eventually allowed us to develop communities of people living together); 40,000 years ago was the beginning of art. Should we have been afraid of fire? Or art?

Our modern society is an anachronism in human life. We do not really want to be "natural." If we wanted to be "natural," we would still have typhoid, bubonic plague, polio, and an average life expectancy, like the African Bushmen, of thirty-five years. If we wanted to be "natural," we would not be going to college, and women would not be pursuing careers and planning to live at least to eighty.

The normal facets of our biology are causing 25 percent of us to be infertile at the age we want to have children. Those who are infertile do not want to suppress the creativity of the human mind to solve this dilemma because of the irrational fear of pessimists, who, in the overall history of humankind, have always been proven to be wrong. Fertility treatment and IVF are the creative human solutions to the growing problem of infertility, which is a natural part of our human condition.

CHAPTER 3

# Beating Your Biological Clock: Antral Follicle Counts

Now that you know how pregnancy is naturally achieved and why humans so often have trouble conceiving, it is time to evaluate whether you should be concerned about your potential to conceive now or later. Since the fertility of all women declines over time, knowing how many years of fertility you have left can make all the difference in planning for your future.

## Age-Related Decline in a Woman's Fertility

### *Most Infertile Women Were Once Fertile*

Most infertile women were fertile when they were younger. In their early twenties, less than 2 percent of women are infertile. But by their late twenties, 16 percent are infertile, and by their midthirties (when, in the modern era, most women will first begin to think about having a child), almost 30 percent are infertile. Nonetheless, some women remain fertile into their forties, while others lose their fertility early in their twenties. At some point in time, as the biological clock ages, no matter how much you spend on sophisticated treatment (other than donor eggs), you will no longer be able to get pregnant and have a baby. You need to figure out at what age this will occur for you, and how you should plan your life. Whether you are a young woman in her early twenties who has just finished college and wants to pursue a career, or whether you just want to learn more about relationships and grow further emotionally before you finally settle down, this inexorable biological clock, which you have heard so much about, will become perhaps your major conflict in life.

The common fear of women in their late teens and early to

midtwenties is an unwanted pregnancy, which is often solved by terminating the pregnancy, or by more diligent use of birth control methods. Just ten or fifteen years later this previously fertile woman and her husband may find themselves going to the doctor because now that she finally is ready for children, she ironically finds that she can't have them. She may begin to feel guilty with self-recrimination, fearing that either the pregnancy termination that she had in her youth, or her decades of being on birth control pills, have in some way caused her current state of infertility.

Of course, that is rarely the case. Whether a woman has been taking contraceptives for a long time or previously became pregnant and terminated that pregnancy, or even if she has just abstained from sex, the decline in her ability to have a child as time passes is inexorable. There will be no shortage of advice (and badgering) to get married and have a child by her mother and father, her doctor, her friends, consumer groups, and professional societies. With a condescending admonition not to disregard her biological clock, they will urge her to hurry up and have children while she can.

In fact, nobody wants her biological clock to tick out, and most women want to bear children eventually. Since the majority of women are still fertile even in their midthirties, many are caught in the dilemma of whether to give up life plans, or to constantly live with the fear that when they are ready to have children, they won't be able to do so. In fact, at some point in a woman's declining fertility, even the most advanced and the most expensive infertility treatment (short of using donor eggs) will not help her.

For example, a twenty-eight-year-old happily married woman (who had had an abortion as a teenager) had been trying to have a baby for approximately two years and finally conceived without seeking treatment. However, she miscarried within the first three months and then sought medical attention. Her miscarriage was caused by a classic chromosomal abnormality, as are most miscarriages. Despite the woman's relatively young age, this fetal chromosomal abnormality was just part of her ovarian aging process. Her infertility and her miscarriage were inevitable and predictable consequences of the low number of eggs with which she was born. When she attempted to undergo in vitro fertilization, only two follicles developed and only one egg was obtained despite stimulation with very high doses of hormones. She had a very dismal chance of ever becoming pregnant with her own child. She had simply run out of eggs prematurely and would go into menopause sometime in her early thirties. Yet ten years earlier she had been quite fertile.

On the opposite side of the spectrum is a forty-four-year-old woman from Europe who was married late in life to a man who had been vasectomized. Her husband had his vasectomy reversed and had only a moderately good sperm count postoperatively. Yet within three months of that surgery, without so much as a single infertility treatment or test, the woman became pregnant and went on to deliver a healthy baby boy.

### *Where Are You on Your Biological Clock?*

Although we know that the biological clock is inexorable, the dilemma that most women face is not knowing just where they personally happen to be on that time scale. Women in their late twenties can be infertile, and women in their early forties can be fertile. Although all women undergo an eventual decline in fertility, the big question for every individual woman is just when that will be. If the forty-four-year-old woman could have known twenty years earlier that she would retain her fertility into her midforties she might have avoided two decades of worry and fear. If the twenty-eight-year-old woman had known she would run out of eggs so early in life, she and her partner might have planned their lives differently as well.

But women no longer have to guess and wonder. Although many tests have been developed in previous decades to diagnose infertility or give a prospective accounting of how much time a woman has left to be fertile, infertile women are painfully aware of how inadequate and completely misleading most of these previous infertility tests have been. Thankfully, there is now a reliable and simple method that allows you and your doctor to take measure of your biological clock, to objectively assess when you should or should not worry about having children, and even to predict how old you will be when you go through menopause.

This simple test can be administered at the time of the yearly Pap smear to all young women who need counseling about their future. Yet there are very few gynecologists who are using it for routine yearly counseling of their patients, let alone for infertile women about to undergo treatment. This chapter will give you a firm basis for understanding how your fertility future can be determined, as well as some simple tools for telling your doctor how to help you discover where you are on your biological clock.

## Age-Related Decline in Fertility Is Due to Loss of Your Egg Supply

### *Evidence That It Is Your Ovary, Not You*

Awareness of the natural and normal age-related decline in a woman's fertility was first made startlingly clear to medical professionals in an article in 1982 in the *New England Journal of Medicine*, resulting from a huge study conducted by a large federation of infertility physicians from France. In this study, 2,193 women who were married to husbands who were azoospermic (had no sperm whatsoever in their ejaculate) had chosen to undergo artificial insemination with donor sperm on a monthly basis until they became pregnant (or gave up). The significance of this study is that there was no male-related contribution to the infertility problem, because normal donor sperm was being used to inseminate all the women. Furthermore, there would be no reason to suspect any infertility problem in any of these women, as all of their preliminary testing for classical, conventional diagnoses of infertility had been either treated or ruled out. Moreover, there was no possibility that insemination might have occurred sporadically during a time of month when the woman was not fertile, as could be the case with random intercourse. Thus, it was the first controlled, reliable study to demonstrate a clear, age-related decline in the fertility of apparently normal, fertile women unrelated to the sperm count or fertility of their husband. After a full year of monthly insemination with high-quality fertile donor sperm, only 40 percent of women over thirty-five years of age were able to become pregnant, whereas twice that many women in their twenties were able to conceive.

In 1996, a British study of IVF demonstrated that the medical diagnosis for which IVF was being used, whether endometriosis, tubal disease, ovulatory dysfunction, or cervical factors, had no effect on the success rate. Pregnancy rates with IVF technology were in no way related to any of the conventional diagnoses that had been used to try to advise and counsel women about their future reproductive potential. The only factor that mattered was the age of the wife and the duration of years that the couple had been trying to get pregnant prior to treatment. This study mentioned nothing about the number of eggs that were available from the wife's ovary, the so-called ovarian reserve. Yet just as important as the woman's chronological age in predicting her future fertility is the number of eggs remaining in her ovaries.

It has become apparent that technology can only go so far in correcting the inexorable age-related decline in a woman's fertility, and that 25 percent of women in their thirties (and 60 percent by the time they reach forty) will not be able to get pregnant without expensive treatment, even though ten or twenty years earlier they might have been quite fertile. Throughout this book, my emphasis will be on what a woman can do to plan her life as it fits her own particular biological clock, without guesswork or admonitions from well-wishers who only create more anxiety. None of the technological advances in infertility treatment will be as important to you as the personal assessment of where you are on your own biological clock.

### *What IVF Pregnancy Rates Tell Us About How the Ovary Ages*

All certified IVF programs are required to report their pregnancy rate (as well as live delivery rate) results to a government agency. As mentioned in the preface, this was originally an attempt by a well-meaning senator to prevent incompetent programs from continuing to flourish without consumer awareness. But unfortunately it has led to a kind of marketing competition between many IVF centers to see which ones can boast the highest pregnancy rates and, thereby, lure the most patients. (In fact, such usage of the reporting data for marketing purposes is strictly against the law that requires the data.) The official government admonition is, "a comparison of clinic success rates is not meaningful because patient characteristics will vary from clinic to clinic." Younger women with many eggs have better results than older women with only a few eggs. The purpose of this section is to avoid comparing results of one IVF program to another, and simply to point out that good IVF results are obtained in women with a high ovarian reserve, while poor IVF results are obtained in women with a low ovarian reserve.

In good IVF programs in the United States, the overall delivered pregnancy rate per treatment cycle for women under thirty-five is about 50 percent. For women ages thirty-five to thirty-seven it is less than 36 percent, for women ages thirty-eight to forty it is only about 25 percent, and for women over forty it is less than 15 percent. However, these results also depend on the woman's ovarian reserve as determined by how many follicles develop (seen on ultrasound) when she is undergoing stimulation with hormones. Even for young women (under age thirty-five) who should be in a favorable category, many programs that boast these high pregnancy rates cancel about 18 percent of IVF cycles because of what is called a "poor ovarian response." The ovarian response, i.e., the number of follicles developing from hormonal stimulation, is related to the total number of eggs in the woman's ovaries.

We have broken down the pregnancy rates per treatment cycle in our IVF program, not only according to the age of the woman, but also according to the number of eggs that can be harvested at the time of her IVF procedure. The overall pregnancy rate for the last nine years has been 45 percent, and for the last four years, it has been 51 percent. Most programs are very excited to have pregnancy rates in this high range, but a closer look shows that pregnancy rates depend upon the age of the woman and the number of eggs that are retrieved (see table 3.1). Women under thirty who had fewer than ten eggs had a 44 percent delivery rate per cycle, and women who were under thirty who had more than ten eggs had a 61 percent delivery rate per cycle. The pregnancy rate and delivery rate went down dramatically in women over age thirty when fewer than ten eggs were retrievable because of a low ovarian reserve. However, the pregnancy rate remained very favorable in women *who had more than ten eggs, despite advancing age.* For women age thirty to thirty-five with fewer than ten eggs, the delivery rate went down to 30 percent, but for those with more than ten eggs, it only went down to 46 percent. Even women over forty years of age (who normally have IVF delivery rates of less than 10 percent) with more than ten eggs had a pregnancy rate per cycle of 47 percent and a delivery rate of 26 percent. Despite advancing age, the pregnancy rate per monthly cycle with IVF was consistently better in women with more eggs. Thus, the deleterious effect of age in the woman is markedly attenuated if she started out with a large storehouse of eggs.

Studies on repeat IVF cycles in our program, as well as carefully documented studies coming out of Oxford, England, demonstrate that roughly the same number of eggs are retrieved repeatedly from any given woman in consecutive IVF cycles. Thus, with an optimal ovarian

**TABLE 3.1**

**Assisted Reproductive Technology (ART) Pregnancy and Delivery Rates (per treatment cycle)**

| | FEWER THAN 10 EGGS | | 10 OR MORE EGGS | |
|---|---|---|---|---|
| Age | Pregnancy | Delivery | Pregnancy | Delivery |
| <30 years old | 50% | 44% | 66% | 61% |
| 30–35 years old | 44% | 30% | 56% | 46% |
| 36–40 years old | 33% | 19% | 48% | 33% |
| >40 years old | 19% | 10% | 47% | 26% |

stimulation program, keeping dosage constant, a given woman at a given time in her life will have a repeatable and predictable number of eggs that can be retrieved in her IVF cycle. It is not just a matter of variability from month to month — it is a constant feature of each woman at every particular stage of her life.

Furthermore, IVF studies over the last dozen years have proved beyond a doubt that the decreased fertility of older women compared to younger women, except in a few instances, is strictly related to her aging ovaries. Although it is true that the obstetrical management of older women in their forties and fifties must be more assiduous because of the somewhat increased risk of high blood pressure, diabetes, and early labor, these are all manageable problems and have nothing to do with the receptivity of the aging uterus. When older women use eggs donated from younger women, the pregnancy rate is not any lower than for younger women undergoing IVF. Thus, we know from IVF studies that the declining fertility of a woman as she becomes older is strictly related to the aging of her ovaries, and not to the rest of her system.

## You Can Freeze Your Eggs (and Even Your Ovary) for Later

There are two reasons why you should know just where you are on your biological clock. The first is that you can plan your life better if you know when you need to worry. The second is that if you find you do not have much time left, you can actually have your eggs (or even one of your ovaries) retrieved and frozen for later use. Thus, despite the otherwise inexorable ticking of your biological clock (the major cause of infertility in the modern era), you can now preserve your fertility for when you are truly ready to have a baby.

Although embryo freezing has been around for decades, up until recently egg freezing has been very problematic. I will describe more fully the whole process of egg and embryo freezing in chapter 10. But for now you should know that if tests show that you will lose your fertility early in life, you can actually do something about it other than just having a baby before you really wish to have one.

This is briefly how it works: 70 percent of the human body is water. The only reason we cannot freeze living organisms (like us) and hold them in suspended animation indefinitely is that the water in our cells would become ice, which crystallizes and expands (like milk in a freezer) and would destroy the integrity of every cell. That is how freezing to death occurs. But if we can avoid that formation of ice crystals inside the cells, then lowering the temperature to –196 degrees Celsius just suspends all metabolic processes, and can do so indefinitely without harm.

Individual cells (like white blood cells and embryos) can be frozen quite successfully on a routine basis by a process called "slow freeze," in which the water content of the cell is removed and antifreeze solution (like in your car's radiator) replaces it.

There are three components of this slow-freeze process. A cryoprotectant antifreeze solution contains sucrose, a sugar that osmotically pulls water out of the cell. At the same time the antifreeze solution itself (either dimethylsulfoxide [DMSO] or propylene glycol) penetrates into the cell just like in your car's radiator. Finally, this antifreeze solution, which contains the embryos, is placed in a computer-controlled freezing machine that lowers the temperature slowly (–0.3 degrees Celsius per minute). That way, as ice crystals form preferentially outside of the cell, the concentration of solutes increases on the outside, gradually drawing more and more water out of the cell by increasing osmotic pressure. Thus, by using these three separate processes, the embryo can be more or less freeze-dried, usually without harm.

However, eggs have rarely survived this slow-freeze technique that worked so well for embryos in IVF patients and for stem cells in cancer patients. The reason is that mature eggs have their chromosomes lined up very precisely on a delicate platelike structure called the spindle, and are therefore much more sensitive to temperature drops. A cell that has completed cell division (with a discernible nucleus) has its DNA in a much more stable arrangement than either a mature egg or any cell in the process of dividing. Therefore, the slightest residual intracellular ice formation can kill the mature egg, even though it does not kill an embryo.

A new technique called vitrification avoids this damage not by trying to pull every molecule of water out of the cell, but by using such a super-high concentration of antifreeze that the water inside the cell never becomes ice no matter how low the temperature. This is a rapid technique that completely avoids the use of a slow-freezing machine. Most important, because the temperature drops so quickly and no intracellular ice at all is allowed to form, this technique finally makes freezing eggs a viable way to preserve fertility. The specific procedure was developed in Japan, and thus far is yielding remarkably good results. However, an even better approach is now feasible.

An entire ovary can also be preserved, an approach that may even surpass egg freezing in efficacy. The reason for the poor success of egg freezing in the past is that the eggs retrieved through normal IVF-type processes are undergoing chromosomal division. The chromosomes of retrieved eggs are highly organized on a complex spindle, which is very susceptible to minor crystal damage from freezing. However, "resting" eggs in primordial follicles within an unstimulated ovary are undergoing minimal cellular activity and have no such complex spindle formation. Therefore, these immature, resting eggs are not easily damaged during an appropriately administered freezing procedure. Furthermore, all these resting eggs, called "primordial follicles," are located in the thin outer one-millimeter crust of the ovary. Thus, we can remove an entire ovary, perform bench microsurgery to remove the inside (to allow successful diffusion of the cryoprotectant into the outer crust), and then successfully freeze this ovarian tissue in the same way we have been freezing embryos for decades (see fig. 3.1). The frozen ovary can be stored safely for many years, and then can be transplanted back and function normally.

In 2004, in St. Louis, we performed the first whole-ovary transplant using this technique, and a young woman who was prematurely menopausal began to have normal periods, conceived several months later, and is now able to have her own genetic offspring. This landmark case proved that an ovary can be transplanted back and forth through a

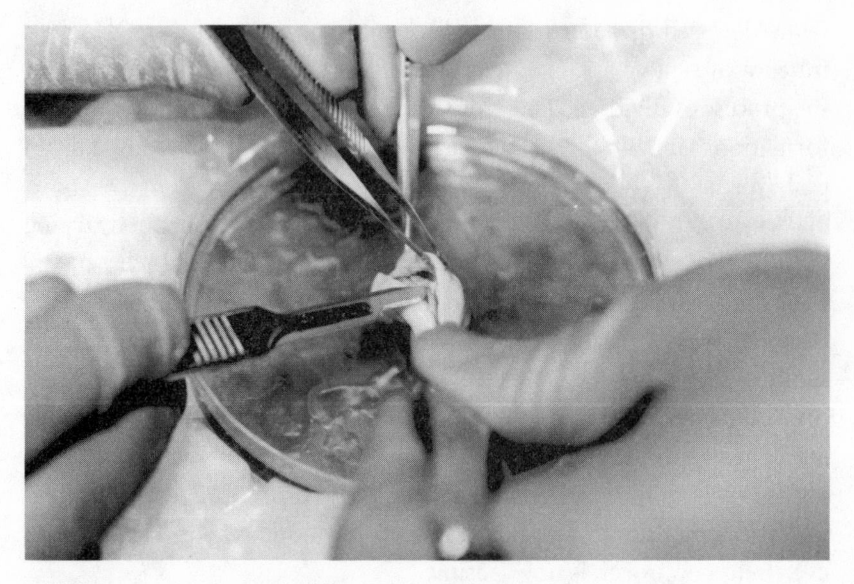

**FIGURE 3.1**

An ovary being prepared for freezing and preservation from a young woman about to undergo radiation and chemotherapy for cancer.

minimally invasive outpatient procedure, completely restoring normal fertility, as well as hormone production, to an otherwise sterile, menopausal woman. This means that women can now put off childbearing until later years, keeping their ovary young until they decide later to have it transplanted back. Thus, menopause can be delayed and reproductive life span lengthened.

The actual procedure to remove the ovary, as well as the procedure for transplanting it back, has been refined to a one-day outpatient approach using a very minimal invasive incision. The reason this is possible is the same reason it is possible to freeze an entire ovary. All of the eggs are located in the one-millimeter outer shell (called the cortex) of the ovary. The entire inside of the ovary contains only blood supply, with no real structure, and is completely dispensable. Therefore, the thin outer shell of the ovary can be placed on any raw surface, just like a routine skin graft, and survive and function normally. This simplicity allows both the ovary removal and the ovary transplant to be performed through a tiny incision on an outpatient basis.

This technology can be used not only to preserve a woman's declining fertility until she is finally ready to have a baby, but also to prevent young cancer patients from becoming sterile as a result of chemotherapy and radiation. We can actually take out a cancer patient's entire ovary and freeze it for grafting back later, or we can retrieve and freeze her individual eggs before she receives an otherwise sterilizing treatment.

Until recently it was feared that breast cancer, the most common malignancy in women, would not be amenable to IVF and freezing of eggs or embryos, because of the increased estrogen level resulting from ovarian stimulation. The fear was that the breast cancer would be accelerated by that brief elevation in estrogen. However, by taking tamoxifen during the ovarian stimulation and IVF cycle, the breast can be protected from this brief estrogen surge. Then the eggs (or embryos derived from fertilizing those eggs with the partner's sperm) can be frozen. Immediately thereafter, the woman can undergo her chemotherapy and radiation, which has at least a 50 percent chance of rendering her sterile. But she will now have frozen eggs or embryos that can be returned to her once she is cured so that she can still have her own genetic child. Alternatively, the embryos could be transferred to a surrogate who could carry her baby for her.

If there is not sufficient time (four to six weeks) available to stimulate the ovary and retrieve eggs before going on chemotherapy or having radiation, the woman can have her ovary removed and frozen safely without delaying her treatment. In fact, since 1996 we have been freezing and saving ovaries for young women who have undergone potentially sterilizing chemotherapy or radiation for a variety of different cancers. If careful examination of sample tissue from the ovary reveals no cancer cells, then at some time in the future the ovary can be transplanted back to restore their fertility.

## Tests for Ovarian Reserve

Since the decline in fertility as a woman passes into each decade of life is strictly related to the aging of her ovaries (and consequently her eggs), considerable effort has been made in the past to try to develop tests to determine ovarian reserve. "Ovarian reserve" simply means the number of eggs your ovary has in reserve. The greater your ovarian reserve, the more time is left on your biological clock. I will briefly discuss those tests that have been demonstrated to be inadequate before going into great depth about the tests that really work.

### *Day Three FSH and Estradiol*

The most commonly used test to estimate an infertile woman's ovarian reserve is the so-called day three FSH blood test. This test was popularized in the late 1980s under the naive assumption that as the egg supply (ovarian reserve) of women diminishes, it results in a decreased inhibitory signal from the ovary to the pituitary gland (as explained in chapter 1) and, therefore, an increased level of FSH (follicle-stimulating hormone). FSH is the pituitary hormone that increases during menstruation on day one of your cycle, and stimulates the formation and growth of the dominant follicle, resulting in ovulation at midcycle (see fig. 3.2).

The FSH level varies throughout the cycle. It increases on day one, and then gradually goes down over the next twelve days as the dominant follicle grows larger and larger, and secretes more and more estrogen. The increased estrogen production from the dominant follicle causes a slow decline in FSH secretion from the pituitary until midcycle, when the very high estrogen level arising from the mature, preovulatory follicle triggers a release of LH. This hormone (LH) then causes the follicle to ovulate. Fourteen days after ovulation the estrogen and progesterone levels precipitously decline if the woman is not pregnant, menstruation occurs, and the FSH once again goes up in response to the declining estrogen level, beginning a new cycle.

A low day three FSH was thought to be indicative of a high ovarian reserve, i.e., a large number of eggs in the ovary. This has not turned out to be true. Of course, when a woman is very close to her menopausal years, at the extreme end of her ovarian follicle supply, her day three FSH will be high, as FSH production goes into overdrive to stimulate the remaining follicles. But for most of her reproductive life, the day three FSH does not correlate with her ovarian reserve and is not at all predictive of when she will lose her fertility.

Nonetheless, the day three FSH test, despite its lack of utility, has become almost an institution in virtually every IVF program. The problem with this test is not so much the variability of FSH levels between day two and day five of the menstrual cycle, but simply that the FSH level only becomes elevated at the extreme end of a woman's fertility, long after it has ceased to be very useful for her planning.

The next attempt to determine ovarian reserve was the so-called day three estradiol level. It was suggested that if the woman's estradiol

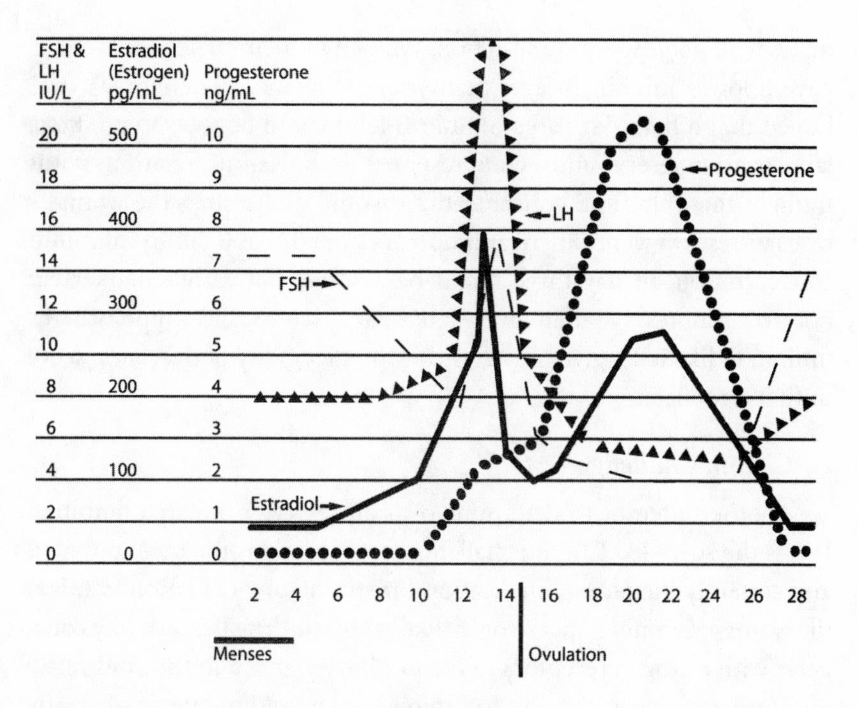


**FIGURE 3.2.** Hormonal control of a normal menstrual cycle.

(estrogen) level by day three was greater than eighty pg per milliliter, she was likely to have a lower ovarian reserve. However, this increased day three estrogen level is simply caused by the increase in FSH experienced by older women. Therefore, the information gained by measuring the blood level of estrogen on day three is not much different from what would be gained by the day three FSH. Furthermore, many studies have found no difference in day three estradiol concentrations in regularly menstruating women between the ages of twenty-four and fifty. Therefore, day three estradiol levels also cannot be used to assess ovarian reserve.

### *Day Three Inhibin B Level*

Another blood test that was used to try to assess ovarian reserve is the "day three inhibin B level." Inhibin B is the very infrequently talked about hormone released along with estrogen from the granulosa cells that surround the follicle, and it seems to have no function other than to inhibit the pituitary's release of FSH. This same inhibin B is secreted from the Sertoli cells of the male testes, thus inhibiting FSH secretion in males with good sperm production. Women in their forties, on average, have a lower inhibin B level than younger women. Therefore, it was hoped that a high day three inhibin B level could be used to predict a large ovarian reserve and a good response to ovarian stimulation. It was thought that inhibin B concentrations would diminish as the woman's ovarian reserve went down, and doctors hoped that a fall in inhibin B concentration on day three might be a somewhat earlier marker for poor ovarian reserve than an elevated day three FSH. Disappointingly, inhibin B, like FSH, gives relatively low predictability of ovarian reserve until it is too late.

### *Clomid Challenge Test*

Another attempt to determine ovarian reserve prior to attempting IVF is the so-called Clomid challenge test. Clomid is the most popular, and certainly the oldest, medication for stimulating ovulation in infertile women. Clomid is an estrogen-like synthetic drug that actually competes with estrogen receptors in the pituitary gland, and thus indirectly diminishes estrogen's ability to inhibit FSH secretion by the pituitary. This increased FSH secretion by the pituitary stimulates ovulation.

The ability of Clomid to stimulate FSH secretion can be used as a "challenge test" to see how much it causes the FSH to rise. Theoretically, if the FSH level rises too much, it is indicative of the ovary's diminished ability to secrete inhibin B and estradiol, thereby inhibiting the pituitary's secretion of FSH. If a woman's FSH does not rise dramatically after Clomid, then, theoretically, her ovary has a good supply of eggs. As you can gather, this is a convoluted and indirect approach to estimating where you are in your biological clock. FSH levels after Clomid administration have shown a wide cycle-to-cycle variability. Thus, the Clomid challenge test is still only an indirect measurement and (like day three FSH and estradiol) is not a very good indicator of ovarian reserve until it is too late.

### *Antral Follicle Count*

None of the previously described tests achieve the accuracy, simplicity, and reproducibility that we have found with ultrasound-performed *antral follicle counts* for ascertaining where you are on your biological calendar. The rest of the chapter will explain this test. The ultrasound determination of antral follicle count is the same at any time during the cycle, is independent of birth control pill usage or other hormone administration, and is very easy to have performed by any radiology center or gynecologist with a relatively modern ultrasound machine. The best preparation for this test is to have a very good understanding of just how your ovary works, how your eggs are formed, how they die and diminish over your reproductive life span, and just what it is that the radiologist, or the technician, or the gynecologist, will be looking at when he or she performs, during a routine ultrasound examination, your antral follicle count.

The procedure is extraordinarily simple for any doctor or technician to perform, but only if they are aware of its significance — *most are not.* Any woman can obtain an easy estimate of when she should or should not begin to be concerned about her biological clock. But she will have to understand and be able to explain to her doctor just what it is that she wants.

## How Does the Biological Clock Work?

### *What You Were Born With*

Remember, women are born with all the eggs they are ever going to have, and they don't make any new eggs during their lifetime. Women are born with approximately two million eggs in their ovaries, but about eleven thousand of them die every month prior to puberty. As a teenager, a woman has only three hundred thousand to four hundred thousand remaining eggs, and from that point on, approximately one thousand eggs are destined to die each month. This phenomenon is completely independent of any hormone production, birth control pills, pregnancies, nutritional supplements, or even health or lifestyle. Nothing stops this inexorable death of approximately one thousand eggs every month regardless of ovulation, ovarian inhibition, or stimulation. Whenever the woman runs out of her supply of eggs, the ovaries cease to make estrogen, and she goes through menopause. Despite a lot of journalistic hype, there is no similar phenomenon in men. Men continue to make sperm and testosterone at virtually the same rates, with only a very modest diminution as they age.

Many population studies have demonstrated over several decades that the average fertile woman becomes infertile by age forty or earlier, and undergoes menopause by age fifty. The mean age of the end of female fertility (according to all the early population studies of fertile women) precedes menopause by about ten to thirteen years. The end of fertility for an otherwise normal, fertile woman, and the age of the onset of menopause, correlates strictly with the decline in the number of eggs remaining in her ovary.

The average female life expectancy in the Western world is currently about eighty-four, whereas in 1900, the average life expectancy was fifty, and in 1850, it was only forty-two years of age. Meanwhile, the average age at which young girls start menstruating in the modern world has decreased from age thirteen or fourteen to age ten or eleven. Neither the overall life expectancy, nor the age of menarche (the beginning of menstruation) has any effect on the average age of menopause. In fact, the average age of menopause in almost every population studied over any period of time and in any era has remained constant at around fifty. Although some women go through menopause in their twenties (because of POF, i.e., premature ovarian failure) and some go into menopause in their late fifties, the timing does not appear to depend upon any specific element in their lives other than the number of eggs with which they were endowed at birth.

It is this wide variation in endowment of eggs from woman to woman that will determine whether you will lose your fertility early (late twenties or early thirties), or whether you'll be one of the lucky women who is able to have children into her mid- or even late forties. To recap, the average woman will have three hundred thousand to four hundred thousand eggs at the time of puberty. An average of one thousand will die every month, and only one of those thousand every month is destined to ovulate. By age thirty-seven, the average woman will be down to only about twenty-five thousand remaining eggs. When only twenty-five thousand eggs remain in the ovaries, menopause will occur in approximately thirteen years. Thus, the average woman begins to become infertile by age thirty-seven or earlier, when her ovarian reserve goes down to about twenty-five thousand eggs, and at age fifty, she will go through menopause. But there are wide variations from this average. What you need to know, in order to plan your entire life, is where *you* fit on that curve (see fig. 3.3).

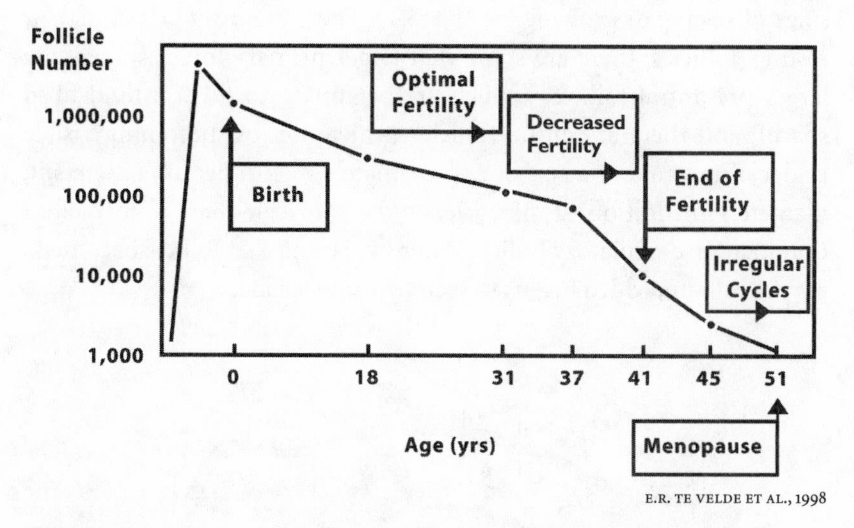


**FIGURE 3.3.** The decreasing follicle pool and age-related decline in female fertility.

### *Antral Follicles and Your Ovarian Reserve*

To understand how an antral follicle count ultrasound can tell you where you are on your biological clock, remember that approximately thirty to thirty-five eggs die every day. That is where the number of one thousand per month comes from. They die only because they have initiated their emergence from the resting pool of eggs and have begun their long, three-month development toward becoming an egg that is capable of ovulation. Only one every month, out of the one thousand that tried, will ever make it. In other words, every day thirty or so eggs that are otherwise safely resting in your ovary, protected from the ravages of age by being in a quiescent phase, emerge by some signal that scientists still don't understand into a very long (approximately three-month) developmental process that is completely dissociated from your menstrual cycle or your ovulatory cycle. Once that three-month growth has reached the antral stage, when the follicles finally become sensitive to the hormones of your monthly menstrual cycle, they will rapidly die and disappear if they are not rescued by FSH. Here is how it happens:

Each egg in your ovaries is enclosed within a resting follicle. Every day, thirty to thirty-five of these resting follicles begin their eighty-five days of development toward eventually trying to ovulate. At any time, a view into your ovary reveals follicles (with their enclosed eggs) in every stage of resting or growing (see fig. 3.4). There are early primordial, or resting, follicles; there are somewhat larger primary follicles; there are larger pre-antral follicles (which are beginning to form a fluid-filled space); and there are antral follicles, which are just becoming visible under ultrasound at a size of approximately one to two millimeters in diameter. In addition, at midcycle, on day fourteen, there is normally a dominant pre-ovulatory follicle. After ovulation, that follicle becomes a corpus luteum, which begins to secrete progesterone.

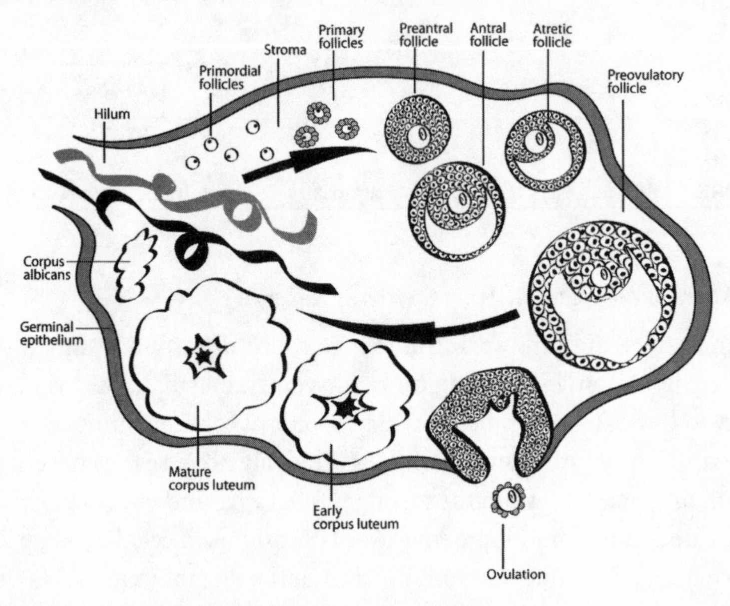


**FIGURE 3.4.** Various stages of follicles in the human ovary.

It is often erroneously thought that just one follicle develops during every month, during the first two weeks of the cycle, ultimately culminating in a large, twenty-millimeter follicle from which the egg is ovulated at approximately day fourteen (in a typical twenty-eight-day ovulatory menstrual cycle). Development of this single, dominant follicle every month with its increasing production of estrogen, and the entire regulation of the monthly cycle via the pituitary hormones of FSH and LH, only gives a tiny part of the picture; it only shows what is happening to one egg in an ovary that contains, in a fertile young woman, as many as 200,000 eggs. That one egg that was destined to ovulate developed as the single dominant follicle out of the thirty or so much smaller pre-antral and antral follicles, which had been developing in the ovary for as long as seventy days prior to the beginning of the current twenty-eight-day menstrual cycle (see fig. 3.5).

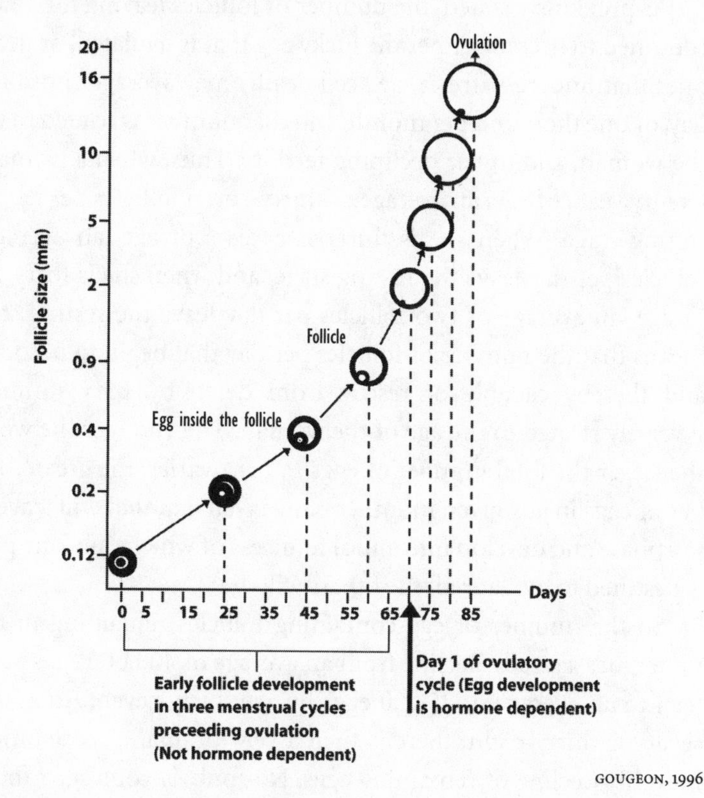


**FIGURE 3.5.** Eighty-five days of follicle development.

Most of the ovaries' 300,000 to 400,000 follicles are quiescent and doing nothing during any given month, but out of that primordial pool a certain number (an average of thirty to forty) will begin to develop each day. By approximately seventy days of development, these follicles will have grown to approximately two millimeters in size, and at that size they are readily visible with modern, high-quality ultrasound scanning. During the first seventy days of a follicle's development, it is completely independent of any hormonal influence. FSH and the monthly hormonal cycle have no influence yet. Sometime between 0.2 millimeters and 2 millimeters in size, these so-called antral follicles begin to become sensitive to stimulation by FSH from the pituitary gland. Prior to the time when these tiny follicles finally become ready to enter the current menstrual / ovulatory cycle, they are completely unaffected by whatever hormonal events have been taking place in the previous cycles.

As previously stated, the number of follicles leaving the resting pool (destined to become either the lucky egg that is ovulated, or the unlucky ones that undergo atresia, i.e., cell death) may average about thirty per day, or one thousand per month, and that number is related to the age of the woman, and to her declining fertility. Thus, when a woman is only twenty years of age, an average of thirty-seven follicles per day leave the resting stage. When she is thirty-five years of age, an average of ten follicles per day leave the resting stage, and when she is forty-five years of age, an average of two follicles per day leave the resting stage. This means that the number of follicles per day that begin to become antral, and thereby capable of rescue from death by FSH stimulation, is inversely related to the age of the woman. The younger the woman and the larger the total number of eggs in her ovaries, the greater the number of eggs in any given month, or any given day, that will leave the resting phase and develop into antral follicles (of which only one per month is destined to ovulate; all the others will die).

So the number of egg-containing follicles remaining in the ovary undergoes a steady decline from an average of 400,000 eggs at age eighteen to an average of 25,000 eggs by age thirty-seven. After age thirty-seven or thirty-eight, there is then a very dramatic acceleration of the monthly decline of remaining eggs. Not only is your egg / follicle pool already down because of a steady decline over the previous twenty years, but the rate of the decline after age thirty-seven becomes even steeper than in prior years (see fig. 3.6). The number of follicles per day that leave this resting pool and begin the three-month developmental path toward being available for future ovulation diminishes dramatically in direct proportion to the number of eggs that are left in the ovary. When the antral follicle first becomes large enough (one to two millimeters) to be visible on ultrasound it also becomes susceptible to hormonal stimulation, and the number of visible antral follicles is directly proportional to ovarian reserve. Therefore, the antral follicle count as determined by ultrasound will give you an accurate read on how many eggs are left in your ovaries.

The antral follicle count also tells you the number of eggs that can be retrieved in an ovulatory stimulation cycle for IVF. To understand this,

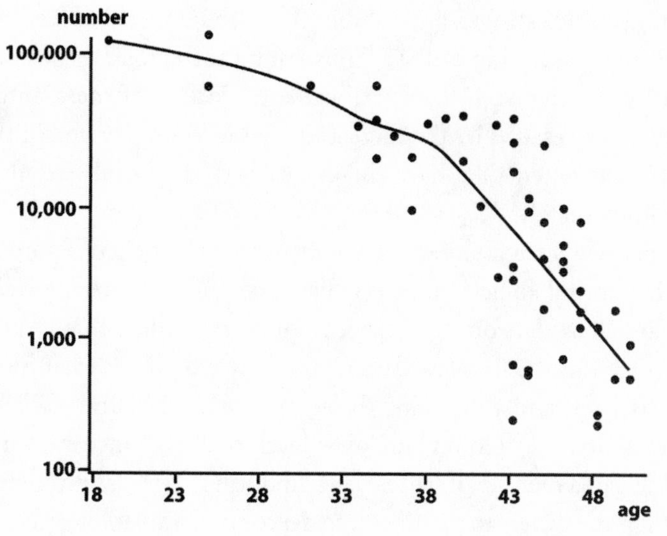


**FIGURE 3.6.** Number of eggs in the human ovary in relation to age of woman.

we will quickly review the normal menstrual cycle with the ovulation of a single egg (from chapter 1) and explain what happens when we give FSH injections to stimulate multiple follicle development for an IVF cycle. Remember that the number of eggs we are able to retrieve in an IVF cycle, regardless of age, is the most important determinant of your likelihood of pregnancy; it is also the most important determinant of any age-related decline in your natural fertility.

### *Emergence of the Dominant Single Follicle During a Normal Ovulatory Monthly Cycle*

At the time of your menses (menstruation), as a result of the rapid fall in estradiol (estrogen) and progesterone secretion from the ovulated follicle of the previous month, the uterus sheds the lining that had built up during that month in preparation for pregnancy (see fig. 3.2). This sudden drop in estrogen causes the FSH secreted from the pituitary gland to rise dramatically around day twenty-six of the previous twenty-eight-day cycle. So, two days later, on day one of your menstruation (the beginning of your next cycle), this elevated FSH stimulates only the development of follicles that had left the resting pool 70 days earlier, and that are now antral. As these antral follicles grow in response to FSH, they secrete estrogen and inhibin B, which in turn suppress further the pituitary secretion of FSH. Thus, as the antral follicles become more mature (by day six), the FSH begins to decline. If these antral follicles were not rescued by the increased FSH level on day one of the menstrual cycle, when they have finally reached the antral size, they would die immediately.

A competitive struggle then ensues between all of these approximately thirty antral follicles to see which one will become the "lead follicle" that will ovulate on day fourteen. The antral follicle that is most sensitive to FSH in the first few days of your cycle becomes even more sensitized to FSH, and thus gains the lead over all the other follicles (which die off because of lower and lower levels of FSH). Once the dominant follicle gains the lead, it will never relinquish it, because it requires less FSH than the others to get the same degree of stimulation. Because FSH continually declines toward the middle of your cycle just prior to your ovulation, all the other antral follicles that month (which have finally become hormone dependent after almost three months of non-hormone-related growth) will die. When they reach this stage of development, the follicles are completely dependent on FSH for survival. Once the estrogen production exponentially peaks, around day twelve or thirteen, it stimulates a dramatic rise in LH from the pituitary gland, and that rise in LH is what prepares the one remaining follicle for ovulation.

In preparation for IVF, FSH injections are given in the early part of the cycle so that the FSH level never declines, as it would normally. This sustained elevation of FSH, which is all that the administration of ovulatory stimulation hormones amounts to, sustains almost all of the thirty or so antral follicles so that no single follicle can gain dominance over the others. Therefore, the number of eggs retrieved in a hormonal stimulation cycle for IVF is directly reflective of your antral follicle count, and your antral follicle count is directly reflective of your total remaining number of eggs.

## Antral Follicle Count Studies

### *Antral Follicle Count and Number of Eggs Left in Your Ovary*

Most of the important clinical work regarding antral follicle count began in the Netherlands. The idea was first introduced by Dr. Bart

Fauser's group in Rotterdam in 1990, and later by Dr. E. R. te Velde's group in Utrecht. Their results have been confirmed by studies in Finland, Taiwan, Vienna, and Hong Kong, and by our group in St. Louis. The procedure is not yet very widely known or practiced, because of the inevitably slow pace of dissemination of new discoveries. For example, the first IVF baby was born in 1978 after ten years of extensive animal research, but IVF did not become very popular until ten or more years later. In a similar vein, antral follicle count will give young women the foreknowledge they need to plan their future reproductive life and will help infertile couples decide how quickly they should begin their treatment — but only after patients start asking their doctors to perform it.

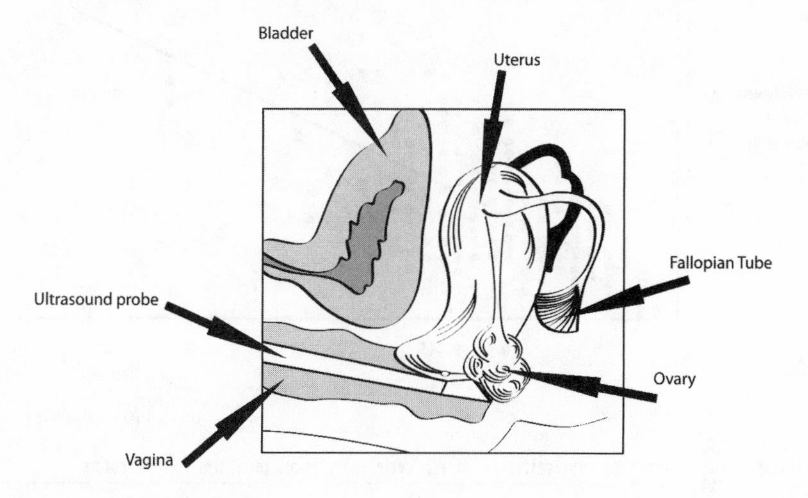


**FIGURE 3.7.** Side view of ultrasound probe in vagina during routine pelvic exam.

Transvaginal ultrasound is a simple, routine procedure (available everywhere) for viewing the ovaries, utilizing ultra-high-frequency sound waves. A probe (which is smaller than the speculum used for your standard pelvic exam and Pap smear) is placed in the vagina, and a clear image of your ovaries and uterus can be plainly seen (see fig. 3.7). In 1990, Dutch doctors found that no matter when they performed ultrasound in the monthly cycle there was no significant difference in the number of small follicles (one to two millimeters in diameter). They followed these follicles during the course of the menstrual cycle in normal fertile women in order to see which one of these early follicles became dominant, how it became dominant, and what happened to the small follicles that were not "recruited" to be ovulated. They found that as the small follicles grew from two to ten millimeters, the follicle that reached greater than ten millimeters in diameter first became the dominant one, and all the other follicles receded and died. Thus, a size of ten millimeters (one centimeter) acts as a threshold whereby one can predict the fate of all the other ovarian follicles in that particular month. Once that size, the dominant follicle (or follicles, in rare cases) will continue to grow, whereas the nondominant follicles will begin to recede.

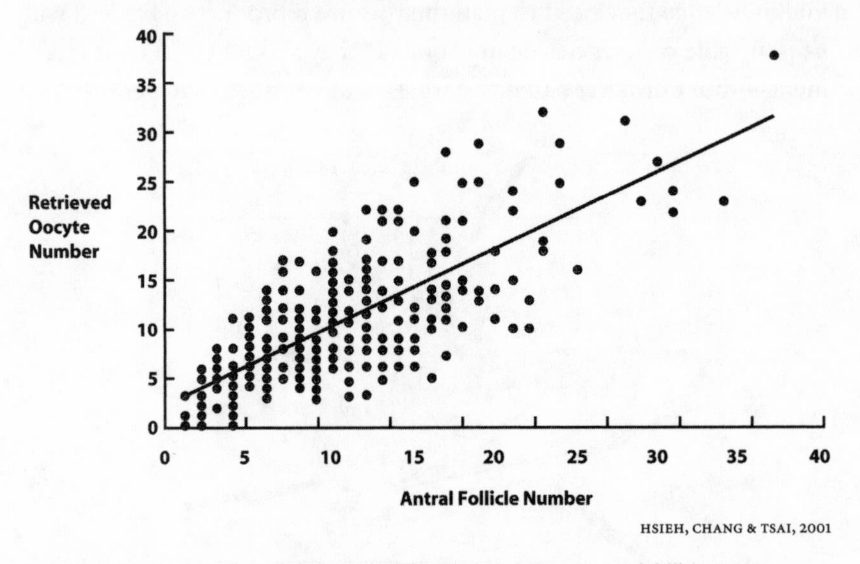


**FIGURE 3.8.** Number of eggs retrieved in IVF cycle in relation to antral follicle count.

The much bigger concept of using the antral follicle count to predict success rate with IVF came from other Dutch investigators and was confirmed in 1997 and 1998 in Finland and in Taiwan (see fig. 3.8). The number of antral follicles present before ovarian stimulation was a better predictor of the outcome of IVF than any other factor, including age. The age of the patient alone is a very weak predictor of ovarian reserve and responsiveness to IVF stimulation. No pregnancies were achieved in patients who had low antral follicle counts, whereas very good pregnancy rates were achieved in patients with higher antral follicle counts. The best pregnancy rates were achieved in patients with the highest antral follicle counts.

### *Antral Follicle Count and Your Age*

The Dutch then went a step further in 1999, when they reported a truly landmark study of 162 fertile women with normal menstrual cycles, ages twenty-five to forty-six years of age. They correlated the decline of antral follicle count with increasing age and with the decline in the number of eggs remaining in the ovary. Their study showed that the number of primordial follicles in the ovary decreases throughout childhood and adult life, eventually leading to ovaries that are almost devoid of follicles at the age of menopause. It also revealed that the antral follicle count is a simple and easy way to measure that decline in any woman (see fig. 3.9).

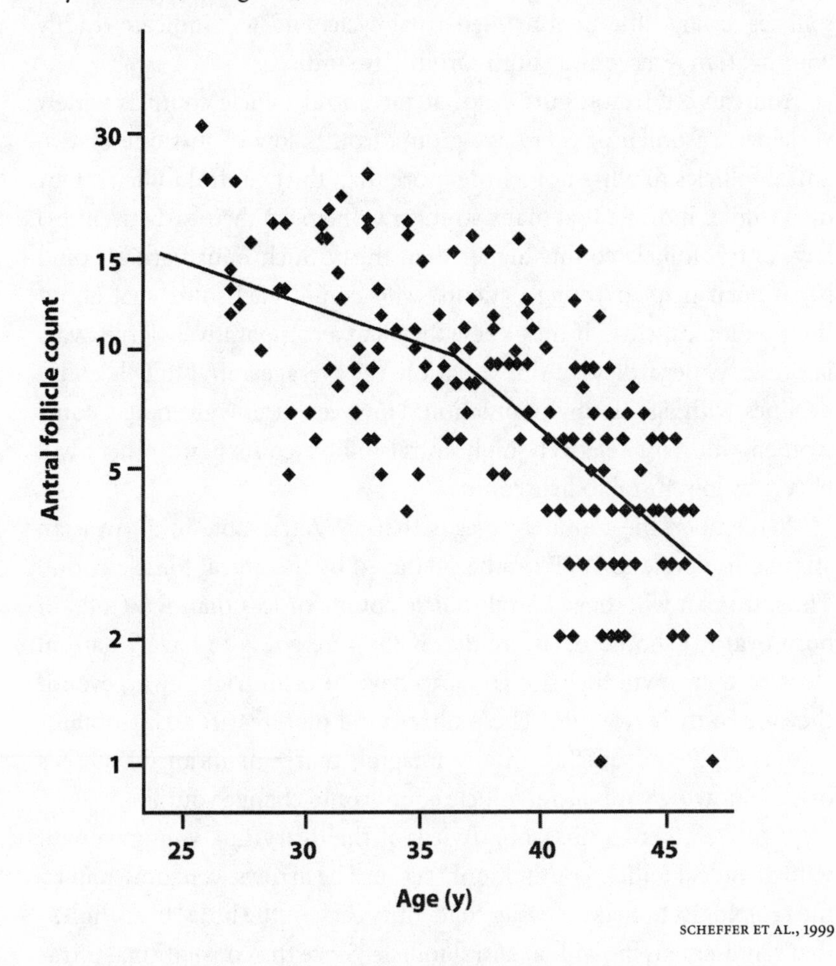


SCHEFFER ET AL., 1999

**FIGURE 3.9.** Decline of antral follicle count with increasing age of woman.

Even before that, the great French biologist François A. Gougeon, as well as English biologist Roger Gosden and Australian mathematician Malcolm Faddy, had conducted ovarian tissue studies demonstrating that the total number of follicles remaining in the ovary decreases every year with age. They showed that the total reserve of primordial resting follicles is correlated with the number of growing follicles at any time in the cycle. Therefore, as the primordial follicle reserve declines, so does the size of the antral follicle cohort that enters each monthly ovulatory cycle. This phenomenon manifests as a reduction in the number of follicles developing (from what were antral follicles before stimulation) as a result of ovarian stimulation for IVF. Transvaginal ultrasound can thus provide an accurate measurement of the total number of antral follicles at any time in your menstrual cycle, and will indicate readily your ovarian reserve and your reproductive future.

You can see from figure 3.9 that the antral follicle count is widely variable in women of every age group, from a low of just one or two antral follicles to a high of a little more than thirty antral follicles. Our own studies indicate that many younger women (in their early twenties) have antral follicle counts higher than thirty. Such information would be of great help to young patients, who could relax somewhat about their biological clock if they knew they had a comparatively large ovarian reserve. Regardless of this variation, the average antral follicle count declines with age in any population. However, at any given age, some women will have relatively high antral follicle counts and others will have very low antral follicle counts.

Remember, the number of eggs that are retrievable in an ovarian stimulation cycle for IVF can be predicted by the antral follicle count. Thus, women who have antral follicle counts of less than ten (total of both ovaries) should be aware that if they are going to have a natural child of their own, they are going to have to begin right away, even if they are in their twenties. These ultrasound pictures are easily obtainable, cheaply and quickly, in any imaging center or in an OB-GYN's office. Knowing your antral follicle count could change your life.

Figure 3.10 is an ultrasound view of the ovary in a young woman with an antral follicle count of only seven. The arrows were drawn in by the radiologist to make it easier to identify each of the little "black holes" that represent an individual antral follicle. Since the conventional ultrasound is only a two-dimensional view, a single photograph often does

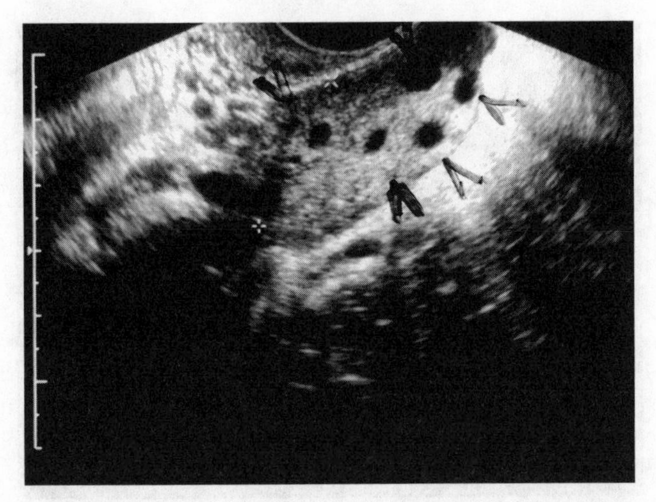

**FIGURE 3.10.** Ultrasound cross-sectional view of an ovary with seven antral follicles.

not show you what the total number of antral follicles is in the volume of an ovary. That is why with conventional ultrasound the radiographer has to gently move the probe from one side of the ovary to the other and count these little black holes throughout the entire substance of the ovary, not just in one view. However, in a small ovary like this, with a low antral follicle count, a single two-dimensional view is usually reflective of the rest of the ovary.

You can see for yourself how easy it would be for any technician, radiologist, or gynecologist to quickly count your antral follicles within a matter of minutes. This woman, with an antral follicle count of seven follicles in one ovary (and seven follicles in the other ovary), has a total antral follicle count of fourteen, which is quite low for a woman in her midtwenties. If for some reason one of her ovaries were ever removed, such as for a cyst, her antral follicle count would be reduced to seven, and her chances of ever conceiving (if she did not do so very soon) would be extremely low. As it is, she needs to know that she does not have a great antral follicle count for a woman in her midtwenties, and she may wish to accelerate her timetable for having a family.

Figure 3.11 shows an ultrasound view of an ovary that has been stimulated for IVF, with more than fourteen mature follicles ready for aspiration. It would appear at first glance that the follicles are located within the substance of the ovary, but in fact, all of these follicles originate from the outer perimeter of the ovary, not from within its sub-

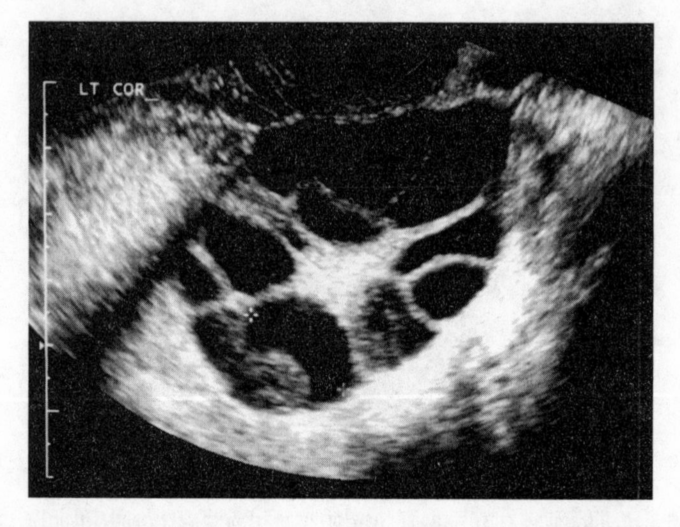


**FIGURE 3.11**

Ultrasound of stimulated ovary with mature follicles ready to be aspirated for IVF.

stance. Keep that in mind when we talk a little later in this chapter about the types of foolish infertility surgery that can reduce your ovarian reserve rather than enhance your fertility.

### *Antral Follicle Count and Your Remaining Years of Fertility*

The reliability of antral follicle count is completely independent of the menstrual cycle. Unlike hormone evaluations, the ultrasound evaluation of antral follicle count can be used on any day of the menstrual cycle to show those follicles that have left the resting state and have reached the antral size. This is a daily event that occurs independently of all the other monthly variations in the menstrual cycle.

Antral follicle count can, of course, be used for counseling infertile women about to undergo IVF so that they will know what their chances are for a successful result. However, it is also extremely useful for all women who are thinking about getting pregnant either sooner or later, and who need to know if it is risky for them to put this decision off. It is even possible to predict at what age menopause will occur (see table 3.2).

Fertile women who have an antral follicle count of twenty to forty, regardless of age, can anticipate becoming infertile within ten to fifteen years and will likely reach menopause about ten years later. An otherwise fertile woman whose antral follicle count is ten is likely to become

**TABLE 3.2**

**Number of Antral Follicles Represents Reproductive Age and Gives the Following Approximate Predictions:**

| ANTRAL FOLLICLE COUNT (PER OVARY) | MEDIAN YEARS TO LAST CHILD | MEDIAN YEARS TO MENOPAUSE |
|---|---|---|
| 20 | 14.8 | 24.0 |
| 15 | 9.3 | 18.4 |
| 10 | 4.2 | 12.9 |
| 5 | — | 7.3 |

FADDY ET AL., 2003

infertile very soon, and to have menopause within about thirteen years. Women who have antral follicle counts of less than five are very unlikely to be able to get pregnant with or without infertility treatment, and they are likely to have menopause begin sometime within the next seven to eight years. Of course, these are average and median figures, and cannot predict exactly for each individual patient. But it can be concluded that even younger women with antral follicle counts of less than ten (total from both ovaries) have no time to waste if they want to have children.

In fact, as the number of eggs diminishes to such low levels, the rate of further egg loss actually accelerates. The proportion of follicles leaving the pool of primordial follicles actually increases with advancing age, just as the total number of primordial follicles in the pool of resting follicles declines. In other words, the ovary is performing a "salvage operation" in order to squeeze whatever it can out of the declining follicle pool as it diminishes. Therefore, follicle counts of less than five or ten are even more alarming because we know that the ovary is pushing out whatever it can in the face of a very difficult situation where very few eggs are left.

Thus, transvaginal ultrasound, which should be a simple and readily available tool in most gynecologists' offices and certainly in any radiology imaging center, can provide an accurate and reproducible measurement of the total number of antral follicles throughout the menstrual cycle, which is indicative of the woman's ovarian reserve and her reproductive future.

## Is There Anything That Can Preserve the Declining Follicle Pool in Your Ovaries?

The question that will naturally come to the mind of every young woman who is contemplating putting off childbearing is whether there is some way of slowing down the rate of emergence of eggs from the resting follicle pool into the antral state, thus keeping her eggs quiescent, so that they will not undergo atresia and die. A primordial follicle is safe until it leaves its resting state and becomes destined to enter an ovulatory cycle (whether it is the dominant follicle that ovulates three months later, or whether it is one of the many follicles that will become antral but then decay). The inexorable loss of eggs with age might be prevented if you could somehow keep the eggs in their primitive, resting state, preventing the natural emergence of one thousand or so eggs each month (thirteen thousand per year) into that three months of growth that will eventually lead to the death of all but one.

If the hormone FSH were in some way necessary for the early development of these eggs from primordial to the antral state, then presumably the administration of birth control pills in high enough doses would reduce the FSH level, delay menopause, and lengthen the period of time in which you retain your fertility. On the contrary, if you undergo hormonal stimulation to retrieve many eggs from multiple follicles in a given month, does that in some way reduce your ovarian pool of eggs and hasten the day when you will run out of eggs?

Most authorities who have done extensive research in this area do not believe that FSH has any effect on the follicles leaving the resting pool prior to their becoming larger and entering the pre-antral phase. There are no receptors for FSH in the resting follicles. Furthermore, we have found that young women who use birth control pills for a long period of time have antral follicle counts indistinguishable from those who have not been on the Pill. Likewise, women who have been on strong hormonal suppression (with Lupron) for as long as half a year to suppress endometriosis have similar responses to ovarian stimulation as a matched group of women who have not been on prolonged suppression with birth control pills. Thus, we see no evidence that either antral follicle count or ovarian reserve can be preserved by maintaining low FSH levels by using birth control pills. Furthermore, stimulation with FSH in multiple cycles of IVF in the same woman causes no reduction in antral follicle count or ovarian reserve.

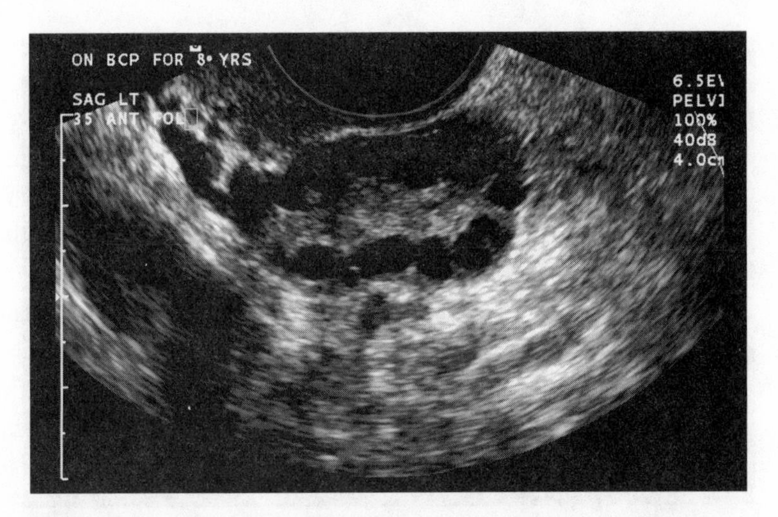


**FIGURE 3.12.** Antral follicle count: twenty-three-year-old on birth control pills eight years.
Total number of follicles (all planes, both ovaries): 66
right ovary: 31, left ovary: 35

Let's give some actual examples with ultrasound pictures of antral follicle counts. First you must understand that a single picture cannot show all of the antral follicles. When there are many antral follicles, we have to move the probe into different positions in order to visualize the entire ovary in three dimensions rather than two. A single picture underestimates the antral follicle count. The count (which is three-dimensional) cannot be based on reading a single film. Figure 3.12 demonstrates a single picture of the antral follicle count of a twenty-three-year-old woman who had been on birth control pills for eight years, and is sufficient to show that she had a very good ovarian reserve. This young woman had a total of thirty-one antral follicles in the right ovary and thirty-five in the left, for a total of sixty-six. She will not have to worry about her biological clock for many years. Figure 3.13 is from a fertile thirty-seven-year-old woman who has a total of thirty-five antral follicles, fifteen on the right and twenty on the left. She also does not have to worry about her biological clock, despite being thirty-seven years old. However, the twenty-three-year-old woman with only seven antral follicles (fig. 3.10), indicating a very low ovarian reserve despite her young age, will need to start trying to get pregnant very soon.

Birth control pills do not suppress antral follicles. Being on birth control pills neither suppresses the antral follicle count nor interferes with the ability to determine a woman's ovarian reserve (which would

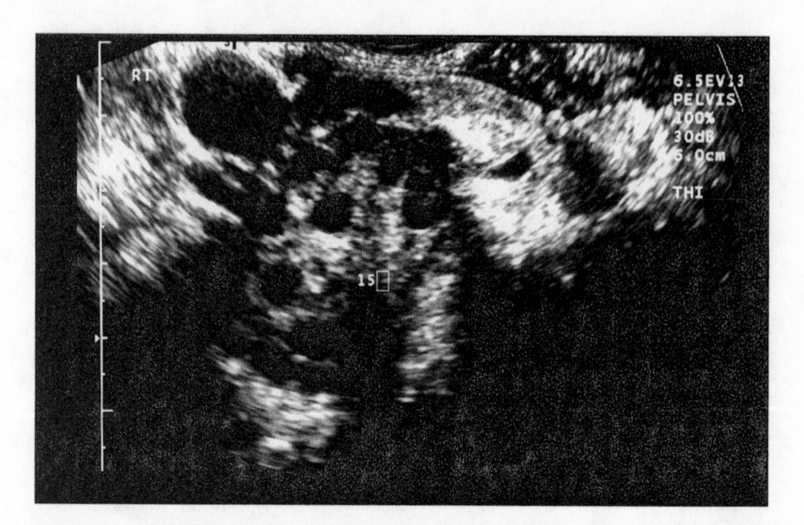


**FIGURE 3.13.** Antral follicle count: fertile thirty-seven-year-old.

Total number of follicles (all planes, both ovaries): 35
right ovary: 15, left ovary: 20

be a problem with any kind of hormonal testing like day three FSH or estradiol). Birth control pills work by suppressing the pituitary secretion of FSH and LH. This prevents ovulation by halting the further development of follicles beyond the antral stage. However, it is clear that it does not prevent the formation of antral follicles, which, at least until the early pre-antral stage, are not hormone dependent. Thus, we have found that even young women on birth control pills can rely on routine antral follicle count testing to give them a prediction of their ovarian reserve, and birth control pills do not slow down the biological clock.

From the opposite point of view, ovulatory stimulation does not deplete the ovary of eggs. FSH shots administered in a stimulatory cycle for IVF simply allow us to retrieve approximately fifteen to thirty eggs out of the one thousand that will have reached the antral stage and allow them to continue developing and not die. So hormonal stimulation does not cause you to lose more eggs, nor does hormonal suppression (birth control pills) prevent the loss of eggs with age.

Thus, you do not have to be concerned about routine birth control pill usage, but you shouldn't be uplifted by the possibility that using birth control pills might spare you an early menopause. For practical purposes, the use of birth control pills will have no significant effect on your reproductive future, or on our ability to make predictions for you using the antral follicle count.

## Aggressive Ovarian Surgery Can Hurt Your Biological Clock

There are two ways in which you can become infertile prematurely. As we have discussed, your biological clock can cause you to run out of your inherent supply of eggs, with one thousand eggs dying every month until none are left. However, there is another way in which you could wind up with a low ovarian reserve, and that is either by inappropriate surgery that inadvertently destroys many of your eggs or by having to go through chemotherapy or radiation for cancer.

A forty-three-year-old man who was married to a thirty-three-year-old woman with normal menstrual cycles underwent a vasectomy reversal and had a perfect result postoperatively, with fifty million sperm per cc and more than 50 percent motility with excellent morphology. There was no doubt that he was fertile after his surgery. Unfortunately, his wife saw a physician who diagnosed her with endometriosis. He performed a laparoscopy with an argon laser and literally burned the entire surface of her ovary in an effort to "control the endometriosis." When she first saw us five months later, to get our opinion, her hysterosalpingogram (HSG) films showed the uterus was perfectly normal, but her right ovary had been removed, along with her right tube, and her left ovary was scarred down to the fallopian tube. Although she had relatively normal menstrual cycles of twenty-six days, her day three FSH level was over twenty, her antral follicle count was only two, and, despite being only thirty-three years old, she obviously had a terribly low ovarian reserve, owing to surgical removal and inadvertent destruction of eggs on the ovarian surface.

Figure 3.1 depicts the dissection of the ovary of a cancer patient, in preparation for freezing it so that it can be transplanted back once she is cured. The thin but tough fibrous outer shell of the ovary contains all of its eggs. Many gynecologic surgeons are not aware of the critical importance of preserving the outer shell when they operate. Any operation in which portions of this seemingly innocuous outer shell are removed would also remove most of the eggs. All mature follicles arise from the surface of the ovary. Follicles do not arise in the middle of the ovary and push their way to the outside. The inside of the ovary is nothing more than a loose network of connective tissue and blood vessels; your reproductive future is located on this thin one-millimeter outer membrane.

Nothing can accelerate the ticking of your biological clock faster than surgery for ovarian cysts or for endometriosis. Benign ovarian cysts are usually nonthreatening and are very common in young women. It breaks my heart whenever I talk to patients who as young women had operations on their ovary to remove simple cysts or other benign lesions, and then suddenly found themselves infertile with low ovarian reserve. Then they often go through even more surgeries because of a misinterpretation that the reduction in ovarian reserve caused by their previous operations can somehow be corrected by another operation.

Occasionally, young women do have what we call "complex" cysts that do need to be removed because of the possibility of a low-grade tumor. However, it is rare that the entire ovary needs to be removed, and even so-called salvage surgery is often performed in such a way that the surgeon inadvertently and unnecessarily removes huge numbers of eggs from the resting pool.

Kathy, thirty-two, and her husband, thirty-four, had been trying for ten years to get pregnant, and she had gone through multiple unnecessary surgeries. This began when she was only fifteen years old, when she was diagnosed with an ovarian cyst. Surgery to treat the cyst involved the removal of her right ovary, and her doctors mistakenly told her and her parents that this would have no effect on her fertility because they were leaving the left ovary intact. What the doctors did not realize is that they were removing 200,000 of her 400,000 eggs. Thus, as a teenager, her ovarian reserve was cut in half in one fell swoop. This did not mean, as one might think, that she would enter menopause as early as age twenty-five, because the ovary engages in a sort of "salvage operation" to squeeze more eggs out even when its resting pool has declined greatly. However, there was no question that she would be infertile earlier as a result of this procedure and would have an earlier menopause. To make matters worse, her infertility doctors found a cyst on her remaining ovary and decided to remove that cyst as well, supposedly "salvaging" the left ovary.

Perhaps even worse, if a woman has little bits of "endometriosis" that are visible on the surface of the ovary, the doctor may just burn them off with a laser or electrocautery, thinking he or she is curing her endometriosis. Sometimes physicians will perform ovarian "drilling" (using a laser or cautery to burn holes in the surface of the ovary) to restore her ovulatory function, but this procedure really doesn't cure anything. Instead, the surface of the ovary is damaged, reducing the total number of eggs. Whenever you reduce the total follicle pool, you decrease the number of antral follicles that are visible at any time, and you reduce the number of eggs that can be retrieved in an IVF cycle. This drop in ovarian reserve hastens the day when a woman will need infertility treatment, and even causes her to have an earlier menopause.

Ovarian cysts, even if associated with lower abdominal pain, are remarkably common, as is surgery to remove these cysts (or to remove the entire ovary), and it is up to the patient to say no. If there is any fear on the part of the surgeon that the cyst might be a low-grade tumor, an effort should be made to remove only the cystlike tumor itself, leaving the ovarian cortex (the thin outer encasement) intact. Of course, this caveat doesn't apply to older women with a complex cyst larger than five centimeters. But in younger women, the most important goal is to save the egg supply.

Lest we conclude this section in too depressive a tone, I should tell the story of a patient who came to us because nobody else was willing to attempt IVF with her. She was thirty-nine years old and had had a lumpectomy for breast cancer seven years earlier. This was a very early breast cancer, and her cancer physicians, who were quite good, felt that she was cured and that there was no reason for her not to try to get pregnant. However, what they did not realize is that her two years of chemotherapy and radiation after the lumpectomy had obliterated most of her egg supply. Even the day three FSH, which is only elevated in women near the end of their reproductive life, was elevated. So we put her on very high doses of FSH and were able to retrieve only one egg. This one egg was injected with her husband's sperm (which had to be retrieved from his testes because he had no sperm in his ejaculate) and fertilized. It was a single, slowly developing embryo. Amazingly, she became pregnant and delivered a completely healthy child. We had warned her that her chances of pregnancy with IVF were probably less than 2 percent, but this is the kind of case that inspires us to do the best we can even in the most severe situations, when pregnancy rates can be expected to be extraordinarily low.

In summary, the bigger the pool of eggs you start with, the longer you will be able to stay fertile and the later your menopause will occur. Birth control pills do not help put this off, and surgery on the ovaries can make matters worse by further decreasing your supply of eggs.

## Antral Follicle Count and Older Women

### *What If I Have Already Had a Child but Want More?*

We see countless patients who had no difficulty getting pregnant years earlier, having had one or even two children, but who now find themselves inexplicably unable to get pregnant again. They wonder how they could suddenly have become infertile. This is only confusing if you think there is a specific diagnosis that explains the cause of infertility, as though it were a disease that could be characterized and then treated like other illnesses. The problem is that most cases of infertility (though of course not all) are simply related to the decline in ovarian function, which is an inescapable result of the years going by.

We saw a forty-one-year-old woman who had no difficulty getting pregnant thirteen years earlier, when she was twenty-eight years old. At age thirty-seven she attempted once again to have more children and, indeed, got pregnant but miscarried. She got pregnant again three years later, but miscarried again. She got pregnant again once more later that year and again miscarried. Subsequently, she was not able to get pregnant at all. These recurrent miscarriages in women who were once fertile and are now older (assuming no intervening uterine problem) are almost always related to declining ovarian reserve. The ovary performs its salvaging function of pushing out whatever eggs it can. Many of these eggs are from the bottom of the follicular pool and, therefore, have a higher incidence of chromosomal errors. Her miscarriages were caused by chromosomal errors in the egg maturation process (to be explained fully in later chapters) and were just a danger signal, warning her that she had already run extremely low on her follicular reserve several years earlier. Infertility and recurrent miscarriage are different expressions of the same problem of declining ovarian reserve.

You may still be fairly young, with no history of difficulty getting pregnant when you were even younger, and still have age-related secondary infertility. A twenty-nine-year-old woman had had her first child with her husband four years earlier, when she was twenty-five, and never dreamed she would become infertile. She had perfect, regular, twenty-eight-day cycles, but a routine infertility evaluation by another clinic found that her husband had a low sperm count (seven million sperm per cc, with only 10 percent motility). When she was four years younger, she had no problem getting pregnant despite the low sperm count, but now, to have more children, she needed infertility treatment.

The fact that you have had children in the past and therefore assume yourself to be fertile does not mean that you should not continue to have regular antral follicle count monitoring to help you make your decision about when you and your husband should try to have your next child. If your antral follicle count is below ten or fifteen, you may have to consider doing this sooner rather than later.

### *Antral Follicle Count and Counseling Older Infertile Patients*

Nowadays, most older women seeking to have a child and planning to undergo IVF recognize that they are in a poor prognostic category even with IVF, but they may not fully understand the reasons why. More important, many couples are torn about whether to go through an expensive treatment that carries a very low success rate for their age group or to seek other approaches, such as using donor eggs or attempting to adopt. Once a woman undergoes ovarian stimulation, it will be possible to determine (by how many follicles develop) whether the couple is in a high prognostic category or a low prognostic category. With an antral follicle count we can advise older women of their prognosis with IVF before they undergo ovarian stimulation.

I met with a forty-two-year-old couple who had had a diagnostic laparoscopy just a year before, believing this would give them an idea of why the wife wasn't getting pregnant, or what her prognosis would be. They were hesitant to attempt the one procedure (IVF) that might give them a chance of getting pregnant, mostly because they were questioning its cost effectiveness and potential for success. During the consultation, I could see unfolding before me an incredible tension between husband and wife, because she was quite ready to try anything, and to spend the money to go through an IVF cycle if there was any chance whatsoever. However, her husband was definitely not interested in spending ten to fourteen thousand dollars if the chance for pregnancy and delivery of a baby was only 5 percent. This is a dilemma that confronts many couples who are looking carefully at their pocketbook and at their emotional ability to handle severe disappointment. Several years ago, they would have been in an unresolvable conflict and probably never would have gotten treatment. However, now we could perform a simple antral follicle count with ultrasound. The wife had a total of nineteen antral follicles. We were, therefore, able to tell her that she was very fortunately endowed at birth, and despite being forty-two years old, she would fall into a more favorable prognosis category. This considerably relieved their tension and allowed them to make a rational decision to have IVF.

On the same day, I reviewed the case of a very young couple. He was thirty years old, and she was twenty-eight. They had suffered from infertility for only two years. The husband had a moderately low sperm count, and a urologist had recommended a varicocelectomy (which would have been useless). The wife's obstetrician told her "not to worry" about trying to get pregnant yet, and that she and her husband would not need any treatment because she was still young (even though she had irregular periods). But an antral follicle count hadn't been performed, so the obstetrician had no evidence to justify telling her not to worry. Indeed, she did have a low antral follicle count (eight), and she did need to have treatment right away. The fact that a woman is still under age thirty is no reason to tell her just to wait a few more years — it is possible that those few years could result in a considerable decline in her chances for pregnancy if her ovarian reserve is already low.

## How Is a Woman's Endowment of Eggs Determined at Birth?

Let's review for just a minute. The supply of follicles (eggs, or oocytes, surrounded by granulosa cells) is established very early in fetal life. There are about one thousand to two thousand of what we call primordial germ cells in the early embryo that are eventually destined to become either the sperm-producing cells in the testes (if the fetus turns out to be a male), or the oogonia, which will become eggs arrested in their earliest stage of development (if the fetus turns out to be a female). These primordial germ cells, therefore, can become either sperm or eggs, completely depending upon whether the organ to which they migrate in the first six weeks of fetal life turns out to be an ovary or a testis. Primordial germ cells originate in what is called the yolk sac at the far end of the embryo, and they can be identified as early as three weeks

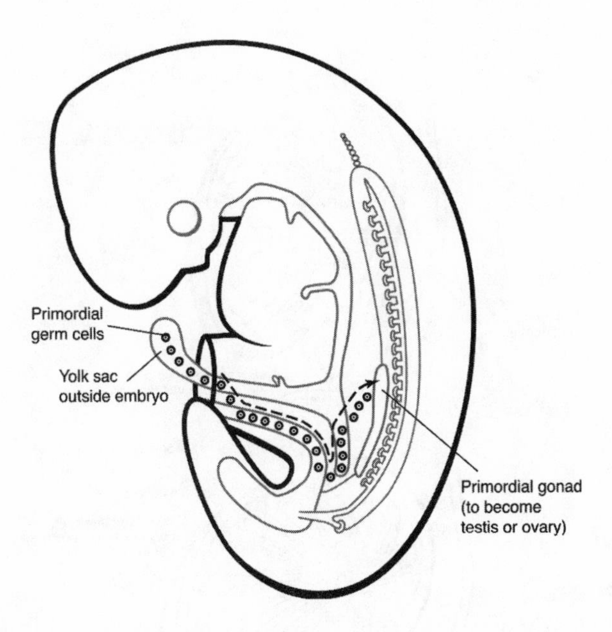


**FIGURE 3.14**

Migration of primordial germ cells (future sperm or eggs) to future testis or ovary in a three-week-old embryo.

after fertilization. These cells clearly originate outside of the body of the embryo (see fig. 3.14). They will not survive unless they are capable of migrating by week five into the embryo to a region called the genital ridge, which will develop into either an ovary or a testis, determined by whether it was an X sperm that fertilized the mother's egg (in which case it becomes an ovary) or a Y sperm (in which case it will become a testis). At this stage, the primitive gonad on the genital ridge (which receives and collects these migrating germ cells) is neither a testis nor an ovary.

The commitment for this indifferent gonad to become either a testis or an ovary is completed between six weeks and nine weeks of fetal life, respectively. If this primitive gonad is going to become a testis, cords (which will eventually become the seminiferous tubules of the adult testes) begin to form by about forty days, and the testis is fairly complete in its structure by about seven weeks of fetal life (see fig. 3.15).

The indifferent germ cells, if left alone, would be genetically programmed toward becoming eggs rather than sperm. That is, in the absence of any other signals, these germ cells will go into early meiosis and become eggs. However, the development of a testis allows these

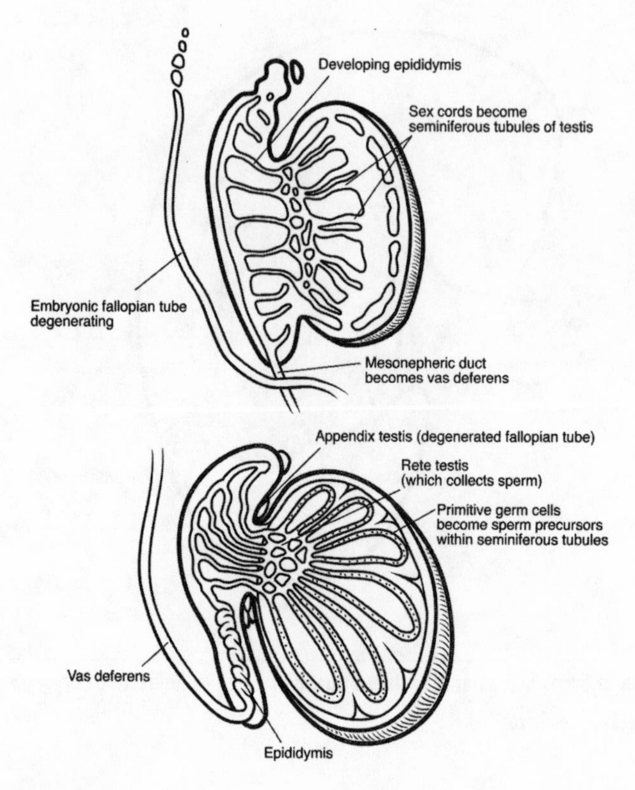


**FIGURE 3.15**

**In the male, primitive germ cells become sperm precursors in seminiferous tubules of embryonic testis.**

spermatogenic cords to encase the indifferent germ cells. In a sense, the Sertoli cells and the seminiferous tubules of this seven-week-old fetus are imprisoning the germ cells and preventing them from becoming eggs, which would otherwise be the normal course of development. If there are very few germ cells that have managed to migrate to the genital ridge of the male fetus, these early seminiferous tubules, with their Sertoli cells, will still develop completely normally. But the seminiferous tubules will have very few, or perhaps no, spermatogonia, and this male child will grow up to be sterile (see chapter 7).

The ovary develops in a female fetus about three weeks after a testis would have developed if it were a male. In embryos destined to be female, the primitive gonadal ridge does not become an ovary until germ cells have migrated into the tissue, between six and nine weeks of fetal age (see fig. 3.16). The egg precursor, or oogonia, is really just a

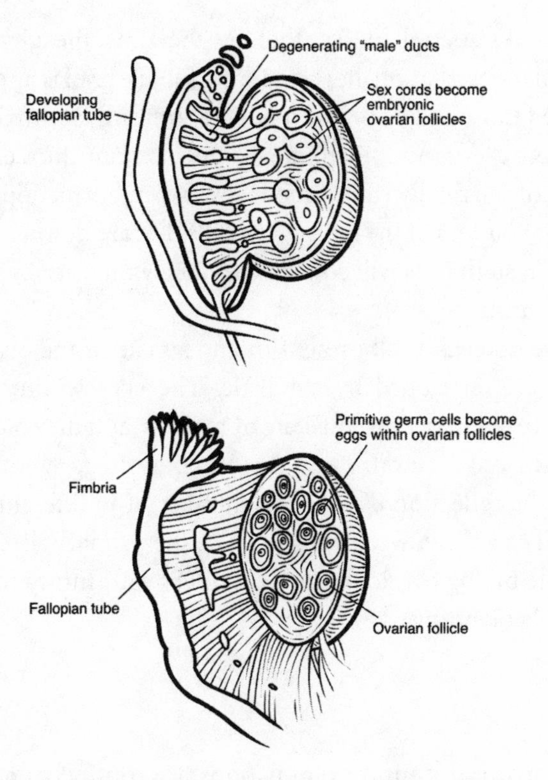


**FIGURE 3.16.** In the female, primitive germ cells become eggs in embryonic ovarian follicles.

primitive germ cell that did not become encased by seminiferous tubules several weeks earlier, because a testis did not form. These oogonia also degenerate if they are not surrounded by granulosa cells of the early follicle. Remember that regardless of their genetic constitution, these primitive cells could become either eggs or sperm depending upon whether the primordial gonad they migrate to becomes a testicle or an ovary. In any event, the germ cells are programmed to become eggs in the absence of any testicular modification, but these eggs will die if they are not eventually enveloped by what will become an ovary.

By eight weeks of fetal life, cell division (mitosis) increases the total number of oogonia from the original one thousand or two thousand to as many as six hundred thousand. By twenty weeks of fetal life (five months of development), the ovary will contain about six or seven million eggs on average. From this point until birth, there will be a relentless and irreversible attrition, and at the time of birth, only one or two million of these eggs are still left in the ovary. This atresia continues throughout prepubertal life so that by the time the girl undergoes puberty with menstruation, her remaining follicle pool is approximately four hundred thousand eggs. From puberty onward, approximately one thousand eggs every month will die (a loss of about thirteen thousand per year) until she finally runs out of eggs and enters menopause. There is no such similar loss of the male germ cells that are destined to become sperm. Sperm stem cells will continue to renew themselves throughout the male's lifetime.

There are no eggs at all present in any female in the ovary at birth unless they are enveloped by a follicle. The eggs within the resting follicles are frozen in the earliest state of meiosis, and they have no capability for stem-cell renewal. Thus, the number of eggs with which you were born — a reflection of the total number of indifferent germ cells that you had as a three-week embryo — is the primary determinant of your ultimate biological clock, and will direct your future reproductive life and family planning.

## Summary

Transvaginal ultrasound examinations are routinely performed by gynecologists, obstetricians, and IVF doctors, as well as in radiology imaging centers, but no one has bothered before to pay close attention to the small one- to two-millimeter follicles present in the ovary because no thought was given to their great significance. Thus, you will probably have to understand the scientific detail that has preceded this summary in order to explain to your physician what you would like to have done. I am sure that in the next five years we will see a revolution in the counseling of young women so that in addition to their yearly Pap smear, they will have this simple ultrasound exam to guide them in their reproductive planning. But it is not just a routine exam that I am suggesting — it is a specific counting of the number of one- to two-millimeter follicles, the so-called antral follicles. This number is constant throughout your menstrual cycle and gives a true measure of your reproductive outlook.

The antral follicles (the small one-millimeter to two-millimeter follicles located on the surface of the ovary) should be abundant in number, certainly greater than twenty. Your antral follicle count is the same at any time during your menstrual cycle and is unrelated to any hormone-dependent aspect of your monthly cycle. This makes sense because the follicles are not visible to ultrasound until they reach the size at which they first become hormone dependent. Thus, there is a continuous daily process of antral follicle formation that began nearly three months earlier (seventy days) with the emergence from the resting follicle state.

There are problems with all the other methods of trying to determine ovarian reserve. The day three FSH, the day three estradiol, and even the Clomid challenge test have been shown to be very faulty and to reveal a problem only if you are near the extreme edge of the reproductive lifetime. Ovarian volume and overall physical fitness have no relationship to the number of eggs you were endowed with at birth. Normal twenty-eight-day cycles and ovulation detection kits are also of no use whatsoever. Even women who are in their forties, with very few follicles left, can have normal twenty-eight-day cycles and ovulate. However, the quality of those eggs is reflective of not only her age, but also her ovarian follicle pool. Her results with IVF (if that is what she has to do) are affected by her age and her total ovarian reserve, not by whether she ovulates or whether she has normal twenty-eight-day cycles.

So how do you get an antral follicle count performed? First, you must explain it to your doctor, because he may not be aware of what to do. Warn your doctor that he or she will have to literally count one by one each of those tiny follicles, located circumferentially around the ovary. The ultrasound probe must be moved gradually from one side of the ovary to the other while your doctor carefully counts, because as one plane of follicles appears, the other will disappear. Whether you are on birth control pills or other hormones should not make any difference. If you are unsure of the interest of the doctor or whether the technician is doing this properly, you may have to get a second exam at a different institution.

The antral follicle count can then be used to determine when you will be likely to have your last naturally conceived child, and even when you are likely to go through menopause. Of course, a high antral follicle count does not guarantee that you are fertile. You may have a diagnostic problem such as blocked tubes or ineffective sperm in your partner. However, the age-related decline in fertility that people are most worried about in making their life decisions can be determined by the antral follicle count. It will be a rational basis for your family planning and decision making.

CHAPTER 4

# Are We Infertile? Simpler Treatments

## How Long Does It Normally Take to Get Pregnant and How Do We Know When to Look for Help?

Couples who have been infertile for many years clearly know they have a problem and need medical help. But what about the couple that has been trying to get pregnant unsuccessfully for just six months, or for one year? When should they begin to worry? Even for those who are not infertile, pregnancy does not usually occur in the first month of trying. When my wife and I decided to start our family, it took a full six months before she finally conceived. We know people who were not able to achieve pregnancy for several years, never bothered to consult a doctor, and eventually had children. So when should you begin to worry that you might not be able to have children?

To a great extent this question can be answered by the antral follicle count ultrasound described in the previous chapter. Nonetheless, even a woman with a high ovarian reserve, when trying to get pregnant, may wonder if there is a particular time beyond which she should seek medical attention. All potential parents-to-be will need a little lesson in statistics to understand the similarity between becoming pregnant and rolling dice. That's the only way you will know when to start worrying.

Getting pregnant is basically a game of odds. Some couples are simply likely to get pregnant sooner than others. If couples had three hundred years in which to breed, it seems almost certain that eventually most wives would become pregnant without any treatment. But the usual breeding period for families is no more than fifteen years, and so the odds need to be considerably improved. When a couple has waited as long as six months to a year without achieving pregnancy, they will probably begin to fear they are infertile, and are likely to become frantic.

Yet many of these couples may have no physical basis for infertility, but may merely be victims of statistical chance, having no less likelihood of pregnancy occurring with each given month than the couple that was fortunate enough to get pregnant with their first attempt. So how do we decide if treatment is needed?

### *Probability of Conception per Month in Fertile Couples*

What is the probability in any given month of a normal, fertile couple's achieving a pregnancy? Many years ago I posed this question to several population authorities. At that time most of them considered it a very difficult question to answer with accuracy. Yet it is critically important to understand the natural incidence of pregnancy month by month in a fertile population, so that the couple having difficulty with conception can understand whether or not they really have a problem.

A century ago we knew from studies in England that young women get pregnant sooner and more easily than older women. The incidence of infertility in women twenty-five years of age was 7 percent, and the incidence of infertility in women thirty years of age was approximately 18 percent. At thirty-five years of age, 25 percent of women were unable to have children. By age forty, the majority of women were unable to get pregnant. Modern statistical data are remarkably similar to these ancient studies. The age-related decline in a woman's fertility has been well explained to you already. At this juncture, you will want to know how long you should wait before seeking treatment.

About 40 to 50 percent of women achieve pregnancy within the first four months of trying. Are the women with high ovarian reserve who are not yet pregnant after four months of trying any less fertile than those who have already conceived? After two years, about 9 percent of fertile women still have not yet conceived. Are the 9 percent of women who are still trying to get pregnant after two years of trying a hard-core group with severe infertility problems, or do they just represent a statistical inevitability that may be erased with the next monthly cycle? How many couples who have not yet gotten pregnant are really worrying for nothing? In how many "infertile" couples would just waiting and doing nothing result in a pregnancy without the expense and trouble of medical treatment? On the other hand, when is complacency as the wife keeps getting older likely to be tragic because of a problem that won't resolve itself without treatment?

Think of fertility in these terms: If a man were to flip a coin three times in a row, and it landed on tails each time, he might think that his particular coin is more likely to land on tails again the next time. Of course, this is not true. Each time the coin is flipped there is a fifty-fifty chance of its landing either heads or tails, regardless of the past history. Therefore, a couple should not be concerned too early about a few unsuccessful flips of the coin.

Modern studies have shown that with the most fertile population of patients (those who eventually went on to raise large families) there was only about a 20 percent chance in any given month of the wife's becoming pregnant. If she was not pregnant after six months, the chance that she would become pregnant in the seventh month was still 20 percent. Studies of artificial insemination with donor sperm done by Dr. Robert Schoysman in Belgium in the 1970s have shown that with each succeeding month the chance for pregnancy is no less in normal women who have not yet conceived than in those who were lucky enough to become pregnant in the very first month. This should be of some comfort to "fertile" couples who simply have not yet achieved pregnancy. But there must be some point beyond which the couples who have not become pregnant are a "selected" group who are less fertile than those who got pregnant earlier. Instead of a 20 percent chance each month, they might have a lower chance, perhaps 5 percent or 1 percent per month. At what point do we identify these couples who might need help?

### *After What Period of Time Does Not Getting Pregnant Mean We're Infertile?*

Studies from Belgium in the 1970s and 1980s with 632 fertile young women whose husbands were azoospermic (had no sperm at all in the ejaculate) helped to clarify this question. Very fertile donor sperm was used to inseminate each female just prior to ovulation each month until she became pregnant. In the first month, 130 of the 632 women became pregnant (20.57 percent). In the second cycle, 103 more women became pregnant (16.29 percent). In the third monthly cycle, 81 more women became pregnant (12.81 percent). Thus, a total of 49.67 percent of the 632 women achieved pregnancy within the first three months. In the fourth month, 54 more women became pregnant (8.54 percent). In the fifth month, 40 women became pregnant (6.32 percent). By six months, a total of 73 percent of the patients had become pregnant. It is at this point (six months) that the other 27 percent might have been tempted to give up. But that is just mathematical naïveté.

In the tenth month, only 3 percent of the total women starting this program became pregnant, but the pregnancy rate among the women who were actually inseminated that month was still 20.21 percent. By that time there were only 94 women out of the original 632 who had not yet achieved pregnancy. But in that month, 19 women, or 20.21 percent, conceived. In the eighteenth month after the beginning of this study, 5 women (less than 1 percent of those originally entering the study) became pregnant. However, by that time, only 23 women were remaining who had not yet achieved pregnancy, and the 5 who became pregnant that month represented 21.75 percent of those remaining.

Thus, it would appear that even though the majority of fertile women became pregnant within the first six months of trying, and only a tiny minority required as long as eighteen months or two years to become pregnant, each normal young woman still had a 20 percent chance of becoming pregnant with each succeeding month. When women who required many months to conceive by donor insemination came back to have their second child, many became pregnant within just a few months. In addition, some women who had achieved pregnancy very early with their first child required a much longer time to become pregnant with the second child, despite no obvious change in their fertility. If the conception rate in a large group of normal young women trying to achieve pregnancy in a given month is 20 percent, it is a mathematical certainty that a small number of them will not obtain their goal until several years have passed.

The problem with drawing broad conclusions from this study is that these were young women who should have had an extremely low risk of infertility, and the donor sperm was extremely fertile. But what about women in their late twenties or thirties who are using their husband's sperm (of unproven fertility)? If they have not achieved pregnancy after a year, what is their chance of ever getting pregnant in subsequent months without any help?

Although young couples with normal sperm may have reason to keep on expecting a 20 percent chance of pregnancy for up to several years, eventually what is left are those patients who have a very low expectation of pregnancy with future attempts. In older patients, in their thirties, this hard-core group of truly infertile couples with a lower chance of pregnancy per month might be revealed after only a year or less of unsuccessful attempts at getting pregnant. If they have a low antral follicle count, waiting for that year could be devastating to whatever chance they might have otherwise had.

Dr. Charles Westoff of Princeton University, using a similar mathematical approach, worked out many years ago the probability of conception with each month for "fertile" couples of various ages (see table 4.1). For women in their early twenties — and presumed to be highly fertile — the monthly probability of conception is thought to be between 20 and 25 percent, in the absence of contraception. For somewhat less fertile women, in their late twenties and early thirties, the monthly probability of conception is lower: between 10 and 15 percent. Around 72 to 86 percent conceive within a year. By four months, about 50 percent of women in their early twenties will have achieved pregnancy, and about 94 percent will be pregnant within the first year. For women in their late twenties and early thirties, however, only about 70 to 85 percent will achieve pregnancy within the first year. However, those who have not become pregnant within the first year might still have the same 10 to 15 percent chance of becoming pregnant in each succeeding month. If their antral follicle count is high, they should not worry simply because they did not become pregnant in the first year.

**TABLE 4.1**

**Likelihood of Pregnancy in Fertile Women — How Long Should It Take?**

| AGE | PROBABILITY OF CONCEPTION PER MONTH | AVERAGE TIME TO CONCEPTION | PROBABILITY OF CONCEPTION WITHIN A YEAR |
|---|---|---|---|
| | (percent) | (months) | (percent) |
| Late thirties | 8.3 | 12 | 65 |
| Early thirties | 10 | 10 | 72 |
| Late twenties | 15 | 6.7 | 86 |
| | 20 | 5 | 93 |
| Early twenties | 25 | 4 | 97 |

For women in their early twenties — and presumed to be highly fertile — the monthly probability of conception is thought to be between 20 and 25 percent, in the absence of contraception. For somewhat less fertile women in their late twenties and early thirties, the monthly probability of conception is lower, between 10 and 15 percent. Around 72 to 86 percent conceive within a year.

However, as women get older (in their thirties), the monthly chance of conception is much lower, and for them numbers like 8 percent per cycle are very theoretical. In this older age group, a failure to get pregnant after a year is likely to mean their monthly chance of natural conception is so low that waiting any longer without treatment would be foolish. This discussion of pregnancy rates in "normal" fertile women demonstrates that fertility is not an absolute, easily definable quality.

So when should the couple begin to worry and when should they seek medical attention? It is difficult to know whether a particular couple's conception probability per month is 20 percent, 15 percent, 10 percent, or 1 percent. The older the couple, the greater the likelihood that a year of infertility means a much lower chance of future conception. Most important, for women with a low antral follicle count, waiting for any period of time could be tragic.

## Proper Timing of Intercourse

Some people who complain of infertility have a simple problem: infrequency of sex at the appropriate time in the cycle. Simply improving the timing and techniques of intercourse may be sufficient to allow pregnancy, without medical intervention or therapy. Animals, of course, always know just when to time their intercourse, because the periodic rise in estrogen in females, just prior to ovulation, is what induces their desire to have sex. Humans cannot be assured that they will automatically want to have sex at the precise moment when it is most likely to lead to pregnancy.

However, scheduling of sex to solve this problem can create other problems. Many couples are so anxious about having intercourse at exactly the right time that they may abstain for a whole week or more prior to the evening when the wife thinks she should be ovulating. The doctor is usually the culprit in this overrigorous scheduling of sex, and the wife may feel that they must abstain until the gynecologist gives her the go-ahead. This kind of overattention to regulating intercourse can create so much anxiety that ovulation itself may be delayed by the emotional distress and its effect on the primitive region of the brain that regulates ovulation.

A long time ago, a somewhat frantic man came to my office and begged that I see him as a patient. He simply couldn't take the strain anymore and was hoping there was something I could do to help. He and his wife had been trying to have a child for a year. Six months earlier she had consulted her gynecologist, who had her monitor her basal body temperatures. Then he told her to abstain from intercourse for five days before her temperature went up; only after her temperature went up was she to have sex with her husband. As I will explain in chapter 7, this is the method you use to avoid getting pregnant. Worse yet, when she was given this directive, her cycles became totally unpredictable, lasting twenty days one month and forty-five days another. Her basal body temperature charts were difficult to interpret, and the couple tried to read into each little temperature elevation the possibility that she was about to ovulate. They did not realize that what the chart was showing was that she had stopped ovulating altogether. She had no idea what was happening but was still trying to pinpoint ovulation. Her original over-anxiety about not conceiving during the first six months coupled with the rigidity of their sex life during the next six months (not to mention its infrequency) was about to lead to a divorce.

I have seen quite a few patients who are able to have sex only on the weekend because of heavy work schedules during the week, often involving traveling. The penalty of success in a career is sometimes a schedule that is so busy that intercourse, in an otherwise workable marriage, either is sporadic or, at best, takes place once a week. It takes no particular medical education to calculate that in these patients the chance of having sex at the fertile preovulatory day is one-third that of couples who have sex three times a week. Furthermore, to be mathematically accurate, if the woman's cycle has a duration of twenty-eight days, then she is likely to be ovulating on the same particular day of the week in any given month. Thus, she may be unfortunate enough to be regularly ovulating on a Wednesday, once every four weeks, when her husband is always out of town. Of course, many couples who have sex only on the weekends have no problem impregnating, because the wife's ovulation may be occurring at that time.

Sometimes the problem with infrequent intercourse is not just a business schedule that keeps the partners apart at the appropriate time of the month, but rather a lack of interest in having intercourse more frequently. An example is a couple who had been trying unsuccessfully for several years to have children but were only having intercourse once every two weeks. I explained to them that this was considerably less than average, and they were a bit surprised. The husband was a very hardworking fellow who usually got home too tired to think about anything but a little quiet conversation and going to sleep. They increased the frequency of intercourse, and the woman became pregnant.

A rigid schedule for intercourse is unrealistic and anxiety provoking. Thus, I do not recommend timing intercourse, unless it's a last resort because of the couple's hectic schedule. For the vast majority of patients, it is much smarter to pay no particular attention to the time of ovulation. Happy, relaxed couples whose lives are not terribly overcluttered tend to have sex somewhere from two to three or more times per week spontaneously and joyously. If you have sex at that frequency, and if your ovulation and cervical mucus are normal, then there is always likely to be some sperm available in the fallopian tube for fertilization.

## Clomid (Clomiphene Citrate)

For ovulation to occur, it is not sufficient for the pituitary gland merely to produce its stimulatory hormones FSH and LH. It must produce these hormones in a specifically synchronized, properly timed fashion. The first requirement for proper ovulation is an adequate amount of FSH stimulation in the very beginning of the menstrual cycle. If there is not an adequate production of FSH by the pituitary gland on the first day of menstruation, the early follicle may not get an adequate growth start, and this sets the stage early in the cycle for poor ovulation. Clomid is a very mild ovulatory stimulant. The object of administering Clomid is to increase the pituitary's production of FSH so that the follicle gets a good boost in the early stage of the cycle. The way this happens is quite fascinating. Clomid is an antiestrogen, which blocks the pituitary's recognition of your body's own naturally circulating estrogen. It gives the pituitary the false message that your ovary is not making estrogen, and this causes the pituitary to increase its FSH production dramatically. If the follicle gets this necessary boost by an early increase in FSH, it will develop properly and release enough estrogen around midcycle to trigger the pituitary gland on day fourteen to release LH, which causes the follicle to rupture and ovulate. A high level of early FSH production by the pituitary gland, stimulating the follicle to grow in the early portion of the menstrual cycle, is the key to successful ovulation.

Clomid has traditionally been given only on days five through nine in the cycle. Some doctors prefer days three through seven. Clomid is needed only during the first five to eight days, when maximum FSH stimulation is necessary. After that, it has already done its job and has set the stage for the proper subsequent hormonal clockwork to take place.

Because Clomid is an antiestrogen, it blocks the effect of estrogen on the cervix and frequently makes the cervical mucus too sticky to allow sperm penetration. The basic problem with Clomid is that it does not have a "clean" effect. On one hand, it stimulates ovulation by increasing FSH early in the cycle. On the other hand, it counteracts the effects of estrogen on the cervix and the endometrium, and possibly on the egg itself. Thus, if Clomid does not result in a pregnancy by four months, it is best to stop using it.

The benefit of Clomid is that it is such a mild drug that it can be prescribed without the need for close monitoring. The incidence of twins in clomiphene-treated women is only about 6 percent. Triplets, quadruplets, and quintuplets are extremely rare with this relatively gentle and mild fertility agent. It is a safe, easy-to-prescribe drug. Clomid is probably the most popular drug used for enhancing fertility because it is so simple to administer, and patients can take it with very little supervision. It is passed around like popcorn to millions of infertility patients as a first line of treatment.

But it is certainly overused, and many patients have been on Clomid for years and years with no pregnancy. The doctor may add an HCG injection at midcycle, or perform artificial insemination with the husband's semen. But if Clomid does not produce a pregnancy in the first several months, it's not likely to do so over the next several years. It is a very mild agent that is not adequate for most cases. But if it does work, it will work right away.

## Parlodel (Bromocriptine)

Very occasionally a lack of ovulation is caused by increased levels of a hormone called prolactin. This condition is very much overdiagnosed. Prolactin directly stimulates the breasts to make milk and is normally released by the pituitary after the delivery of a baby. It also prevents ovulation. Breast-feeding then stimulates the pituitary gland to secrete more and more prolactin. Normally, prolactin is only secreted in large amounts during breast-feeding. It prevents ovulation by inhibiting the release of FSH and LH.

In some patients a small and often undetectable pituitary tumor may cause the prolactin level in the blood to be increased in a non-breast-feeding woman, thereby making her infertile. A drug called Parlodel (bromocriptine) dramatically suppresses the pituitary's production of prolactin in these cases, and ovulation ensues promptly after its administration. Parlodel is not useful in other cases of infertility and is not a cure-all fertility drug. This drug has been vastly overprescribed in the past for all kinds of infertility and even for male impotence. In truth, it is only occasionally appropriate to prescribe it.

Parlodel can have some aggravating side effects, such as nausea, dizziness, headaches, and tremors, if given in normal doses too rapidly, without a gradual buildup. It is a nasty drug. Therefore, the patient is started on a low dose of one half of a 2.5-milligram tablet once a day; she then goes to a full 2.5-milligram tablet once a day and then, finally, to two full tablets per day, one at night and one in the morning. But it still is not without unpleasant side effects.

Prolactin, like testosterone and virtually all the hormones secreted during the menstrual cycle, normally rises at the time of the LH surge. Often the prolactin level may seem to be at the upper limit of normal only because it is supposed to go up at midcycle, when estrogen, LH, FSH, and even testosterone also peak. Giving Parlodel to "normal" women to prevent this normal midcycle surge of prolactin enjoyed some faddish popularity for a while as a possible overall fertility enhancer, but this is no longer in style, and this unpleasant drug should be reserved only for the occasional true, constant elevations of prolactin level.

## Endometriosis

Among some doctors, endometriosis is considered a major cause of infertility. Endometriosis has enjoyed unprecedented popularity as a diagnosis, and surgery for it has built many fine homes for doctors who are enthusiasts for operating on this condition. In truth, endometriosis is a more controversial condition than some would contend, and although it is an extremely frequent diagnosis associated with hospital and surgery bills for infertility-related procedures, its relationship to infertility is highly mysterious and the treatment of it is very questionable.

### *What Is Endometriosis?*

When a woman menstruates, the lining of her uterus is shed and most of the blood is extruded through the cervix, which opens up at the time of menstruation. At the same time that the menstrual blood is shed out into the vagina, a small portion of it is shed backward through the fallopian tube into the abdominal cavity. This is called retrograde menstruation. If the endometrial tissue, or menstrual flow, that goes back into the abdomen catches hold and endometrial cells start growing in the abdominal cavity, that is the beginning of endometriosis.

There have been dozens of theories offered for how the presence of endometriosis might cause infertility. Most of these reasons are quite mysterious and unproven. Its proponents claim that the presence of endometriosis in a woman's pelvis creates a "hostile" pelvic environment that prevents pregnancy. Under this assumption, a doctor who sees the smallest lesion of endometriosis in an infertile woman may want to surgically remove it or put her on some sort of drug that will cause the endometriosis to dissolve. But this is foolish. Controlled studies have demonstrated that women who are treated for "moderate" or "minimal" lesion endometriosis have no greater pregnancy rate than similar women who go with no treatment at all. So does endometriosis actually cause infertility, or is endometriosis in some way caused by other factors associated with infertility? If that were the case, then removing the endometriosis would do nothing to improve the woman's fertility.

Women always notice that their otherwise heavy or painful periods become much lighter and usually more comfortable after going on birth control pills. The reason for this is that most birth control pills contain more progesterone than estrogen. This formulation causes a softening of the uterine lining without a great deal of estrogen buildup, so the periods are very light. This is why women who have been on the Pill have a much lower incidence of cancer of the endometrium later in life than women who never took it. In the same respect, women who ovulate normally have a lower incidence of cancer of the endometrium later in life than women who didn't ovulate. The simple point is that the progesterone secreted normally in the second half of the ovulatory cycle causes the endometrial tissue to soften up for a clean bleed and prevents endometrial tissue from developing an estrogen-mediated overbuildup. For this same reason, progesterone deficiency is associated with a greater incidence of endometriosis.

In fact, one of the old treatments for endometriosis was to place the woman on high doses of progesterone, and this treatment was actually quite effective. Over a prolonged period of time, progesterone eventually causes endometrial lesions to disappear. It is for this same reason that women with endometriosis were told, ironically, that their condition could be best cured by getting pregnant, since pregnancy produced super-high levels of progesterone for nine months.

Hundreds of millions of operations have been performed to remove these little endometriosis lesions, and hundreds of thousands of women are being placed on drugs like Lupron to shrink up their lesions. Such treatment has not caused any higher pregnancy rate than no treatment at all.

### *Drug Treatment for Endometriosis*

There are two types of therapy for attempting to shrink endometriosis — medical (drugs) and surgical. For many years, medical therapy meant the continual administration of birth control pills, which resulted in a strong "progesterone effect" that eventually caused the endometriosis tissue to become more "secretory," shrink up, and disappear. This treatment became less popular in the late 1970s and 1980s, however, with the development of the heavily marketed drug Danocrine.

Danocrine was actually not much more effective than progesterone in shrinking up endometriosis lesions. Progesterone was said to have produced an "artificial pregnancy" effect, which caused lesions to shrink up over a long period of time, while Danocrine was said to have produced an "artificial menopause effect," which caused the lesions to shrink up more quickly. Danocrine is simply a male hormone, a testosterone-like derivative, which had only a mild male-hormone effect. By giving Danocrine to a woman you inhibit her pituitary gland from making FSH and LH, and this puts her into an artificial menopause. By causing the ovary to cease functioning, and removing the estrogen that is stimulating the continued development of endometrial tissue, the woman will cease menstruating and her endometriosis will gradually shrink away. Danocrine had some very unpleasant side effects, because of its male hormone–like effect. Women complained of oily skin, acne, increased appetite, and weight gain.

Now Lupron has become the popular drug for endometriosis. Lupron directly turns off your pituitary, preventing the secretion of FSH and LH. It produces a clean, artificial menopause that causes your uterine lining and endometriosis lesions to shrivel up. You cannot get pregnant as long as you are on any of these drugs, and it could take a full year to shrink your endometriosis. While on the drug you feel like you are in menopause, and I doubt this treatment will increase your chance of pregnancy. In the long term, Lupron causes nasty menopausal-type hot flashes and a loss of calcium from the bones. I don't recommend it being used for more than a few months.

### *Surgery for Endometriosis — WATCH OUT!*

Surgery for endometriosis is extremely popular. In fact, in the late 1970s and 1980s it would be very difficult for a woman to show up at a fertility clinic asking for infertility help without getting a diagnosis of endometriosis and, subsequently, some sort of surgery for it. It was overdiagnosed because insurance companies would readily pay for the procedure without any questions. An endometriosis lesion as tiny as one millimeter was actually given the respectable label "minimal lesion endometriosis." Lesions so minuscule that they were almost (and sometimes actually) imaginary were signed out on the hospital chart as "endometriosis." Many women underwent an unnecessary, major, open-abdominal operation to remove these little endometriosis lesions. Today these endometriosis lesions commonly, and usually harmlessly, are ablated with electrocautery or with a laser through the laparoscope. However, this is not a harmless procedure when the surface of the ovary is inadvertently cauterized, destroying many eggs (all located in the thin, outer ovarian capsule). Many women have gone through laparoscopy after laparoscopy to "ablate" these endometriosis lesions, causing far more scarring and damage than the original endometriosis.

With these comments I will not earn any friends among doctors treating endometriosis, but most scientifically minded doctors in the field of infertility will verify that the endometriosis craze has finally run its course. The treatments for endometriosis, used in an effort to supposedly cure infertility, are as farfetched in benefit as they are commonly and popularly overprescribed.

## Surgery for Blocked Tubes and Pelvic Scarring

In about 5 percent of infertile couples there is scarring of either the outside or inside of the fallopian tubes causing complete blockage. Scarring on the outside, referred to as adhesions, can "tie the tube down" and make it difficult for it to pick up the egg from the surface of the ovary at the time of ovulation. Such scarring is usually caused by previous pelvic infections from venereal disease, a ruptured appendix, or bowel disease. If the infection causing these adhesions was very severe, it could result in total blockage, usually at the fimbriated end. This total blockage of the tube at the fimbriated end means that the tubal secretions can no longer flow out into the abdominal cavity, and the tube tends to balloon with fluid. This condition is the most common cause of tubal blockage and is referred to as hydrosalpinx. Surgery through the laparoscope or by opening up the abdomen was popular in the past to treat this type of infertility problem.

However, when the end of the fallopian tube is actually blocked, this is usually associated with fairly severe damage to the inside lining of the tube, and the ability of the tube to pick up the egg from the ovary and nourish it is severely inhibited. Therefore, despite very nice surgical operations for opening up the end of the tube and creating a new, beautifully flowered fimbriated end, the pregnancy rate after solving this kind of obstructive problem is very poor. It was actually this low pregnancy rate with surgery for hydrosalpinx that initially led to the clinical development of in vitro fertilization, completely bypassing the need for a fallopian tube. Nowadays, surgery to free up the adhesions around the fallopian tube or to open up its scarred closed end is usually performed as an outpatient, laparoscopic procedure. However, because of the expense and the low pregnancy rate with surgery for these conditions, IVF is the preferred treatment today.

One type of surgery for blocked tubes that is quite effective is reversal of tubal ligation. In this case there has been no damage to the inside of the tube by infection, and microsurgical reconnection of the blocked ends of the tube should usually restore the woman's fertility. The procedure is easy on the patient but must be performed by someone with expertise and microsurgical dexterity.

## Conclusions

The purpose of this chapter has been to review what I consider to be conventional infertility treatments (including just watchful waiting, for those people who are younger and whose infertility has not been of terribly long duration). Some of these conventional approaches, such as Clomid, Parlodel, or surgery, are going to help certain patients get pregnant and need to be understood. On the other hand, it is important not to spend too many years using ineffective treatments such as varicocelectomy, different drug treatments for improving sperm count, ablation of endometriosis, years and years of Clomid or Parlodel in women who don't have elevated prolactin, or withholding intercourse until ovulation occurs, which can lead to tremendous emotional pain and cost and still not get a couple closer to getting pregnant. Many people wait too long before embarking on more modern procedures that would have given them the highest pregnancy rate, until they've finally reached a point of emotional and economic exhaustion.

CHAPTER 5

# Figuring Out What's Wrong: Tests on the Female

Now that you know some of the conventional treatments for infertile couples, you may want to know what tests your physician or clinic might be performing in order to find out what exactly is wrong with you or your husband. As you may have already surmised, despite all of the testing that is available, you may never really find out why you're not getting pregnant. Since getting pregnant is such an incredibly complex process for the body to achieve, the real question is, how does anybody ever get pregnant at all?

In 1980, we thought, perhaps smugly, that we had diagnostic tools for discovering the cause of infertility in most couples. In fact, many couples got pregnant with the conventional treatments we had available at that time, which were applied according to the "diagnosis" of their problem. But many simply did not get pregnant with the inadequate methods that were available at that time.

Those inadequate methods of treatment were based upon the misconception (pardon the double meaning) that a specific problem in the couple had been pinpointed and that solving that specific problem should result in the woman's getting pregnant. This was merely an illusion fueled by the general view in most fields of medicine: First you make a diagnosis, and then you apply a specific treatment. The fact is that the process of human reproduction is so incredibly fragile that a myriad of things can go wrong, and current diagnostic testing will only reveal the most obvious and gross abnormalities. Thus, even after physicians and scientists "figure out what's wrong," there is a very good chance they will be wrong about it. Because treatment today is so much more effective, the extensive and convoluted diagnostic testing of the past is completely unnecessary and confusing, not only to you, but to any honest fertility specialist.

In this chapter, I will outline some of the diagnostic testing you may go through, excluding tests on the husband's sperm (which will be covered in chapter 7). You should realize, however, that in the majority of women even if these tests come up with a "diagnosis," in most cases it does not represent a definitive reason why you're not getting pregnant. Therefore, if the treatment of a specific diagnosis does not result in pregnancy, you should not delay for too long. If you're in your mid- to late thirties (or if your antral follicle count is below fifteen), you should go right to IVF, which bypasses not just one problem but all of the problems that can crop up in this complex reproductive process. Ironically, the cost of IVF is actually less than many of the older, conventional methods of treatment that are erroneously based upon some specific diagnosis.

I'll never forget many years ago seeing a couple who were requesting a vasectomy; they had three children and were now in their midthirties. They did not want to have any more children. Although the man had a normal semen analysis, I had never seen a more clearly infertile-looking woman in my life. She was overweight; her menstrual history was quite irregular, incompatible with any kind of regular ovulation; and she had oily skin with facial hair indicative of very high testosterone levels and severe hormonal imbalance. I was so fascinated by this couple that, despite the fact that they were coming in for a vasectomy (which I willingly performed), I did a complete infertility evaluation on them just as though they had come in complaining that they had not been able to get pregnant.

Daily hormone evaluations of the woman showed lack of ovulation, elevated male hormone levels, and no progesterone production. Whenever I saw her she had lots of clear cervical mucus but showed no sign of ovulation. This was clearly an "infertile" woman by any of our sophisticated hormonal testing, but she had three children. They had a very regular sex life, and I have to assume that their three children were the result of the few times in her whole life that she ovulated. But when she did ovulate, there were always sperm continually moving up from her cervical mucus to the fallopian tube so that on her lucky day of ovulation, the sperm were ready.

When we perform fertility testing on women whose fertility has been clearly demonstrated by prior pregnancy and who have a desire to go on birth control, we often come up with the same diagnoses that in childless women we would have incorrectly determined to be the "cause" of infertility. Going through expensive and sometimes painful tests without a clear understanding of what the tests are going to accomplish is an intimidating experience that a woman may sometimes be afraid to question. This should not be the case. The purpose of this section is to explain what tests are actually needed. A large number do not give any information that helps in treatment, and many are expensive and uncomfortable. Fertility testing should be simple and not overly expensive. Let's look at some of these tests and see what they really do and do not tell us.

## History and Physical

### *Irregular Periods and Oily Skin*

An abnormal menstrual history is the best clue to ovulation problems. When a girl's periods first begin, a stage in life known as menarche, they are naturally very irregular. However, by age fifteen or sixteen they should have stabilized so that they come about every twenty-eight days, are of four to five days' duration, and tend to be a bit heavier the first or second day, tapering off to just a little spotting on the last day. There is a precise hormonal clockwork that regulates the development of the follicle, secretion of estrogen, buildup of a thick lining in the uterus prior to ovulation, the pouring out of large quantities of clear cervical mucus, the LH surge that induces ovulation, and the conversion to a soft lining in the uterus after ovulation when the ruptured follicle starts making progesterone. If this intricately synchronized clockwork of hormonal events is out of tune, the periods may be irregular. In a fertile woman, the normal buildup of a firm, thick lining in the womb, followed by a lush softening of that lining in the second half of the month, leads to an even and neat flow of menstrual blood. The uterus has a fresh start with each new cycle. However, if there is no ovulation, the lining of the uterus builds up unevenly, and bleeding can occur irregularly.

When the number of days between menstrual periods varies too greatly, this is a sign of error somewhere in the clockwork that regulates proper buildup of the lining of the womb and may be associated with either lack of ovulation, poor ovulation, or some deviation from the normal pattern of hormonal regulation. Certainly, women with irregular periods can ovulate and get pregnant, but if they are ovulating, they may be ovulating late or not ovulating every month. Some women may ovulate only twice a year and have very mixed-up periods in between. If the husband has a very high sperm count, the woman may very well get pregnant the one time she does ovulate.

The reason that more regular cycles indicate ovulation is that progesterone, which is secreted only after ovulation has occurred, softens up the lining of the uterus so that a more complete and clean shedding of it will occur at the end of the cycle. When ovulation has not occurred, and progesterone has not been produced, the lining of the womb is somewhat tougher and flakes off in bits and pieces. Periods may not be heavy until several months' worth of this inadequately shed lining has built up. Irregular periods indicate a step-by-step peeling off of the lining rather than a heavy shedding of its entire thickness, and indicate hormonal and ovulatory irregularity.

Extremely painful periods have been thought to be a sign of endometriosis in which some of the tissue lining the inside of the womb is located inside the lower abdomen or pelvis. Thus, when the lining of the womb begins to shed, supposedly similar shedding occurs in the abdomen and causes pain. As discussed in the previous chapter, endometriosis is probably not a cause of infertility in most cases but rather a result of it. But the major myth to be shattered here is not that the treatment of endometriosis is needed but that painful periods are a result of endometriosis. Painful periods are not usually an indication of endometriosis, or any other specific infertility problem.

Using birth control pills will generally make irregular periods regular, because the pills artificially control the buildup and shedding of the lining of the womb. With the Pill, a much thinner lining develops and the periods are much lighter. The woman who has had uncomfortable periods is thus relieved of all of her menstrual discomfort when she goes on the Pill.

Some women feel several hours of pain called *Mittelschmerz* at the time of ovulation. This is a sharp, crampy sensation felt on one side or the other, depending on which ovary is extruding the egg. For reasons we don't understand, most women do not feel this pain. Those who do feel this pain can tell exactly when they are ovulating.

Most women who do not ovulate regularly have a slightly increased amount of male hormone. It is not clear whether the increased production of male hormone is causing them not to ovulate, or whether their inability to ovulate is upsetting their hormonal clockwork to the point where too much male hormone is being produced. Regardless, there is frequently a definite increase in male hormone output in women who are not ovulating regularly. For this reason it is important to check for subtle signs of increased male hormone production. A small amount of hair on the breast, a slightly denser than usual amount of hair in the midline of the lower abdomen, a small amount of fuzzy hair around the anus, or even hair on the great toe are all signs of slightly elevated male hormone production.

Another sign of excess male hormone, which often turns up in the late teens (the significance of which is not realized until ten or fifteen years later when a woman is unable to get pregnant), is acne. Very frequently, acne that persists beyond the midteens in a girl is a sign of elevated male-hormone production associated with lack of ovulation. Oily skin has similar connotations. Thus, menstrual irregularity, abnormal body-hair distribution, oily skin, and acne can be clues to an ovulatory disturbance.

### *Too Fat or Too Thin*

There is a fascinating hormonal explanation for the association of being either overweight or extremely underweight with infertility. The fat cells in your body absorb and slowly release the female hormone estrogen. Therefore, if a woman is obese, she has a lot of estrogen stored in her body that is slowly and gradually released constantly in a noncyclical fashion from places other than her ovaries. At the time of menstruation (day one of the cycle) she will not get as rapid and as high an increase in FSH production from her pituitary gland, because the estrogen constantly coming out of her fat cells is actually suppressing her pituitary gland. Without that early burst of FSH from the pituitary, the ovarian follicle gets a slow start, and all of the hormonal events leading up to preparing the egg's chromosomes for ovulation and fertilization can be out of synch.

I had a very pleasant patient who happened to be 130 pounds overweight and had been infertile all of her married life. She had been through all of the testing performed at several fertility clinics and was now requesting that we perform IVF since no other cause of infertility had been determined. I explained to her that I preferred not to treat her (if she agreed) with a procedure that involved even "minor" surgery unless she lost a hundred pounds, thereby becoming a safer operative candidate. I recommended her to several weight-loss programs that have had good results with the problem of massive obesity and told her to return after she had lost the weight; then we would evaluate whether IVF would be an appropriate procedure for her. She called one year later to tell me that after losing this significant amount of weight, her periods had become more regular, and she was now pregnant.

Being overweight and having this storage of estrogen not only can hurt fertility but can also increase the risk of getting cancer of the uterus later in life. It is well known by physicians that overweight women have a much higher risk of developing this cancer than women of normal weight. The reason for this increased risk of cancer of the uterus is that these women have an excess of continued estrogen release from their fat cells unopposed by any cyclic ovulatory production of progesterone. Thus, they continue to build up the hard, thick uterine lining that is typical of the first two weeks of the menstrual cycle, and this buildup can cause cancer.

Ironically, there is one health benefit caused by obesity and related to excess estrogen levels. As you may already know from popular articles, if women do not receive estrogen hormone replacement after menopause, their bones thin out severely and they will usually develop a condition called osteoporosis. Without estrogen secretion in the female (or testosterone in the male), calcium is gradually leached out of the bones and they become extremely weak and brittle. This leads to the classic "dowager's hump" seen in women in their sixties and seventies who have not been on estrogen replacement, and to the frequent incidence of broken hips that occurs much more commonly in postmenopausal women than in men (who never really go through a hormonal menopause). Women who are fat have a much lower risk of osteoporosis because their fat cells continue to release estrogen even after menopause.

Excessive skinniness is also sometimes associated with infertility in the woman, but suggesting that a woman gain a few pounds is not necessarily the right approach. You'll remember from the previous chapter that the primitive region of the brain called the hypothalamus releases brief pulses of the hormone GnRH at ninety-minute intervals throughout postpubertal life. These ninety-minute pulsatile releases of GnRH are what permit the pituitary gland to secrete the FSH and LH, which in turn regulate the ovarian menstrual cycle.

There is a condition called anorexia nervosa in which strong emotional problems interfere with the functioning of the hypothalamus, and the pulsatile release of GnRH does not occur. This condition is also associated with an inappropriately decreased appetite. The appetite center of the brain is very close to that same area in the hypothalamus that releases the GnRH. Thus, in some extremely skinny women with eating disorders, there is sometimes an inadequate pulsatile release of GnRH from the hypothalamus resulting in inadequate secretion of FSH and LH, and a poor menstrual cycle. However, skinniness itself is *not* a problem at all. It is only if you suffer from anorexia nervosa or other eating disorders that there is a fertility problem associated with being extremely thin.

## Am I Ovulating?

### *Basal Body Temperature (BBT)*

The least expensive method of determining ovulation is to keep a daily basal body temperature (BBT) chart, although this test is becoming unpopular now that simple home ovulation test kits (LH dipsticks) for urine are available. The BBT is taken immediately upon waking up in the morning, before getting out of bed or engaging in any activity whatsoever. Before ovulation, this temperature will always be about one half to one degree Fahrenheit lower than after ovulation. The production of progesterone (which can only occur after ovulation) is what raises the body's basal temperature, so it is actually progesterone production that is being measured. Charts for recording these monthly temperatures are available at almost any pharmacy or from your doctor (see figs. 5.1, 5.2, 5.3, and 5.4).

It seems easy to do, but there are pitfalls and incredible aggravation associated with this inexpensive way of determining ovulation. If the temperatures are not taken first thing in the morning, before you even move to get out of bed, they may give a falsely elevated reading and be difficult to interpret. Every evening before going to bed you must place the thermometer by your nightstand (after shaking it down) within easy reach. If you forget to do this, you will have to get out of bed in the morning to get your thermometer. Even this slight degree of activity can raise your temperature above the basal level and make that day's temperature reading worthless.

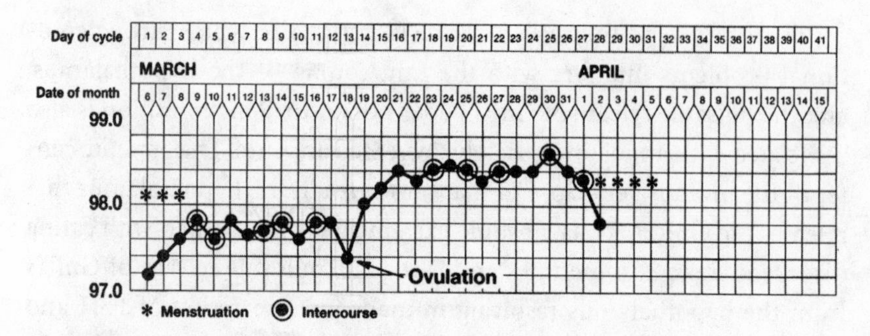


**FIGURE 5.1.** Normal basal body temperature (BBT).

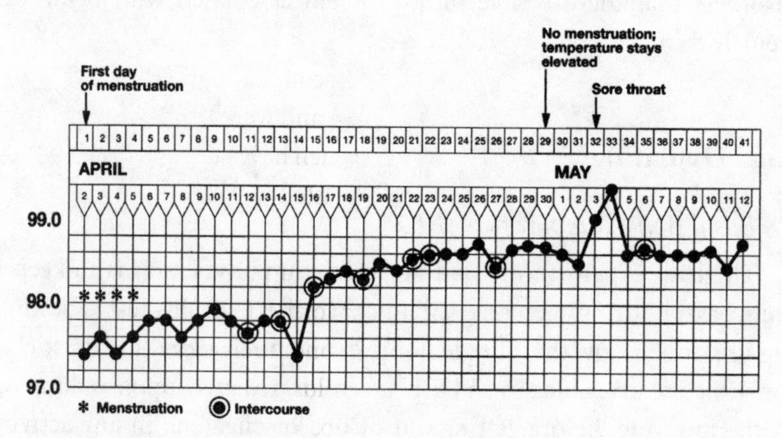


**FIGURE 5.2.** BBT — pregnancy.

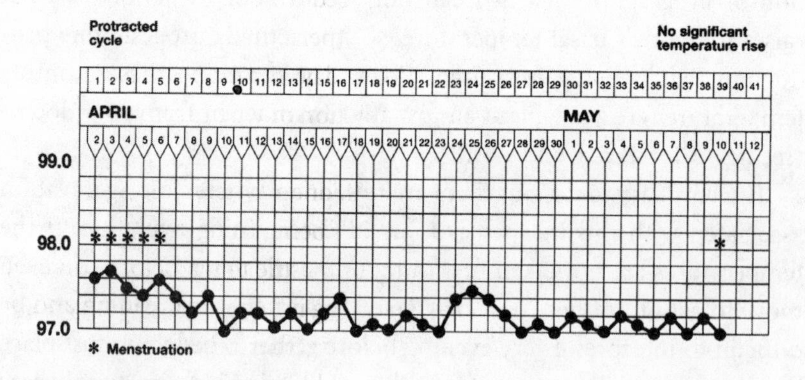


**FIGURE 5.3.** BBT — anovulation.

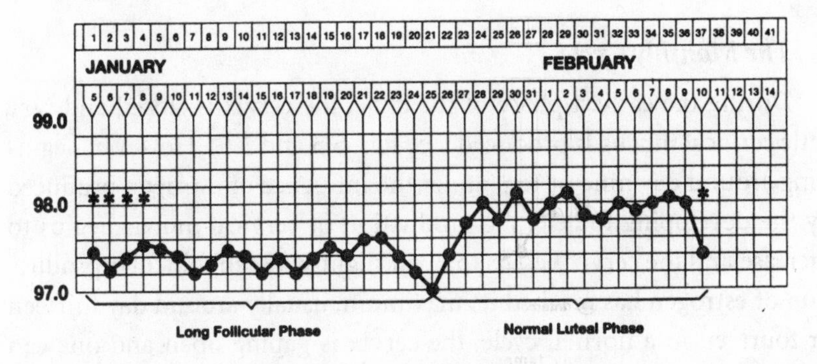


**FIGURE 5.4.** BBT — Long follicular phase and short luteal phase.

Another problem is that it tends to become a daily nuisance, constantly reminding you about your problem and weighing heavily on you emotionally. I can't tell you how many women have called to tell me they finally got pregnant after just getting disgusted with their thermometer and throwing it out the window.

A third problem is that although it gives a picture of progesterone production, BBT is only an indirect indicator. BBT usually must be verified with direct assays of blood progesterone levels since the temperature can be affected by such things as colds, flu viruses, keeping late hours, or even having a poor night's sleep. Remember, the basal body temperature refers to the body temperature after a night of normal, restful sleep. The body temperature normally reaches its lowest levels after all mental and muscular activity has ceased for several hours. That is why the best time to record this basal temperature is upon awakening. Your temperature during the rest of the day is affected by your daily activities and will not be an accurate reflection of whether or not you are making progesterone.

The temperature does not go up until one day after ovulation, and by that time the egg is no longer capable of being fertilized, the cervix is closed, and the cervical mucus has become hostile to sperm. Thus, waiting for the temperature to rise before having intercourse is not a way of maximizing the chances of conception but rather an excellent method of rhythm birth control. Intercourse should take place one or two days prior to the temperature rise, and the basal body temperature cannot predict when you are going to ovulate. You can only show that you have probably already ovulated after it's too late to do anything about it.

### *The Monthly Cycle*

During the earliest phase of the cycle, the cervix is closed and very little cervical mucus is produced (see figs. 5.5 and 5.6). However, beginning around day nine or ten, under the influence of estrogen produced by the developing follicle, the production of cervical mucus begins to increase and the cervix begins to open slightly. When follicular production of estrogen has reached its maximum, usually around day thirteen or fourteen in a normal cycle, the cervix is gaping open and one can actually see into it because of the optically clear, watery cervical mucus flowing out (see fig. 5.7). Then, when the woman ovulates and progesterone is produced, the entrance to the cervix will dramatically close, and the production of cervical mucus will come almost to a standstill.

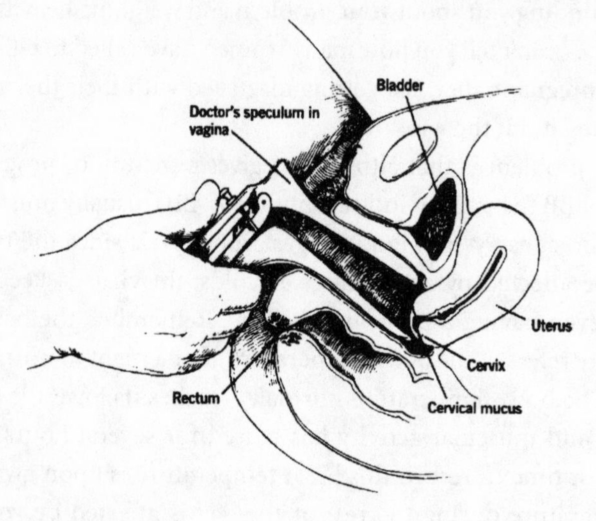


**FIGURE 5.5.** Pelvic examination to observe the opening of the cervix.

What mucus is left will be sticky and tacky and will have lost its optical clarity. At this point sperm would have no chance of invading the mucus. If the physician sees a so-called preovulatory cervix (with a gaping opening and optically clear, abundant mucus) on day fourteen, and then the cervical opening closes within the next day or two, he or she can be fairly certain the woman has ovulated.

Testing the cervical mucus is useful not only as a method for timing when ovulation has occurred, but also for determining whether or not the cervix is receptive to sperm invasion. One of the commonly men-

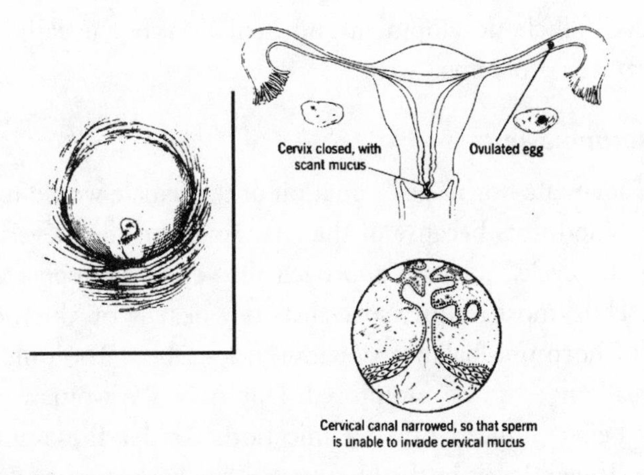


**FIGURE 5.6.** Cervical mucus after ovulation.

tioned causes of female infertility is the cervical factor. This simply means that even at midcycle the woman does not produce an adequate amount or quality of cervical mucus to permit sperm penetration.

Frankly, most of the time, this cervical factor is not really caused by any specific abnormality in the cervix or any particular inability of the cervix to produce good-quality cervical mucus, but rather by inadequate hormonal stimulation in the follicular phase of the cycle. I have found that stimulating the ovulatory cycle with FSH injections not only

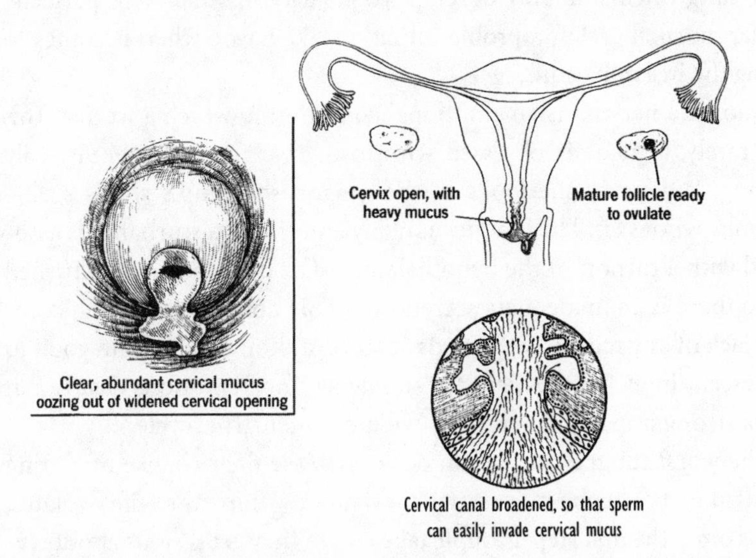


**FIGURE 5.7.** Cervical mucus just before ovulation.

provokes good follicle development and ovulation, but usually solves the cervical mucus problem as well.

### *Blood Hormone Tests*

To do an adequate hormone evaluation of the female would require almost daily blood tests because of the changing hormone levels with each day of the cycle. Such an approach, however, is expensive and impractical. Thus, most fertility specialists rely heavily on the indirect indications of hormone balance previously described. The only time hormones really need to be monitored daily is in the woman whose ovulation is being induced by FSH injections. Under these circumstances, the estrogen levels in the blood must be checked every day (or every other day) in order to determine the proper dose. Otherwise a complicated, daily battery of hormone tests is rarely needed.

### *Effect of the Brain on the Hormonal Cycle*

There are many examples of the impact of emotions on the menstrual cycle. Girls who live together in college dormitories who start out in September having their menstrual periods at random times during the month will, by the end of the college year, adjust their cycles so that they wind up menstruating at about the same time. Women who have been placed on artificial donor insemination programs without proper counseling often suddenly develop irregularity in what were perfectly regular, normal cycles, a problem that wreaks havoc when it comes to timing the insemination.

Anorexia nervosa is an emotional condition in which a woman (or, very rarely, a man) is obsessed with losing weight and eats virtually nothing: Whenever she looks in the mirror, she thinks she is seeing someone who is fat. This unquestionably emotional disturbance is associated with a turnoff of the hypothalamus. The hypothalamus is turned off, so there is an inadequate secretion of FSH and LH, and often complete lack of any menstrual periods at all. So although it does no good to condescendingly tell a patient to "stop worrying," emotions clearly can have a strong impact on a normal ovulatory menstrual cycle.

The worst thing a couple can do to increase their chance of getting pregnant is try to time intercourse to when they think the wife ovulates. This is often the first step a couple takes when they get serious about trying to get pregnant, but it usually creates so much tension and stress in the marital relationship that ovulation is delayed, causing previously regular menstrual cycles to become irregular.

### *LH Urine Dipstick*

The most useful information about the adequacy of your menstrual cycle and your ovulation can be learned at home via the LH dipstick. This technology is available in your local drugstore under brand names such as Ovustick, First Response, and a variety of others from different companies. When these tests first came out, they were laborious and cumbersome and required about an hour of testing time. But now you can get a simple answer in just a few minutes.

LH dipstick tests do not give you the exact quantitative level of LH in your blood, but rather turn a certain color on the day that your LH surges to a high level. If you do this dipstick testing every morning, the test will be negative until the day of your LH surge. If you do the test a day or two later, it will once again be negative. This simple home method for determining when you ovulate has many advantages over the basal body temperature thermometer and cervical mucus testing.

We know from the previous chapter that ovulation should occur within about thirty-six to forty hours of the very beginning of the slight increase in LH production, and about twenty to twenty-four hours after this LH surge reaches its peak. By using the LH dipstick, you can tell the day before you are going to ovulate. However, I must warn that "saving it all up" and abstaining from sex until just before ovulation has no advantage over just having sex three times per week, and not paying any attention to when you ovulate. Therefore, I am very much against couples going out and buying these ovulation detection kits to try to maximize their chance for pregnancy. In truth, it can do just the opposite. Frequent intercourse is a much better, and cheaper, strategy.

### *Ultrasound*

All of the tests for ovulation we have discussed thus far are indirect and fail to positively visualize and clearly prove the occurrence of ovulation. Development of transvaginal ultrasound (a medical application of the sonar used to navigate submarines) allows us to safely view the developing follicle or follicles without fear of radiation damage (a concern when using X-rays). Doctors can actually see the disappearance or reduction in size of the follicle, positively proving that ovulation has occurred. You have already learned something about this in the chapter on antral follicle count.

Of course, this is not a test that you can do on yourself at home. The cost of an inexpensive ultrasound machine is about sixty thousand dollars, and the better ones can cost up to two hundred fifty thousand. Nonetheless, hospitals and clinics use them quite frequently, so the cost of doing a series of examinations for a single cycle can be as low as four hundred dollars. This is a lot more expensive than a forty-dollar dipstick kit and may not be cost-effective for routine evaluation of your menstrual cycle, but it is absolutely essential for monitoring the stimulation of ovulation and is the most precise way of being certain of when ovulation has occurred.

An ultrasound exam can be done in a matter of minutes, without discomfort. It is a very quick examination in which the ovaries, uterus, and developing follicle can be clearly seen by you and your doctor. A physician or technician simply puts a rubber glove over the transducer, with ultrasonic lubricant placed on the tip, and then gently places it in the vagina and looks at the TV screen of the ultrasound machine. This should be no more uncomfortable than a routine pelvic exam. By placing the transducer to the right, left, or center, you can see your ovaries and visualize any developing follicle. You can also see your uterus, either longitudinally, if the transducer is held in one direction, or transversely, if it is held in another. You can even see the endometrial lining building up as the follicular phase progresses in preparation for ovulation.

The ultrasound can also tell you if you have uterine fibroids, ovarian cysts, or tumors. It is the best way to evaluate your egg supply and can tell you when you need to start worrying about your biological clock (see chapter 3). It can fully evaluate your uterus for polyps or any other intrauterine lesions if a small amount of water is instilled to heighten the contrast. (A 3-D ultrasound can do this without the need to instill water.) Furthermore, during the late proliferative stage of your cycle, when the uterine lining is thick, there is no need for 3-D images or water instillation at all. Transvaginal ultrasound is standardly used to nonsurgically obtain eggs from your ovaries for IVF, thus making IVF a completely nonoperative outpatient procedure. Transvaginal ultrasound has completely transformed IVF into a simple, relatively noninvasive treatment, because eggs can be retrieved without surgery of any kind.

### *Polycystic Ovarian Syndrome (PCOS)*

A common condition that always has confused physicians is so-called PCOS, polycystic ovarian syndrome. In the classic condition, the woman does not ovulate and has irregular cycles. Often, the level of male hormone (testosterone) is elevated, the skin is oily and more hairy than normal, and the woman is overweight. Her pituitary hormones have a peculiar shift in that the FSH is low and the LH is high. Although her testosterone level is high for a woman, her estrogen level is also high and her cervical mucus is excellent. Such a woman can easily be induced to ovulate with either Clomid or with a drug called metformin (Glucophage).

Clomid works easily in these cases by just raising the FSH level in the first part of the cycle. Destructive ovarian surgery has been used for decades to remedy PCOS, but no one seems to know why it works. Yet it is one of the most popular treatments for PCOS, to get women to ovulate. Ovarian drilling, or wedge resection, certainly will induce ovulation for a while, and insurance actually pays for this ridiculous procedure. It works by destroying enough eggs that the ovary inhibits the pituitary less, and so the FSH goes up in response to the destruction of ovarian tissue. It would be better to raise the FSH without destroying ovarian tissue and thereby decreasing reproductive life span.

In fact, PCOS is associated with very high ovarian reserve and a long reproductive life span. In a sense, the woman has so many eggs that her FSH is inhibited, and the FSH to LH ratio is therefore lowered. Women with this condition, even if it is untreated, will often start ovulating spontaneously later in life as their egg supply diminishes with age. In that sense, PCOS should not be a frustrating or difficult infertility problem to treat.

## X-ray of the Uterus and Tubes (Hysterosalpingogram)

In some cases the tubes that carry the egg to the site of fertilization may be blocked or restricted in their movement. Thus, failure to conceive might be caused by purely physical factors, even though ovulation may occur normally. The most obvious case in point is a woman who has had her tubes tied, i.e., she has undergone sterilization. However, many women have blockage of the tubes because of previous infections, and sometimes these are infections she never even knew she had. Even a simple case of appendicitis in youth could result in scarring around the area of the tubes, which could interfere with pickup of the egg from the ovary.

One of the clearest ways to determine whether the tubes are structurally intact is through an X-ray called a hysterosalpingogram (HSG), a nonsurgical procedure that does not require hospitalization. However, sometimes it can be very painful, and it must be performed very gently. The woman is given a pelvic examination during which a liquid that is opaque to X-rays (radiopaque) is injected via a cannula through her cervix. An X-ray is then taken, and the doctor can see a perfect outline of the cavity of the uterus as well as the tubes (see fig. 5.8). If the tubes are open without obstruction, this liquid should spill freely into the abdominal cavity, and this is readily seen when the X-ray is taken.

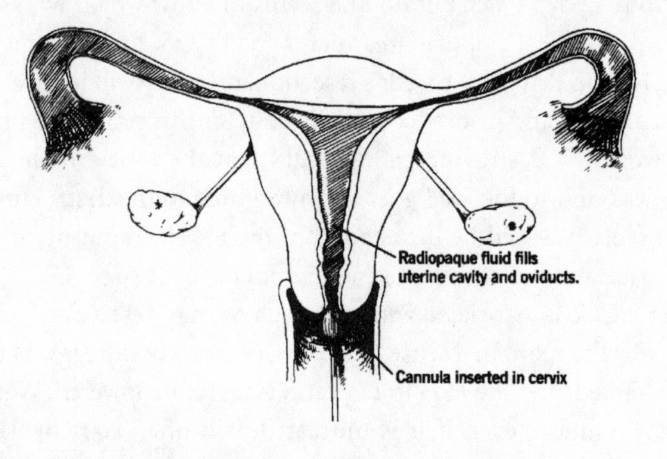


**FIGURE 5.8.** Hysterosalpingogram.

Occasionally the X-ray may give an impression that the tubes are blocked when they really are not. Remember that the tiny canal that connects the uterus to the tubes has a valvelike constricting effect that slows down the sperm trying to get into the tube. Consequently, the X-ray contrast fluid sometimes may not go beyond the uterus simply because of spasms in this area (called the cornu of the uterus).

Performing this test accurately thus requires gentleness on the part of the gynecologist or radiologist, and a full explanation of what is happening. Otherwise, the patient's anxiety itself may interfere with the performance of an adequate X-ray. The radiopaque fluid must be instilled very slowly and gently. This is often neglected by doctors. Just recently I saw a patient who was referred for blocked tubes. However, before we could evaluate whether to operate, she became pregnant, indicating that the X-rays she had had performed elsewhere (which seemed to indicate blockage at the cornu) were erroneous and really just represented temporary tubal spasm. This is a common story.

This test should not be painful if the gynecologist or radiologist administering it is gentle and slow. However, it is often unnecessarily very painful. Any pain at all is simply caused by too rapid an injection, which suddenly increases pressure inside the uterus. Pick a mild-mannered, gentle doctor, and remind him or her to *inject slowly.*

## Laparoscopy

The hysterosalpingogram does not always show scarring around the outside of the tubes or the presence of endometriosis. This type of information can be obtained by actually looking inside the abdomen with a telescope inserted through the belly button (see fig. 5.9). This is called laparoscopy. It is my view that this expensive surgical test (requiring a general anesthetic) is rarely useful.

Laparoscopy can reveal adhesions from previous infection that may be blocking the tubes, as well as more subtle adhesions outside the tubes

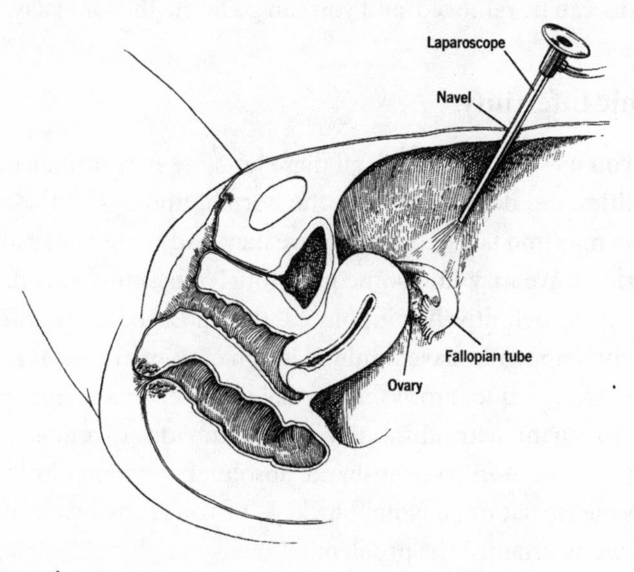


**FIGURE 5.9.** Laparoscopy.

that could interfere with their ability to pick up the egg. Laparoscopy is the only way to make a firm diagnosis of endometriosis. In truth, as I have already discussed, I think the importance of this finding has been vastly overrated.

Some gynecologists feel that if there is any doubt about the appearance of obstruction on an X-ray, laparoscopy can be used to confirm the diagnosis. A blue-colored liquid is injected into the uterus through the cervix, and the doctor then observes through the telescope whether this fluid spills freely through the tube into the abdomen. Some doctors feel that sometimes tubes that appear to be blocked on an X-ray may be shown to be open on laparoscopy. I have found that the HSG X-ray (described previously) is very accurate if performed gently, and laparoscopy is never necessary to make a diagnosis of blocked tubes. In fact, today, laparoscopy as a purely diagnostic procedure is rarely necessary.

However, a skilled laparoscopist can surgically correct, right through the telescope, some of the milder tubal problems that may be found. He or she can cut through adhesions using operating instruments attached to the end of the telescope (or that are inserted through a second or third puncture). This may be all that is necessary for the tubes to be sufficiently mobilized so that their tentacle-like action can grasp the egg effectively. Through the laparoscope, benign ovarian tumors can be removed, ectopic pregnancy can be excised, and even your gallbladder or appendix can be removed, and you can go home the same day.

## Idiopathic Infertility

After you have gone through all these tests, we may or may not find abnormalities, i.e., deviations from the normal findings in the average person. We may find late ovulation or we may find some minimal lesion endometriosis. We may find some mild tubal adhesions. This does not mean we have definitively pinpointed the cause of your infertility. Women who happen to have minimal lesion endometriosis, mild tubal adhesions, or deviations from the normal ovulatory/menstrual pattern often get pregnant with absolutely no treatment. So unless we find absolutely no sperm in your husband, absolutely no ovulation in your cycles, no menstruation, or total blockage of your tubes, we cannot be sure we have ascertained the problem.

In a large number of patients with infertility dating back many years, none of these tests turn up even a dubious abnormality. Frustrated fertility specialists used to vastly underestimate the number of patients in whom they could find nothing wrong. Doctors would go to great lengths to find subtle abnormalities. If subtle abnormalities couldn't be found in the wife and her husband had a sperm count under forty million per cc (as more than 40 percent of husbands do), doctors could simply blame the infertility on him and call it "male factor" infertility. The fact is that we are now admitting more and more openly a high frequency of finding nothing distinctly wrong with either partner after going through all of these tests. We call this idiopathic infertility. *Idiopathic* is a Greek word used in medical terminology to mean "we don't know what causes it."

Idiopathic infertility can usually be explained by age because, as we have discussed in great detail, the older the wife, the lower the pregnancy rate and the higher the incidence of infertility. When you simply feel like throwing up your hands because all treatment for a specific diagnosis has failed, or when no specific diagnoses can be made, then bypassing the whole process via IVF results in a high success rate and usually turns out, in the long run, to be more cost-effective than the years of conventional therapy that may have preceded it.

CHAPTER 6

# Emotions and Infertility (Evidence Based)

## Popular Myths About Emotions and Infertility

To most infertile couples, it is insulting to suggest that their infertility might in some way be caused by emotions. Yet there is clear evidence that the brain has a powerful influence on our hormonal output.

We know from classic studies of college girls in dormitories that although they start their semester with menstrual cycles occurring at various times during the month, by the time they finish the year living together, their menstruation dates become closely synchronized to each other. This synchronization of cycles of women living in close proximity is related to the close association of the pituitary gland and the hypothalamus. The hypothalamus is the primitive region of the brain just above the pituitary gland, that directs the pituitary gland (via GnRH release) to secrete FSH and LH.

An obvious connection between the brain and your menstrual cycle is also apparent in women with anorexia nervosa. Women with anorexia nervosa suffer from an eating disorder related to poor self-esteem. These anorexic women also have hypothalamic amenorrhea, meaning that the hypothalamus is not producing GnRH, and, therefore, their pituitary gland is not stimulated to release FSH and LH, causing failure to menstruate. Thus many circumstantial observations have made it clear that there may be, in some cases, an emotional cause for a couple's infertility.

This has led to a popular myth that infertile couples should "simply adopt a child." That will take off the pressure, and then they supposedly will get pregnant. This belief is very irksome to most infertile couples. In truth, the incidence of infertile couples becoming pregnant spontaneously after adopting a child is less than 4 percent. Nonetheless, whenever this does happen the event sticks in people's minds. In addition, it is not very easy to adopt a child. Costs can range from twenty thousand to sixty thousand dollars and the process may involve trips to Eastern Europe, Russia, China, or South America. There simply aren't many unwanted babies readily available for adoption, and there haven't been for the last thirty years. Thus, trying to adopt becomes just one more source of pressure and anxiety for an infertile couple.

We have systematically studied patients who spontaneously conceived after previously requiring IVF and ICSI to become pregnant. Our findings were remarkable in two completely contradictory ways. In couples where the sperm count is below two million per cc (a severe sperm production defect) who got pregnant with ICSI and the wife was under thirty years of age, 4 percent of them became pregnant again within the next seven years *without any treatment.* This finding was startling and exciting to us because it verified that in young couples, even with extremely poor sperm counts, spontaneous pregnancy can result over time (in a small percentage of cases). The father had the same genetic sperm defect as the infertile son, but he got married at a younger age and his wife was able to get pregnant while she was still in her early to midtwenties. But this study also showed that the rate of spontaneous pregnancy that occurs once the emotional pressure is relieved by having a child is not very high, and probably not related to the relief of emotional pressure.

The other problem caused by the misperception that infertility is simply caused by emotional pressure is that it is just empty reassurance based on no evidence. Reassurance that is not evidence based only increases a couple's anxiety. If you could really tell the patient that examinations and studies suggest they should just relax and wait, then that would be true reassurance. But if the evidence shows that the couple is unlikely to get pregnant if they simply calm down and wait, then every year that they put off treatment is another year that they are less likely to conceive, because the biological clock continues to tick. Although we know that infertile couples are understandably emotional and tense, most of them would argue that their tension did not produce their infertility but rather their infertility has been the major source of their tension.

Nonetheless, certain situations that suggest an emotional link to infertility do occur. Anna was one of the most anxious patients I ever treated. She had already named all her children when she herself was just five years old. She got married at age twenty and planned to have lots of kids. Yet after ten years of marriage, she still was not pregnant. She underwent three IVF cycles at a different center and then three at our center. She had many eggs and great embryo quality in all six IVF cycles, but still she did not get pregnant. She then went to a disreputable center, where the doctors convinced her that expensive immune therapy would work, but it didn't. Finally, after years of effort, she and her husband adopted two children from overseas, and six months later, she got pregnant on her own with no treatment at all. In fact, it might have been the only six months in their entire marriage in which she was not on some type of treatment.

## Does Infertility Cause Emotional Tension, or Does Emotional Tension Cause Infertility?

There are many couples whose marriages are completely destroyed by the pressures and resentments caused by their infertility. The wife is often meticulously checking her ovulation times by observing her cervical mucus, taking her basal body temperature, or using expensive drugstore kits to check her urine every day to see if the dipstick turns blue (indicating she's going to ovulate soon). The couple will often put off intercourse for several weeks or more, waiting for the moment when the woman's urine ovulation test turns positive. But at the right time, the husband or wife may be out of town. A conflict then ensues because he can't fly back home just because she's ready to ovulate, or because she can't fly to where he has business meetings. They finally agree on where to meet, not for the purpose of having a joyous reunion, but so he can inseminate her at the right moment. The emotional tension induced by trying to time intercourse precisely to the moment of ovulation often delays ovulation anyway, and their efforts are therefore of little use.

Carefully observed follow-up studies of families with infertility from both Europe and the United States compared to control groups of families with naturally conceived children have objectively demonstrated that parents of children conceived by IVF express greater warmth toward their child, are more emotionally involved with their child, interact more successfully with their child, and report less stress associated with parenting than couples who have conceived the child naturally. Thus, there seems to be no objective evidence for the hurtful myth that infertile couples are infertile because they have psychological problems. Some argue that, in an evolutionary sense, emotional dysfunction would have negative effects on a child, and that is why it is a cause for infertility. However, evidence that children conceived with IVF exhibit greater psychological health than the population norm favors the opposite view, that infertility is not caused by an emotional condition, but that the emotional tension of infertile couples is caused by the infertility itself.

Nonetheless, evidence is accumulating to suggest that couples undergoing assisted reproductive technology (ART) in order to solve their infertility problem are likely to have better results if they are emotionally calm and capable of dealing with the extreme stress this can place upon them. I will get into the details of those observations later in the chapter, but at the outset I want to emphasize that it is bad medicine to just tell these couples to relax. Usually, such an approach is self-delusional, and the anguish persists even though it may be suppressed and unadmitted.

## Anxiety Caused by Trying to Time Your Intercourse

Perhaps the biggest mistake couples make when they have not been able to get pregnant after a relatively short interval of trying is to work on timing their intercourse to the precise moment of ovulation. Humans are designed in such a way that intercourse is not used solely as a means of getting pregnant. It has perhaps an even more important function of promoting the human family system (based on establishing a pair-bonding-type relationship), which is crucial for the raising of children. Thus, when the husband and wife nervously hold off having sex despite the romantic inclination to do so, until some moment when her urine test turns positive or her morning temperature starts to rise, this couple is confounding nature. Tension created by such an attempt to make every episode of sex count (in terms of getting pregnant) creates so much anxiety that very often ovulation is delayed anyway.

Even if ovulation isn't delayed by the emotions and tension created by scheduling sex, does precise timing actually improve the chance of getting pregnant? Once ovulated, the egg normally has about twelve hours in which it can be fertilized and result in a viable embryo. However, ejaculated sperm migrating up through the cervical mucus may remain motile for up to a week, and they are quite capable of fertilizing the egg for up to three days. Even if you do make it to the bedroom on time, is it of any benefit over random, happy sex that arises out of a good relationship?

Studies going back forty years have shown that couples who do not have an excessively cluttered life, and who are not having marital problems, will have intercourse an average of two to three times per week. If you are having sex two to three times per week, nature works pretty well. There will always be some normal sperm present and available for the egg whenever you ovulate. If, however, you are not having sex two to three times per week, then it's time to examine your lifestyle and think about whether it needs to be changed.

In any event, timing intercourse seems to be of no use unless a couple is so busy that they can only have sex once a week or less. For everyone else it would be better to put aside fears about "wasting" intercourse at a time when it is not likely to lead to pregnancy.

## Anxiety Causing You to Hurry into Worthless and Potentially Damaging Treatment

Anxious couples who rush to get treatment may fall prey to a host of fairly useless infertility procedures that can run up a large bill or, if covered by insurance, can be utilized by physicians with very poor judgment in remarkably ill-conceived ways. For example, a very well-known and intelligent physician couple, who had already had one child, was having trouble conceiving a second child. His sperm count was extremely low, less than one million, and so he saw a local urologist. The urologist, of course, found a varicocele (a varicose vein of the scrotum) on both sides and recommended surgery. As we have stated earlier in this book, varicocele surgery is performed on almost every infertile man who visits a urologist's office, but unfortunately all carefully controlled studies fail to show any benefit of varicocelectomy on either sperm count or pregnancy rate.

The urologist, being well intentioned and recognizing that his patient was also a physician, recommended that a more conservative approach be tried first. So he put this man on HCG injections three times per week for three months. HCG is equivalent to LH and will stimulate the testes to make huge amounts of testosterone. Nonetheless, countless studies have failed to demonstrate that HCG, or any other hormones, improves sperm production in infertile men (unless they suffer from a very rare condition called Kallman's syndrome, which this patient did not have). However, the administration of HCG for three months can have a devastating effect on what little spermatogenesis exists in the infertile male. HCG stimulates the testicles' Leydig cells to produce more testosterone. Some doctors believe that increased testosterone production in the testes will create an improved environment for sperm production. However, the increased testosterone production inhibits the pituitary's release of FSH, and the already poor sperm production, ironically, is further reduced.

This patient, after three months of inappropriate treatment, had no sperm whatsoever in the ejaculate. Dismayed by this result, the urologist decided he'd better go ahead and perform varicocele repair on this patient. At that point the patient saw me, and I discovered that he had no varicocele, but rather a perfectly normal scrotum. I made him stop taking the HCG injections, and three months later he had small numbers of sperm in the ejaculate. The patient then became one of our earliest ICSI cases, and his wife subsequently became pregnant and delivered healthy twins. Nonetheless, in the effort to "do something," this man wound up hurting rather than helping his chances of having more children.

Another ill-conceived treatment, which is very popular and often stupidly covered by insurance just like varicocelectomy, is the laserization of ovarian endometriosis. I performed a vasectomy reversal on a forty-one-year-old man married to a thirty-one-year-old woman. It was actually a difficult vasectomy reversal (partly because his vasectomy had been performed more than a decade earlier), requiring vasoepididymostomy (bypass of blowouts in the more delicate ductwork that conveys sperm from the testes into the vas deferens). The operation went extremely well, and postoperatively he had a perfectly normal sperm count of fifty million per cc with 50 percent motility and excellent-quality sperm. The wife was so excited that she simply couldn't wait to get pregnant naturally. She became convinced by everything she'd read in the popular press and on television that it's difficult to get pregnant without some kind of medical supervision, so she went to see a gynecologist who was all too happy to "do something."

Unbeknown to me, she scheduled a laparoscopy that turned out to be tragic. Her husband's sperm count had come up to normal five months after his operation, and it was only one month later that she rushed into having laparoscopic surgery. It is true that she had a small endometriosis cyst in one ovary, but it was less than four centimeters in size and shouldn't have caused any worry. During this laparoscopy, the gynecologist removed her entire right ovary, thus removing one half of her eggs in one fell swoop. He then cauterized much of the remaining left ovary in an attempt to get rid of whatever endometriosis was thought to be present in the left side. The end result was that this thirty-one-year-old woman who had no previous history of infertility or gynecologic problems was now perimenopausal. She had lost virtually all of her eggs. When she arrived in St. Louis to start an IVF cycle, we checked her FSH level and did detailed ultrasound examination and MRI imaging studies. What we discovered is that she had no ovary on the right and no remaining ovarian tissue on the left. Her FSH level was forty-two (anything over fifteen is perimenopausal), and despite her husband now having a normal sperm count, she would require IVF with donor eggs if she wanted to have a child. This tragedy arose from the overwhelming anxiety that drove her to seek inappropriate early treatment.

Worse than this well-intentioned but disastrous operation for endometriosis is the so-called ovarian drilling procedure, which has been popularized as a method to stimulate ovulation in nonovulatory women. The theory behind ovarian drilling is that a woman may have a condition called PCOS (polycystic ovarian syndrome) in which she has multiple tiny, unovulated cystlike follicles. This is often associated with infrequent ovulation and a somewhat elevated male hormone level. Although this condition is associated with lack of ovulation, PCOS patients have large numbers of eggs and usually do not suffer from a deficiency in ovarian reserve. In fact, the whole problem with stimulating them for IVF or simple ovulation induction is you may get more eggs than you really want, and have to worry about hyperstimulation syndrome. But these women would rarely be deficient in eggs. Ovarian drilling is a laparoscopic procedure in which the doctor uses a laser to drill holes into the ovary so as to "drain" these unovulated microfollicles. This decreases the testosterone level and supposedly allows the woman to spontaneously correct her irregular cycle and ovulate.

In fact, when the well-intentioned gynecologist, via laparoscopy, is cauterizing or drilling holes through the surface of the ovary in order to stimulate ovulation, ironically he or she is actually inadvertently destroying many thousands of eggs. As a result of this surgery, a woman will most likely have an earlier menopause, and may not even have enough eggs for a good prognosis with IVF.

Nobody really understands why ovarian drilling seems to cause women to ovulate for several months after the procedure when they weren't ovulating before. It is likely that so much ovarian tissue is damaged that FSH secretion from the pituitary goes up in response to massive destruction of eggs, giving a bit of a boost for a few months to what is now a deficient ovary. Thus, because of a couple's desire to "do something," they may sometimes be even worse off than if they just did nothing.

We recently saw a forty-year-old woman (married to a forty-eight-year-old man) who had been trying to get pregnant since she was thirty-five years of age. Unfortunately, the first doctors that she saw (before even a year had passed) immediately scheduled laparoscopy. Her prior hysterosalpingogram, performed after only several months of trying to get pregnant, showed a round "filling defect" in the uterine cavity that was clearly an air bubble indicative of an inexpertly performed X-ray. There was really nothing wrong with her uterus. Several months later she underwent "diagnostic" D and C (dilation and curettage), operative hysteroscopy, operative laparoscopy, and ovarian drilling. The doctor then cauterized the inside of the endometrial lining of the uterus through the hysteroscope to remove the so-called polyps that weren't really polyps. This created scarring within the uterus. Because the doctor wasn't sure that he got anything out that was significant, he then did a standard, old-fashioned D and C. Using laparoscopy, he then drilled multiple holes, according to his own notes, ten times through the ovary on each side. After several years of still not getting pregnant following these procedures, she went to a local IVF program, and they were able to get only one follicle with her first IVF attempt and no follicles with her second IVF attempt. As a result of her ridiculous series of surgeries, she was now perimenopausal, probably a decade before she needed to be, and would only be able to get pregnant with donor eggs. Therefore, as empty as the advice of "just relax" is, it would have been better to do nothing than to receive this kind of ill-conceived, aggressive treatment.

Several years ago we saw a very wealthy couple from Latin America who should have had access to the best possible medical treatment anywhere in the world. They were a young couple in their twenties who wanted to get pregnant as soon as possible after marriage and have a large family. The wife did not get pregnant within the first few months, and they were very anxious to "do something." They went to a local doctor, who put the husband on testosterone injections every two weeks. This is actually a very effective method of male contraception, as the testosterone injections suppress FSH and thus reduce sperm production rather than increase it. But since he immediately noticed an increased libido, he assumed that this had to be good treatment. He didn't have a sperm count performed until several years later, and to his disappointment, it showed zero sperm in the ejaculate. He came to us for a TESE/ICSI (testicular sperm extraction/intracytoplasmic sperm injection) procedure to determine if there were any sperm in his testes, and he never told us, despite detailed questioning, that he was on testosterone injections. We did a TESE and found no sperm. It wasn't until we found no sperm that he finally, sheepishly confessed that he had lied about not being on any drugs. He admitted he was just too embarrassed to tell us he had had this stupid treatment. In fact, this couple had been on male birth control for the last five years, only because they were so anxious to hurry into treatment.

Before concluding the discussion about the dangers of hurrying into inappropriate treatment, I should mention the risk of stocking up on nutritional supplements from your local health-food store. A couple in their early thirties was planning to come here for IVF after many years of not getting pregnant with more conventional treatment. His sperm count had always been very high whenever it was tested, between 80 and 120 million per cc with 75 percent motility and good-quality morphology. Despite his high sperm count, the husband wanted to do whatever he could to maximize the chance of success with IVF. So, on his own, he began bodybuilding, doing aerobic exercise, and taking some of the nutritional bodybuilding supplements he was able to find at the local health-food store.

It's important to know that none of these supplements are subject to FDA approval, and you cannot be sure of what's in them. Nor can you trust that the label is correct — there is simply no accountability or supervision. The husband came in on the day of the IVF procedure expecting to be in his best physical condition, which he erroneously thought would improve the result of IVF, and we found he had a sperm count of less than twenty-five thousand sperm, none of which were motile. His hormone levels (FSH, LH, and testosterone) were normal, and so the nutritional supplement he was taking was having no impact on his endocrinal system. It therefore had to be directly toxic to the testes. We directed him to stop taking all nutritional bodybuilding supplements, and six months later he had a completely normal sperm count. His wife eventually became pregnant and delivered a healthy baby.

In order to enhance sales, many of the companies making these so-called natural supplements want them to have some effect. So some are clandestinely spiked with Ephedra, anabolic steroids, or even small amounts of Viagra, all under the guise of being natural. Nutritional supplements cannot improve your fertility, and can be dangerous.

The manufacturers of Proxceed, a heavily marketed nutritional supplement, claim their product can improve sperm quality. It is actually being advertised in medical journals for doctors to prescribe to patients. Yet it is not a drug, requires no prescription, and is under no FDA supervision. In our experience it has been completely ineffective and is just an amino acid supplement. Fortunately, it is not dangerous, but it does no good. But people are buying it in droves. It is no different from the snake oil sold by unscrupulous salesmen in prior centuries. But some people are so wrought with anxiety over their infertility that they are willing to waste money so they can feel like they're "doing something." Far better to just "relax."

## The Effect of Emotions on IVF Success

Our nurses often comment that certain patients they see coming in for IVF are unlikely to get pregnant despite the best treatment, because they seem so anxious and emotionally troubled. Most physicians would view this as non-evidence-based speculation. But we began to notice in our follow-up visits that pregnancy rates were much lower in the patients the nurses classified as "very nervous" as compared to those that seemed to be more "calm." Regardless of the subjective nature of such an observation, it did appear, in retrospect, that the nurses' opinions had very good predictive value. So we began to study the impact of emotions on pregnancy rates with IVF.

Generally, routine ultrasound examination of the uterus doesn't seem to show any obvious activity of the uterine musculature (see fig. 6.1). However, if you videotape the ultrasound over a period of time and then run the tape back at high speed (using time-lapse photography), you can observe a series of very slow, rhythmic contractions in the uterus

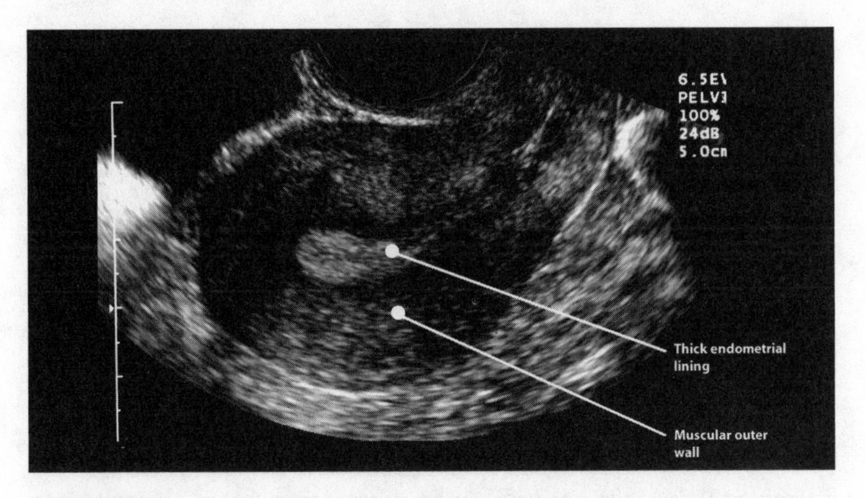


**FIGURE 6.1**

Uterine lining (endometrium) *thick* when estrogen level goes up toward midcycle.

that occur at a greater frequency in the first two weeks of the monthly cycle (before ovulation); after ovulation the frequency of the uterine contractions diminishes dramatically. Thus, although the uterus appears to be calm and immobile, there is a lot of subtle activity going on. In the normal woman this activity is much greater prior to ovulation.

We wondered whether this uterine activity could have something to do with any of the puzzling cases in which the woman fails to get pregnant even though embryos that appear perfectly normal are transferred in multiple IVF cycles. Uterine irritability is a profound impediment to getting pregnant. (In fact, that is how an IUD [intrauterine device] provides contraception.) Indeed, in some women, the pregnancy rate is higher when we put the embryos into the fallopian tube rather than the uterus. The embryo arrives in the uterus naturally without any irritation. The general anesthetic administered in order to do this tubal embryo transfer also completely wipes out uterine contractions (which in nervous women were more frequent than in calm women). Nonetheless, performing a surgical tubal transfer is not as effective as simply paying attention to the couple's emotions in improving the pregnancy rate in women with multiple previous failures.

For example, we saw a thirty-five-year-old woman whose husband needed to have sperm retrieved and frozen because of irreparable blockage, and this sperm was used for the wife's ICSI/IVF cycles. His wife was extraordinarily terrified about any medical procedures and had always had severe phobias of needles and anything medical. In fact, she had originally asked for a tubal transfer only because she knew she would have to have a general anesthetic for it and didn't want to be awake. Ultimately, however, she decided to have a standard IVF transfer into the uterus because she had a low pain threshold and didn't want to wake up to any pain after an operation. When we did her IVF transfer she was very frightened, and it required great sensitivity to complete it because she was so afraid. The nurses predicted that despite the transfer of such beautiful embryos she would not get pregnant, and she didn't.

But she was a courageous woman, and although she was still very phobic, she came back with her husband five months later for another attempt at IVF. Again, beautiful embryos were transferred, this time into her fallopian tube via a tiny minilap incision. Once again she did not become pregnant despite the use of embryos that seemed perfectly normal. Eight months later, the couple returned once more, after having had intensive psychotherapy together over the past year. Our nurses this time observed (and we concurred) that she seemed like a different woman. She explained how she had worked out her fears and how her therapist had helped them both to understand and be aware of these fears. This time we transferred three embryos, which were no different in appearance than what had been transferred in her previous cycles, and she became pregnant with triplets and delivered healthy children.

In another case, a couple, who traveled from the other side of the world after having many unsuccessful IVF cycles elsewhere, had been seeing us for four years, from age thirty-four to age thirty-eight. The woman underwent five IVF cycles during that period, and each time we transferred what looked like perfectly good embryos. This woman was not outwardly nervous, but held all of her fears and concerns inside. By the time she came here for her tenth IVF cycle, she explained that nothing really bothered her anymore because she wasn't even seriously contemplating the possibility of success. She was just going through the motions, because this is what she thought she "ought to do." Sure enough, after four years of frantic effort and when she had finally "relaxed," she became pregnant and delivered healthy twins.

There are countless anecdotes that suggest that a state of calm, which is very hard for an infertile couple undergoing the rigors of an IVF procedure to achieve, may be helpful and conducive to a higher pregnancy rate. This does not mean that the anxiety or emotions caused the infertility, but when you transfer normal embryos in an otherwise successful IVF cycle, there may be a greater chance of pregnancy if the couple is in a state of emotional calm rather than harried and frightened by the complexity of their circumstances. It is possible that this may be related to the increased frequency of uterine contractions observed on time-lapse ultrasonography in women who appear to be more anxious.

## The Effect of Emotional Calm on Your Body

It is well known that certain diseases occur more frequently in patients with severe anxiety, and any modern observer is aware of this mind-body interaction. For example, asthma, stomach ulcers, neurodermatitis (or ectopic dermatitis), spastic colon, and high blood pressure are all physical, somatic ailments that have a strong psychological component. An illness diagnosed as psychosomatic is not necessarily "all in your head." What it means is that emotional difficulties can precipitate adverse physical, or somatic, effects on the body.

Individuals are often unaware of many of the factors that determine their emotions and behavior. These unconscious factors may create great emotional pain or seemingly inexplicable self-destructive behavior. Sometimes this pain takes the form of recognizable physical symptoms, disturbances in mood and relationships, low self-esteem, or even troubling personality traits. It can even cause "slips" in competitive sports, much like the verbal equivalent of the "Freudian slip." Because these forces are unconscious, listening to the advice of friends and family, reading self-help books, or even applying the most determined efforts of willpower often fails to provide help. These unconscious forces are usually the cause of otherwise great athletes getting "psyched out" at specific points in their competitive career. For example, certain pitchers who have incredible abilities all of a sudden lose "control." No matter how good their control had been in their prior games, or how incredible they were as pitchers, they suddenly throw balls so wild you wonder how they ever even got through Little League baseball, let alone became great major league prospects. They simply can't get it right because something deep within their subconscious is preventing them from pitching with control, even though they clearly have the physical ability to do so.

The patient's ability to become almost philosophical about her situation is based on becoming aware of the underlying source of her anxiety. Such self-understanding often requires intensive psychological counseling rather than just a few short, goal-oriented sessions. Not all patients can afford, or have the patience for, intense psychotherapy, and we have found that there are other approaches that work. We employ those approaches in all of our IVF embryo transfers. Using these other approaches, which I'll explain in the rest of this chapter, has given us deeper insight into the role of emotions in getting pregnant.

## IVF Embryo Transfer and Emotions

There is a more dramatic observation we made about the impact of emotions on our IVF patients that doesn't require fancy time-lapse ultrasonography, and that can surely enhance the chance of pregnancy. This observation was made during the actual technique of embryo transfer into the uterus.

By the mid- to late 1990s it became apparent to leading IVF physicians that the delicacy of the seemingly simple embryo transfer has a very high impact on pregnancy rate and is just as important as a good laboratory or a good response to hormonal stimulation. With a traumatic embryo transfer, or even a *seemingly* atraumatic transfer, in which there was a tiny amount of blood noticed on the tip of the catheter after its removal, the pregnancy rate has always been very low. In fact the pregnancy rate was much lower in the era of so-called stiff catheters (which always did this) than in the present era, wherein only the softest catheters are advised. The difference between good programs and bad programs comes down to the last few moments of the whole two-month IVF ordeal: when the embryos are transferred into the woman's uterus. Our observations, made at the time of embryo transfer, have provided enormous information about the role of emotional calm.

What I continually observe when I visit IVF programs around the world (and I am familiar with most of them) is that programs with high success rates have delicate and smooth embryo transfers, while programs with lower success rates relegate the embryo transfer to an inexperienced physician who always seems to be in a hurry because he has so much else to do. In fact, very meticulous follow-up studies have demonstrated that certain physicians working with the same exact laboratory and the same type of population of patients have very high pregnancy rates, while other physicians in the same IVF program have very low pregnancy rates. The difference is repeatable from physician to physician, and the difference in pregnancy rate between physicians performing the embryo transfer is very dramatic.

When talking shop among themselves, IVF and infertility doctors will refer to "difficult transfers" versus "good transfers." A difficult transfer simply means that when the doctor tries to thread the delicate little catheter containing the embryos through the cervical opening into the uterus, he or she encounters resistance. Sometimes it is thought by the physician that there is a stenosis, or scarred narrowing of the cervix, making it impossible to insert the catheter. But this cannot be true, because if a stenosis were present, the woman would not be able to menstruate. Nonetheless, it does seem that in as many as 25 percent of IVF cycles, physicians have difficulty passing the catheter into the uterus. Why should that be?

Of course, it is easy to force a stiff, rigid stylet, or sound, into the uterus via the cervix. A physician can simply guide it in by feel as long as the catheter or stylet is stiff enough that he or she can angle it or push it through. In fact, that is the way the common D and C is performed on a routine basis at hospitals around the world. Dilation is performed by putting a stiff, relatively thick and smooth sound into the cervix, thus dilating the cervix to get into the uterus. But we all know that such an approach irritates the uterus, causes bleeding in the uterine lining, and certainly would prevent pregnancy from occurring. That is why smaller, very delicate catheters must be used to put either sperm (IUI) or embryos (IVF) into the uterus.

However, even the so-called delicate catheters can be stiff enough to create irritation. The most popular catheters over the course of the years had been stiff catheters that had a curve on them that would allow the physician to guide them into the uterus by feel, or even to push them through. These stiffer catheters were very popular and are still used in many IVF centers because they seem to be easier to use. However, programs that use these stiffer catheters always have lower pregnancy rates. Putting in a stiff catheter and irritating the uterus has the same contraceptive effect as putting in an IUD. An IUD works by irritating the uterus and preventing implantation.

The cervix is a four-centimeter (one-and-a-half-inch) canal that leads from the vagina into the interior of the uterine cavity, and it is just a sphincter. When a catheter does not pass easily it is not because of a physical blockage but rather a contraction of the muscles of the cervix just like any other sphincter. The cervical canal is never occluded, only constricted by muscular contraction, which is intensified by stress.

Another misconception is that a difficult transfer occurs because of too sharp a curvature of the cervix. But every cervix has some sort of sharp curvature. Physicians can always straighten the cervix by placing a sharp tenaculum on the cervix and pulling on it. But grasping the cervix with the tenaculum and pulling on it to straighten it out is in itself traumatic and somewhat painful, and will greatly reduce the pregnancy rate. Thus, either using a stiff catheter with a preformed curve (to make embryo transfer easier) or using a tenaculum to pull on the cervix to straighten it out irritates the uterus, disturbs the endometrial lining, and therefore lowers the pregnancy rates.

The reason that many IVF centers do not use a soft, atraumatic catheter is that it seems to be more difficult to put it in, but that is only because it can't be forced in. Some physicians have a very hard time using a soft catheter; however, programs in which the doctors have learned how to use a soft catheter properly have much higher pregnancy rates.

What do I mean by using a soft catheter? The catheter we use (and I won't promote nor do I have any interest in any particular brand) is literally as soft as a wet noodle. It cannot possibly irritate the uterus. However, you can imagine how difficult it would be to guide something as soft as a wet noodle through the cervix. Even sensitive and manually dexterous physicians who use such soft catheters can sometimes encounter difficult transfers, and even they will then regretfully ask the embryologist to reload the embryos into a stiff catheter. They have no trouble getting the stiff catheter in, but they know the pregnancy rate is reduced because the stiff catheter will irritate the uterus. *So what does all this have to do with emotions and IVF pregnancy rate?*

## How to Avoid Difficult Embryo Transfers

Since we have adopted our current approach toward embryo transfer, always using only a soft catheter and never resorting to a stiff catheter, we have figured out the reason for difficult transfers. Our current approach for the last five years was prompted by the observations that anxious patients were much more likely to be difficult transfers and that relaxed patients were much more likely to be easy transfers with a higher pregnancy rate. We were determined never to resort to switching from a soft catheter to a stiff catheter but rather always to figure out how to negotiate the soft catheter without any uterine irritation. With this in mind, we took advantage of the poorly recognized phenomenon that the cervix is truly a sphincter and is as much under the control of emotions as the rectum. Under states of high anxiety, the remarkably thick cervical sphincter (which is a thicker, more muscular sphincter than any other sphincter in the body, including the bladder, the rectum, and the stomach) contracts with great force.

Whenever we noted that the soft catheter was not passing easily through the cervix into the uterus, we talked to the patient calmly in a quiet room and explained what was happening. We told her that we were willing to wait as long as we had to until we could eventually get the soft catheter in, because we did not want to irritate her uterus with a stiff catheter, or by using a tenaculum. In many cases, the nurses noticed that whenever the patient became visibly relaxed, there was suddenly no longer any resistance in the cervix, and the catheter slipped in easily. If this did not happen, we would bring in the anesthesiologist, and the patient would then be sedated. Once the patient was fully sedated, we found it remarkable that the soft catheter always slipped in as the resistance just melted away.

However, we wanted to avoid putting patients to sleep on a frequent basis. All we wanted was the cervical sphincter to be relaxed so that the catheter could pass easily, in just a matter of seconds. We knew that no matter how firmly we would tell a patient to "relax," this was like telling an insomniac to "stop worrying and just go to sleep." So we developed a better method for helping patients relax.

## Relaxation Techniques

We tried a relaxation technique borrowed from the principles of Yoga, Eastern philosophy, and modern behavior-modification psychology. We know that emotions can have a severe, traumatic effect on one's health. We know that anxiety and fear can cause any sphincter to tighten unconsciously. The question is how to get a patient to relax so that her cervical sphincter will also relax. The answer is not to try to downplay her emotions or fears, but rather to explain the simple truth. We have no direct control over involuntary muscles, but we do have control over the voluntary ones. This is the basis of all meditation. One can sit in a contemplative position, systematically think about each muscle group in the body, and relax these muscle groups. You can start from the forehead muscles that cause headache, your neck muscles, your tight and hunched shoulders, and work all the way down to your toes, being aware of all your muscle groups that are tense and voluntarily relaxing them. It does not matter how worried or how fearful you are. You have the ability to relax all of these voluntary muscles and to let your body go limp.

This may sound a little far-out, but our observations are that it works. As the patient is in the humiliating position that women go through on a yearly basis for their Pap smears, we tell her we are aware that this is a difficult time, but that she must simply concentrate on letting her body go limp. We warn her about this ahead of time, before we even go into the embryo transfer room. In an almost hypnotic repetitive way, we systematically ask her to begin with her head and work down to her toes, relaxing all of her voluntary muscles and letting her body just become a wet noodle. Even for what would appear to be difficult transfers at first, once her body goes limp, and she truly relaxes her skeletal muscles, the catheter then slips in with ease.

The reason I mention this in such detail is not only to explain the importance of delicate embryo transfer to a successful IVF cycle, but to try to give you what evidence we do have for the profound effect of emotions on your chances of getting pregnant in any cycle. *Your emotions control the tightness of your cervical sphincter and the frequency of uterine contractions.*

When we perform the embryo transfer, we want the embryos to have a "soft landing" in the endometrium with no disturbance whatsoever. That is why we use a soft catheter rather than a stiff one. However, maintaining a relaxed condition for several weeks after embryo transfer may also enhance the chances of implantation and pregnancy. We recommend that no matter how nervous or worried the patient is about the IVF cycle, or about her whole life, she do simple meditative relaxation exercises on a regular basis. We know this is no magic answer, especially with older women with low ovarian reserve or poor embryo quality, but there is strong evidence that your emotions have a profound impact on uterine contractility, which can affect your chances for pregnancy.

CHAPTER 7

# How the Male Works

## The Male Myth

It is a common misconception that a low sperm count means that the male is the cause of the couple's infertility. But it is not quite that simple. Even men with very low sperm counts can be quite fertile. In fact, 10 percent of fertile men coming to us for vasectomy have sperm counts that are very low (less than ten million per cc). Before explaining what really does constitute male infertility, I will first try to clarify what causes a low sperm count. I will debunk some of the myths regarding low sperm production and explain why, in most cases, treating the wife should not be neglected while the husband is subjected to years of worthless medication and surgery that gets the couple no closer to getting pregnant.

### *Function of the Testicles*

The testicle has two major functions: (1) to make the male hormone testosterone, which is responsible for the development of male sexual characteristics and behavior, and (2) to produce spermatozoa, or sperm, capable of fertilizing the female's egg. The testicle consists of several hundred seminiferous tubules, coiled microscopic tubules in which the sperm are manufactured. These tubules converge and collect into a delta (like the mouth of a river) near the upper part of the testicle. This delta (called the rete testis) then empties out of the testicle through a series of five to seven very small ducts (vasa efferentia) (see fig. 7.1). In between the microscopic seminiferous tubules, which manufacture the sperm, are clumps of Leydig cells, which make the male hormone testosterone. The testosterone-producing Leydig cells are yellow, just like the progesterone-secreting cells of the corpus luteum in the ovary after ovulation.

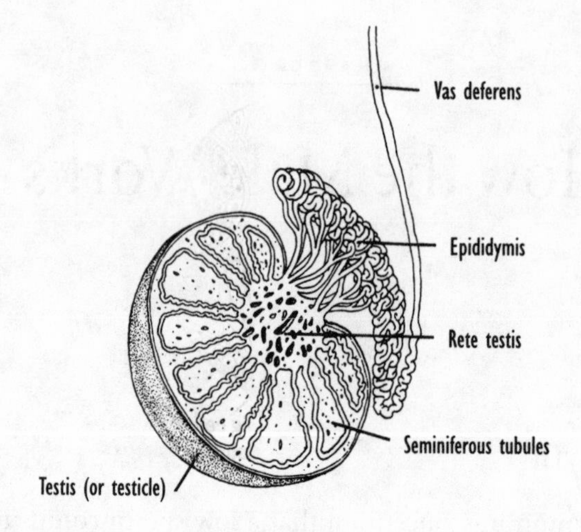


**FIGURE 7.1.** The testicle.

These Leydig cells appear to be sprinkled like pepper throughout the substance of the testicle (see fig. 7.2).

While sperm are carried out of the testicle into the vas deferens to be ejaculated at the time of orgasm, the male hormone manufactured by the Leydig cells is picked up by tiny veins coursing through the testicle, and distributed into the circulation. It is because the male hormone drains into the circulation this way, rather than via the seminiferous tubules and vas deferens, that a man can undergo a vasectomy without altering his hormone production or sexual drive.

Most men with very poor sperm production still make an adequate amount of testosterone. It is very difficult for any sort of illness or disease to interfere with adequate testosterone production. That is why so many men suffer from infertility yet have no lack of virility.

Both the production of testosterone and the production of sperm are regulated by hormones produced by the pituitary gland, which sits just underneath the brain. These pituitary hormones are in turn regulated by a releasing factor — GnRH — produced by the hypothalamus, the most primitive area of the brain. This is exactly the same GnRH that in the female permits the complex menstrual cycle to take place. This driving force from the brain acts no differently in the male than in the female, pulsing at ninety-minute intervals.

The brain then stimulates the pituitary gland to produce and release

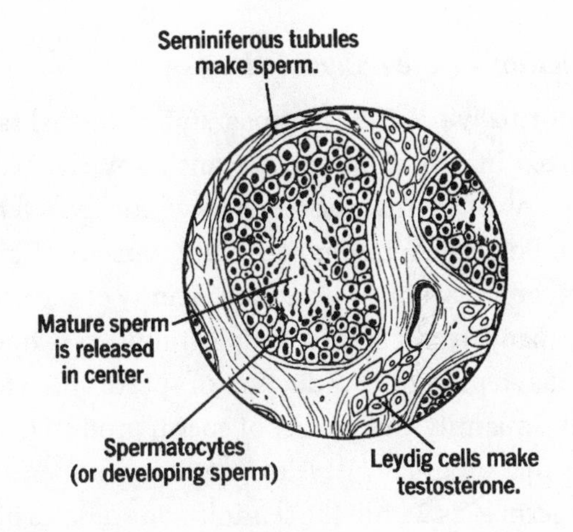


**FIGURE 7.2.** The sperm factory (testicle biopsy).

the follicle-stimulating hormone and luteinizing hormone, just as it does in the female. Without FSH and LH from the pituitary gland, and without GnRH from the brain, the testes in the male and the ovaries in the female would shrivel up and cease to function. The only reason for the constant production of FSH, LH, and testosterone in the male as opposed to the monthly cycle of ups and downs of FSH, LH, and estrogen plus progesterone in the female is that the ovary gives a different "feedback" message than the testicle.

In the male, FSH helps to stimulate and maintain proper sperm production, whereas LH stimulates and maintains production of testosterone. Increased testosterone in turn causes the pituitary gland to make less LH, and then testosterone production is in turn decreased. This feedback mechanism keeps the testosterone level in balance. That is why muscle builders who take steroids always have tiny testicles. The exogenous testosterone they are taking suppresses their pituitary secretion of LH, and so their testicles in turn stop functioning. Likewise, men who have severely damaged testicles (or who have no testicles at all) have extremely high circulating levels of LH and FSH. These pituitary hormones are responding to a deficiency in testicular production of sperm and testosterone in an effort to stir whatever testicular tissue still exists into working at its maximum possible capacity. Thus, when there are very few sperm or sperm precursors in the testicle, the FSH level is elevated.

### *Sperm Production — the Assembly Line*

The testicles normally produce sperm at a phenomenal rate, so that sperm are ejaculated in seemingly extravagant numbers. Think of the unbelievable sperm wastage that seems required for male fertility. Out of perhaps 200 million sperm inseminated with one act of intercourse, only four hundred ever reach the immediate vicinity of the egg. Because male fertility in many respects is a simple numbers game, we will describe the various steps in the production of sperm and what factors, if any, influence the quantity and quality of sperm produced.

All of the cells that eventually develop into normal sperm are called germ cells. These germ cells within the seminiferous tubules of the testes are lined up in an orderly array, with the most primitive early cells lying along the outer edge and the more developed sperm moving toward the center. All of these cells are held in place and nourished by a sort of formless nurturing cell (much like an amoeba) called the Sertoli cell. In fact, the developing sperm sits with its head imbedded within the nurturing Sertoli cell. In the final phase of sperm production, the sperm develops an oval head and a tail necessary for locomotion. The mature spermatozoon is then released from the Sertoli cell into the seminiferous tubule, and is swept along toward the efferent ducts to make its escape (along with millions of others) from the testicle.

The sperm are passed along from one stage of production to another at an absolutely unalterable speed of sixteen days for each stage. The sperm go through four and a half such stages of production. Thus, the total time required to produce every sperm is about seventy-two days. Neither sickness, testicular damage, nor hormonal manipulation can alter the inexorable rate at which the individual spermatozoa are produced. If one can imagine an automobile assembly line with a slow, steady, unstoppable movement from one stage to progressively more complex stages of production until the final car comes out for inspection, then one will have a pretty good understanding of how sperm are produced, and indeed how sloppy the results can often be. In humans, the architecture of this sperm factory is very chaotic compared with that of almost all other animals. In most animals, there is an orderly wave of sperm production that proceeds in a logical fashion across the seminiferous tubule. In humans, sperm production follows no wave at all and is very disordered, indicating just how reproductively fragile we are.

A deficiency in sperm production, causing a low sperm count, does not result from a slowing down of the speed at which the developing sperm proceed along the assembly line. This velocity cannot be changed. Rather, a deficiency in sperm production results from an inadequate number of the earliest precursors of sperm, or from interruption of some stage of sperm production. Interruption at some stage of sperm production is called spermatogenic arrest.

### *What Can Be Done to Stimulate Greater Sperm Production? Nothing!*

Although it is very easy to stimulate the female's ovary to produce large numbers of follicles by administering FSH, or a combination of FSH and LH (or even Clomid, which stimulates the pituitary to release greater amounts of FSH and LH), this same effort in men has failed miserably. This might seem difficult to understand, because we know that sperm production is completely dependent upon the secretion of FSH and LH from the pituitary gland. Why shouldn't we be able to drive the testicles to produce more sperm by increasing FSH, as in the female?

When a woman is given FSH to stimulate the release of more eggs, she is not really making more eggs. She has all the eggs she will ever have when she is born (with about 400,000 left when she is a teenager), and a thousand of those eggs die on their own every month until, by her forties, she completely runs out of them. The FSH in the first half of her menstrual cycle does not stimulate her to make eggs; it merely recruits eggs for ovulation out of the thousand that are programmed to die every month. It allows eggs to be retrieved that would otherwise have died during that month.

This is not what happens with the male. The male is constantly making sperm, as many as one hundred million per day, under the permissive action of FSH and LH. How many sperm the testicles make is determined by that particular testicle's genetic makeup. It cannot be increased by administering more FSH or LH.

There is a very rare condition called Kallman's syndrome, in which the man's pituitary gland does not make FSH or LH. In this case, his testicle is normal, but it makes no sperm and no testosterone because there is no pituitary FSH or LH to stimulate it. In these rare men, administering FSH and LH allows them to begin to make sperm normally, but it cannot increase their sperm production beyond what their testicle is genetically programmed to make. Almost all severely infertile men have normal or high pituitary FSH and LH levels anyway. Giving them more FSH or LH does nothing to increase their sperm production.

Men with low sperm production have an intrinsic testicular defect. Indeed, oligospermia (low sperm count) is a genetically transmitted problem found exclusively in monogamous species like ours because of the lack of sperm competition in our mating systems. As will be discussed in the chapters on genetics, we have localized major areas for controlling sperm production on the Y chromosome and are locating other such areas on the X chromosome. We now have direct DNA proof of what we had postulated more than fourteen years ago: that spermatogenesis is under direct genetic control, and that popular therapies designed to increase the quality and quantity of spermatogenesis are ineffective.

Over the past two decades, countless ineffective tests and treatments were foisted upon infertile men. Infertility specialists would treat male infertility with a variety of hormones, such as Clomid, FSH, HCG, testosterone, tamoxifen, and so on, with completely unsupported claims of success. When scrutinized carefully, all these claims were demonstrated to be invalid. Every kind of hormone treatment that was attempted in infertile men yielded no improvement in either sperm count or pregnancy rates when it was subjected to a proper controlled study. The same can be said of varicocelectomy. Very few infertile men who are referred to urologists ever escape this procedure, despite the fact that no beneficial effect from varicocelectomy has ever been demonstrated in properly controlled studies. Indeed, more than 15 percent of all fertile men on the face of the earth have a large varicocoele, and it is of no consequence.

One of the reasons that physicians have been fooled into erroneously thinking in the past that these various therapies for male infertility worked is a mathematical phenomenon called "regression toward the mean" (see fig. 7.3). Whenever there is a widely fluctuating variable, like the temperature in July, a below-average temperature is likely to go up in a few days, while an above-average temperature is likely to go down. Every fluctuating variable tends to gravitate toward a mean, or an average value. Since sperm counts can fluctuate wildly (depending on variable sperm transport efficiency from day to day), any patient whose first sperm count is very low is likely to have a higher sperm count later. Con-

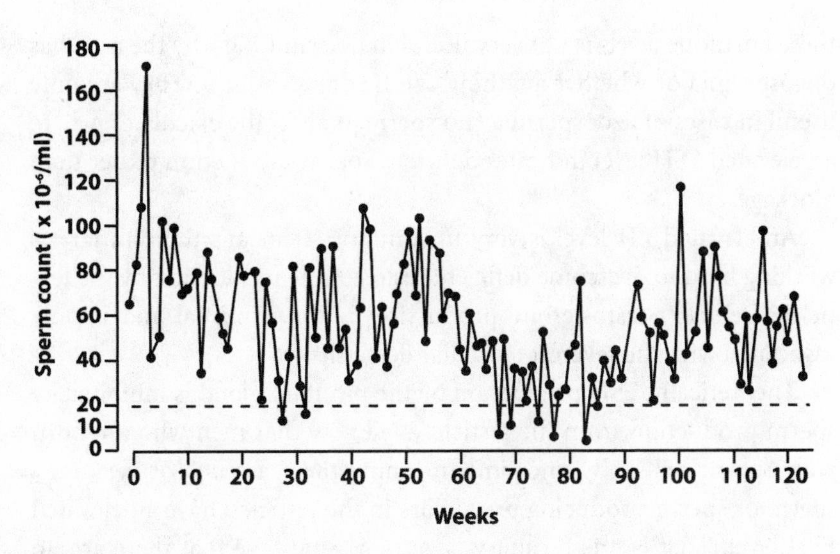


FIGURE 7.3

Variation of weekly sperm count over a two-year period in a single, normal male volunteer (WHO Manual, 1998).

versely, though rarely discussed, any patient whose first sperm count is very high is subsequently likely to have a lower sperm count. Thus, a clinician can easily be fooled into thinking that whatever foolish therapy he or she may be trying is effective. But if the clinician were to try that same therapy (in a controlled study) on men with very high initial sperm counts, he or she might be fooled into thinking the therapy was actually detrimental to sperm production.

A simple understanding of these concepts of sperm production should make the reader depressingly aware of how impossible it is to improve sperm count (or quality) in a man with oligospermia. Many infertile men have been treated in a haphazard and unscientific manner to improve their sperm count or fertility, and none of these regimens have any proven value. That is why the use of IVF and ICSI is much more likely to be effective than the hopeless effort of trying to improve sperm production.

### *Hormone Testing for Men*

If a man with low sperm count sees a urologist, he is certain to have his blood tested for FSH, LH, and testosterone, and in the majority of cases, these levels will be confusingly normal. Most of the time, checking these hormone levels is not very useful in determining why the man has oligospermia or whether anything can be done about it. They are only useful in cases of azoospermia (no sperm at all in the ejaculate), where an elevated FSH level indicates deficient sperm production rather than blockage.

An elevated LH level is very uncommon. It means the pituitary is working hard to overcome deficient testosterone production by the testicles. Deficient testosterone production is very unusual and is only associated with the severest testicular defects.

Theoretically, FSH production by the pituitary gland is inhibited by sperm production from the testicle. We know that men who are born with Sertoli cell–only syndrome, meaning there are no (or very few) sperm or sperm-producing precursors in the testicles, have an elevated FSH level. That is, the pituitary is getting a message that there are no sperm present in the testicles, and it is therefore secreting an excess amount of FSH. Thus, it would seem that if there is low sperm production because of a testicular defect, the FSH level should be high. But this is not always the case.

The fact that so many urologists do not understand this negative feedback system for FSH in the male causes lots of problems. An elevated FSH level does indicate severely deficient sperm production, but a normal FSH does not necessarily mean normal sperm production. Some physicians mistakenly assume that a man with azoospermia, i.e., no sperm in the ejaculate, and a normal FSH has obstruction. They figure that with a normal FSH level, the patient has to be making sperm. They assume that the sperm simply aren't getting into the ejaculate and that the patient must have an obstruction. Going on that erroneous assumption, they often operate on these men to try to correct this illusion of obstruction even though in reality there is no reason whatsoever to do so. The only proof of sperm production is a testicle biopsy, not the FSH level.

Here's why. In approximately half of infertile men with severe oligospermia, there is no deficiency in the total number of sperm-producing precursor cells in the testicle. The problem is with maturation of the sperm precursor (spermatocyte) into sperm. This is the point where meiosis, or reduction division, has to occur so that the sperm precursors with forty-six chromosomes can be transformed into sperm with only twenty-three chromosomes. Remember, this is the same process the egg must go through when the sperm penetrates it, in order to allow fertilization to occur. The number of chromosomes has to be reduced by half for normal fertilization to occur, and this process, called meiosis, is the most difficult part of sperm production (spermatogenesis).

FSH production by the pituitary is not regulated by the number of mature sperm produced by the testicles, but by the total number of sperm precursor cells present within the testicle, including the precursors that never get past the final stages of maturation into sperm. Thus, a man can have a very low sperm count and still have a completely normal FSH level.

## How Sperm Reach the Ejaculate

### *Leaving the Testicles*

There is a remarkable transport mechanism that allows the eager little sperm to exit from the male's genitals and get their crack at the egg. After the completed spermatozoa are released into the seminiferous tubule, they flow into the rete testis, which is like a river delta near the upper edge of the testicle. Sperm are pushed along the seminiferous tubule toward this exit point by contractions of very delicate muscle fibers. After they leave the testicles, sperm are transferred into an amazing structure called the epididymis.

The tiny epididymis is the most common site of blockage causing male sterility. To correct such blockage requires very delicate microsurgery (see fig. 7.1). The epididymis is a twenty-foot-long microscopic tube (1/300 of an inch in diameter) that runs back and forth in loops like a strand of spaghetti. Despite the twenty-foot length, the epididymis traverses a distance of only one and one-half inches. This convoluted microscopic tubule transfers sperm from the testicle into the vas deferens. With its multiple curves and convolutions, the epididymis appears to be many tubules, but it is actually just one very long tiny tubule.

Sperm are propelled along this highly contorted microscopic tunnel by frequent contractions of its thin muscular wall. When the sperm reach the end of the epididymis (the tail), they move up the vas deferens and await their call to be rushed through the vas deferens and ejaculated at the time of orgasm. Actually, very little sperm is stored in the epididymis in the human as compared with most other animals, in which the tail of the epididymis serves as a huge storage depot. Because human males lack this storage capacity in the epididymis, once they ejaculate there is very little sperm left in the next ejaculate until several days have passed.

### *What Happens to Sperm in the Epididymis?*

The epididymal tubule is not just a bridge between the testicle and the sperm duct. A remarkable process occurs here. Sperm that leave the testicle are only slightly motile and are not yet capable of fertilization. As they pass through the epididymis, they obtain their ability to move in a straightforward direction with sufficient velocity to fertilize the female egg. Sperm that were completely unable to fertilize an egg become fertile during this twenty-foot-long journey. None of the sperm located in the earliest regions of the epididymis just after their exit from the testicle are capable of fertilization. Sperm inside the testicle can only vibrate their tails weakly and barely wiggle around. Sperm from the beginning regions of the epididymis can swim, but only in circles. During this seemingly endless journey through the winding turns of the epididymis, the sperm mature their structure, develop their incredible unidirectional swimming ability, and attain the ability to fertilize.

Sperm remain fresh and alive in the epididymis and vas deferens for less than a month. If a sperm has to sit around for more than a month waiting to be ejaculated, it will be of no use. This does not mean that the man who has intercourse only once a month will not have fertile sperm. There are still fresh sperm arriving every day that upon ejaculation will be capable of fertilization. However, a man who ejaculates only once a month will have a much higher percentage of dead, ineffectual sperm in his ejaculate, despite having a higher overall number of sperm stored up. Furthermore, sperm storage in the human is so poor that saving up for such a prolonged period of time is of little help in raising the sperm count.

### *The Ejaculate*

Most of the fluid in the ejaculate does not come from the testicle, the epididymis, or the sperm duct. That is why vasectomy results in the absence of sperm with no noticeable change in the volume of ejaculate. During sexual intercourse, most of the fluid that pushes the sperm out comes from the seminal vesicles and the prostate gland (see fig. 7.4). The seminal vesicles, located behind the bladder, expel their fluid very force-

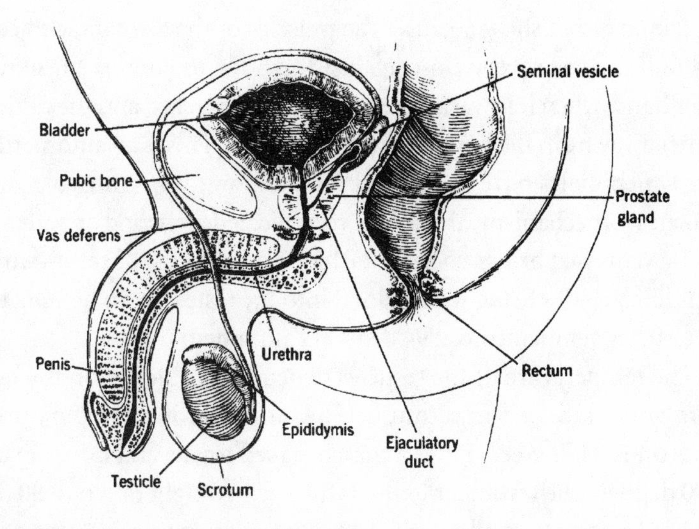


**FIGURE 7.4.** Male reproductive organs (side view).

fully behind the sperm, pushing it into the urethra. The first portion of the ejaculate thus contains most of the sperm. The second portion is from the seminal vesicles, which contract violently and account for most of the ejaculatory fluid. At this time, the internal sphincter of the bladder clamps down powerfully to prevent the semen from accidentally going backward into the bladder. It also prevents urine from leaking forward out of the bladder. The external sphincter, which sits just in front of the ejaculatory duct, then opens up and allows the ejaculate to enter the bulbous urethra, the holding area just near the base of the penis. Finally, the very powerful muscles around the bulbous urethra contract and squirt the ejaculate out of the penis with remarkable force. This highly coordinated symphony of complicated muscular contractions that propel the sperm from the epididymis all the way up through the abdomen and out the penis is what the male subjectively feels as orgasm.

### *Testicular Temperature*

The testicles are located basically outside the body because they do not function properly at body temperature. The testes must remain at a temperature about four degrees lower than the usual 98.6 degrees Fahrenheit maintained in the rest of the body. The testicles are so sensitive to these four degrees of extra heat that if they were inside the body they would not be able to produce sperm at all.

Taking a cold shower causes the muscles of the scrotal sac to contract and pull the testes very close against the body to conserve heat. On the other hand, when it is warm, the scrotal muscles relax, and the testicles fall farther away from the body in order to cool off. This is an automatic reflex over which males have no control. In addition to this muscular thermal regulatory mechanism, there is a complicated network of radiator-like coiling veins that brings cool scrotal blood away from the testes, while surrounding arteries bring warm blood into the testes, again helping to keep the testicles' temperature at 94 degrees Fahrenheit.

The temperature of the testicles depends completely on the temperature surrounding the scrotum. The usual scrotal temperature with pants on is 94 degrees. But if a man is naked for several hours in a room at 70 degrees, the testicular temperature will go right down to 80 degrees or less. The scrotum allows the testicles to adjust to almost any outside temperature without the insulation from temperature change that the body of warm-blooded animals normally provides. In that sense, our testicles are no different from cold-blooded creatures like snakes or fish. In a sense, the testicle is a cold-blooded animal.

Traditionally, men have been advised to avoid tight underwear, hot baths, and steam rooms. Unfortunately, not a single good scientific study has been performed on either normal men or infertile couples to see whether in a controlled, disciplined fashion these kinds of habits can have any impact on sperm count. Whether a man wears boxer shorts or briefs has hardly any effect on scrotal temperature. Basically, as long as underwear or pants are worn, the average scrotal temperature is going to be around 94 degrees to 95 degrees. In the absence of hard data, it is nonetheless still reasonable advice to avoid prolonged hot tubs, steam baths, excessively tight underwear, or anything that might conceivably raise the testicular temperature.

## Sperm Count

There are immense errors and great misinterpretations of the meaning of the simple sperm count. Because of the many pitfalls in interpreting the sperm count, many useless ancillary diagnostic tests are available at andrology clinics. These tests include sperm antibody titers, hamster egg penetration tests, cervical mucus penetration tests, computerized sperm motion analyses, acrosome reaction assays, hormone stimulation tests, electron microscopy, sperm DNA fragmentation, and so on. Various combinations and adaptations of these tests have proliferated in an attempt to crack through the enigma of the male infertility dilemma. These tests are costly, and now, in retrospect, we realize that they have yielded very little useful information. The single best method of determining to what degree the male partner is contributing to the couple's barrenness is still the cheap, old-fashioned semen analysis, or sperm count.

To what extent does the semen analysis actually reflect the male's infertility? In truth, when a couple has been unable to achieve pregnancy over a certain period of time, all we really know is that the couple is infertile. It had been thought in the past that sperm concentrations of under twenty million per cc indicated male infertility. But 11 percent of men with proven fertility (those seeing us for a vasectomy) have been found to have sperm counts below ten million per cc. Low sperm counts (like high sperm counts) may simply occur at the ends of the bell-shaped population curve, and may not necessarily be related to infertility in the couple. It is, therefore, essential to be cautious when suggesting to any infertile couple with a poor sperm count that the husband is infertile. A low sperm count is associated with decreased fertility based on a large statistical population, but it may not be an indication of infertility for that particular male with that particular female. Even if her partner's sperm count is extremely low, a woman may become pregnant without resorting to high-tech treatment. But the higher the sperm count, the greater the chance of pregnancy, and the lower the sperm count, the more likely it is that the man is infertile.

The semen analysis evaluates the number of sperm, the degree of movement of the sperm (motility), and the shape of the sperm (morphology). There have been hundreds of studies attempting to correlate deficiencies in any of these three modalities with the fertilization or pregnancy rates in infertile couples. This test, with all of its faults, is still the most commonly used method for determining to what extent the male's infertility may be contributing to the infertility of the couple (short of actually going through an IVF cycle). We will now spend a little time explaining in detail the process of obtaining and interpreting the sperm count.

### *What Are Sperm?*

Semen is the fluid ejaculated at the time of orgasm, and it may or may not contain sperm. Sperm (or spermatozoa) are microscopic creatures that look like tadpoles swimming about at a frantic pace back and forth

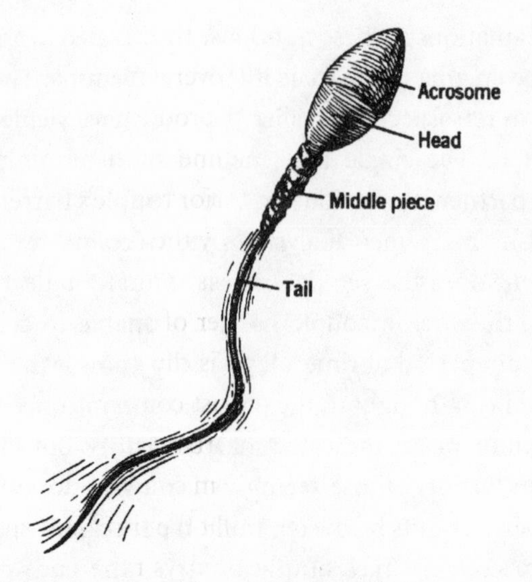


**FIGURE 7.5.** The basic structure of a normal sperm.

in the semen. Each sperm consists of a head, which contains all of the genetic material (DNA) of the father-to-be, and a tail, which lashes back and forth at an incredible speed to propel the sperm along (see fig. 7.5). In the ejaculate of a fertile man there are hundreds of millions of sperm, and they usually move quite rapidly.

Upon first observation of sperm under the microscope, I can't help being awestruck by the massive numbers and by the rapid, gyrating pace of their movement. Perhaps more subtle and important than the apparent frenzy of activity is the purposefulness of the movements. Despite the fact that they are all going in different directions (and so their motion appears to be haphazard and random), each one moves in a straight line with the accuracy of a guided missile. In a normal specimen, each sperm observed under a microscope goes straight across the field without stopping, turning around, or going in a pointless circle, and with no deviation from what appears to be a straight line. It is only the massive number of these sperm all mixed together and each going in different straight lines that superficially makes the motion appear aimless.

### *Does Saving It Up Help?*

No matter how accurately the laboratory does the sperm count and no matter how carefully and consistently the specimen is collected by the patient, there will be huge variations caused by sperm transport fluctuations. Because of these variations, the sperm count should be repeated many times over the course of several months. That is the only way to get a reliable estimate of sperm production. Since intercourse will temporarily deplete the male of some sperm, it is important to abstain from intercourse for a few days prior to collecting the specimen. Otherwise, a low value will be reported by the laboratory, and the husband may mistakenly conclude that he is infertile even though prior counts may have had a very large number of sperm. When the couple have had intercourse the night before, this can reduce the sperm count to one third of its normal level. Since most couples seem to have intercourse two to three times a week, it has arbitrarily been felt that two to three days of abstinence prior to the sperm count will accurately reflect how much sperm is delivered to the wife at the time of intercourse.

Abstaining for more than four or five days rarely results in any significant increase in the sperm count. The reason for this is that in humans there is very little sperm storage in the epididymis. The tail of the epididymis in most animals is a storage depot for huge quantities of sperm. That allows repetitive ejaculations to contain large numbers of sperm. In the human, however, sperm transport through the epididymis is very rapid, and sperm storage is very poor. Therefore, saving it up for long periods does very little good.

In most men, the majority of sperm come out in the early portion of the ejaculate. Subsequent squirts usually contain very few sperm. Thus, if one were having a difficult time getting the specimen bottle into the proper position and spilled an early portion of the ejaculate, the sperm count might turn out to be falsely low. Therefore, to obtain an accurate count, the patient should use a wide-mouthed collection jar, and collect all of the ejaculate into one specimen container. Collection in a condom during intercourse is also unacceptable because most condoms will harm the sperm. Once obtained, the semen should be examined promptly. If the analysis of the specimen is delayed more than two hours, a large proportion of otherwise fertile sperm may have died off or lost a good deal of their motility.

### *How Many Sperm?*

The number of sperm in the ejaculate is determined by looking at a tiny but measured portion of it in a counting chamber under a microscope. Nowadays, many large laboratories are using computerized sperm counting. This saves time and salaries, and makes semen analysis very profitable for a lab. Unfortunately, these computerized methods are woefully inaccurate, especially with very low sperm counts where accuracy is most needed. I completely disapprove of such moneymaking but misleading methods.

### *Motility of the Sperm*

More important than the quantity of sperm are their activity and quality. After the specimen has been counted, the lab will determine the percentage of sperm seen in any microscopic field that are actually moving and the percentage that are not moving. There will always be a certain number of nonmotile (nonmoving) sperm, which are incapable of fertilization, in the ejaculate. Only the moving sperm are able to enter the cervical mucus and ultimately reach and penetrate the egg. After the percent motility is determined, the quality of that motion is observed.

There are four types of sperm movement. *Grade 1* motility means that the sperm are only wiggling sluggishly in place and making very little, if any, forward progression. These are pathetic vibratory-type motions that get the sperm nowhere. Such sperm are usually incapable of fertilizing the egg. *Grade 2* motility means that the sperm are moving forward, but either the speed is very slow or they veer off on a curve instead of moving in a straight line. Such sperm are unlikely to make it in the ferocious arena of the female genital tract. *Grade 3* sperm are able to move at a reasonable speed with straightforward progress. *Grade 4* sperm advance straight ahead as well, but at an extraordinarily rapid speed. Grade 3 and grade 4 sperm are usually capable of fertilization. Grade 1 and grade 2 sperm generally are not.

The average velocity of a grade 3 sperm is about twenty-five microns (a micron equals 1/1,000 of a millimeter) per second. That can best be understood by realizing that the average sperm head is about six microns long, and an entire sperm is a total of about twenty-five microns in length from the front of its head to the tip of its tail. That means the sperm head normally travels forward about four times its own length every second. This may seem fast, and it may swell our male ego to think we have within us creatures that can perform such a feat. But in truth we are relatively pathetic compared with other animals. Horse sperm routinely swim at about three times that speed, and bull sperm finish the race before we even leave the starting gate.

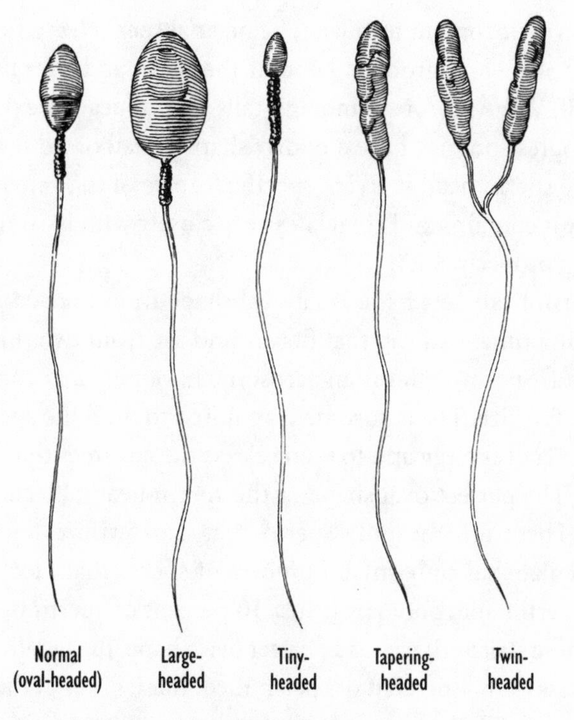


**FIGURE 7.6.** Normal and abnormal morphology of sperm.

### *The Shape (Morphology) of the Sperm*

As important as the motility is the microscopic examination for morphology, or shape, of the sperm. Even in a normal human specimen, as many as 40 percent of the spermatozoa may have abnormal morphology (see fig. 7.6). In this respect, we are pitiful as a species in comparison with most other animals, in which virtually every single sperm has a perfect structure.

There is no relationship between abnormal sperm and abnormal pregnancy. Abnormally shaped sperm simply cannot fertilize the egg. The normal sperm has an oval head with a long tail. Abnormally shaped sperm may have either a very large, round head, or an extremely small, pinpoint head. They may even have two heads. The sperm may be bent at the neck and misshapen, and the tails may have kinks and curls in them. None of these odd-looking sperm (which are present in large numbers even in a normal ejaculate) correlate with any genetic problem in the offspring.

Morphology is at least as important as motility in indicating whether spermatozoa can fertilize. The normal sperm has a head with a perfect oval shape, no crooked bend at the neck, and a straight, long, tapering tail. Very vigorously moving tails that appear to exhibit good forward progression may have a poorly shaped head or none at all. The shape of the sperm head is a very specific feature of the genetic folding of the DNA it contains and correlates very closely with its ability to fertilize the egg properly.

The sperm head gets its normal oval shape from the acrosome, the enzyme-containing warhead that fits around the front two thirds of the sperm's head. Sperm without an acrosome have perfectly round heads and cannot fertilize. The acrosome is required to bind the sperm to the zona pellucida of the egg and to then release the enzymes that cut a hole through it. The perfect oval shape of the sperm head reflects a normal acrosome. These are the only sperm that can fertilize the egg. The human ejaculate has only small numbers of sperm that meet the strict criteria for fertile morphology. If just 10 percent of sperm in an ejaculate meet these strict criteria of a perfect oval shape, the fertilization rate is good. If less than 4 percent of sperm meet these criteria, the fertilization rate is poor. Thus, you need very few normally structured sperm to accomplish fertilization.

### *The Semen*

Most men ejaculate a half a teaspoon to one full teaspoon of semen (2.5 cc to 5 cc), quite a bit less than the full pint that a pig ejaculates. The volume of ejaculate does not indicate the amount of sperm being produced. There are some men who have very low ejaculate volumes of less than a fifth of a teaspoon, but they may have a very high concentration of sperm in that low volume. On the other hand, some men may have a very high volume of ejaculate (and think that they are making a lot of sperm) but have a relatively low sperm concentration.

If the ejaculate volume is less than one cc (one fifth of a teaspoon) and there are no sperm, it could mean ejaculatory duct blockage or congenital absence of the vas deferens, a relatively common cause of obstructive sterility in men (which we can treat today but was considered hopeless only a few years ago). If there is a low volume of ejaculate with sperm present, it is a sign of prostate problems, or it may simply indicate a relatively high frequency of intercourse.

In certain cases there may be no ejaculate whatsoever because all of

the patient's sperm and seminal fluid are being ejaculated bac
the bladder rather than forward out of the penis. This retrogr
lation is a condition caused by diabetes or by past surgery. In
certain patients on medication to control high blood pressure may have backward ejaculation of sperm into the bladder as a side effect. Such a man may mistakenly believe that he is making no sperm at all, but in truth he may be making large amounts; they are simply not getting out. Except in these instances, the diagnosis of retrograde ejaculation is overdone, and usually wrong.

Within a minute of ejaculation, the semen should coagulate into a tapioca-like gel. The sperm cannot be adequately counted or examined while the semen is in this coagulated blob. The main function of this blob is to prevent early leakage of sperm out of the vagina. Within ten to thirty minutes after ejaculation, the specimen should again liquefy.

The semen's alkalinity protects against the harsh, acid environment in the vagina that would otherwise quickly kill the sperm. The early gelatin-like blob of semen prevents early leakage out of the vagina, and the sugar in the semen provides instant energy for locomotion. However, the fluid of the ejaculate is not really designed to keep the sperm alive for very long, only to get them on their way as quickly as possible into the cervical mucus. Sperm that don't make it into the cervical mucus quickly will find after several hours that the ejaculatory fluid is actually a very hostile environment also.

## How Many Sperm Are Necessary for a Man to Be Fertile?

For years doctors assumed that if a man had a sperm count below a certain arbitrary minimum, he was infertile, and that a couple's failure to achieve pregnancy was caused by this male factor. As recently as twenty-five years ago it was thought that a sperm count of under forty million per cc meant the husband was infertile, and urologists actually gave such couples a very poor prognosis for pregnancy. If the wife did become pregnant, the pregnancy was ascribed to whatever useless treatment was being administered to the supposedly infertile husband. We now know that men with very low sperm counts (even less than two million per cc) can impregnate their wives, and that the semen analysis and sperm count can often be misleading.

In many infertile couples in which the husband's sperm count is low, female factors also exist that prevent conception. If the wife were very fertile, she might have become pregnant despite her husband's low sperm count. As far back as 1987, Dr. Rebecca Sokol reported the case of a woman who got pregnant despite the fact that her husband's sperm count was less than fifty thousand per cc and that less than 10 percent of those few sperm were alive. Reviewers were skeptical because this sperm count was so extremely low. However, after the baby was born, careful genetic tissue-typing and blood-typing of mother, father, and baby determined with 99.9 percent certainty that the husband indeed was genetically the father, despite having a count so low that natural conception would seem beyond belief. We have found that if the wife is not over thirty years of age, 5 percent of men with such disastrously low sperm counts eventually father a child without any treatment at all. So, what is "male infertility" and how many sperm are really necessary for a man to be fertile?

Studies done in the late 1970s by Dr. Emil Steinberger's group in Texas revealed that when the sperm count was less than ten million per cc, 30 percent of couples got pregnant without the aid of IVF (which didn't even exist then). But when the sperm count was over forty million per cc, 60 percent eventually got pregnant (see table 7.1). Thus, a very low sperm count is compatible with fertility — the pregnancy rate is simply lower.

**TABLE 7.1**

**Relationship of Sperm Count to Pregnancy Rate among Infertile Couples**

| MOTILE SPERM COUNT (millions per cc) | PREGNANCY RATE (percent) |
|---|---|
| Less than 5.0 | 27.8 |
| 5–10.0 | 33.3 |
| 10–20.0 | 52.9 |
| 20–40.0 | 57.1 |
| 40–60.0 | 60.0 |
| 60–100.0 | 62.5 |
| Over 100 | 70.0 |

The best understanding of the sperm count comes from Dr. Robert Schoysman's study in Brussels (also from the late 1970s) of more than one thousand men with low sperm counts whose wives were awaiting insemination with donor sperm (see table 7.2). At the time of his study, Dr. Schoysman had one of the few large donor-sperm insemination programs in Europe. So at that time, couples in which the husband had either no sperm or a very low sperm count often had to wait for many years before being able to be inseminated with donor sperm. Some of these wives became pregnant before their turn came to undergo donor insemination, and this gave a very clear picture of what the chances would be for a woman whose husband was extremely oligospermic to get pregnant with no treatment whatsoever over a period of time. The wife underwent no treatment because it was assumed to be strictly the "husband's fault." Even when the sperm count was less than one million per cc (as low as 100,000 per cc), there was almost a 4 percent chance of pregnancy occurring with no treatment within five years and close to a 10 percent chance of pregnancy occurring in twelve years. When the sperm count was in the range of ten to twenty million per cc (still considered a low count), more than 50 percent of the patients became pregnant within five years despite receiving no treatment.

**TABLE 7.2**

## 1,327 Oligospermic Men

| MOTILE SPERM COUNT | PREGNANCY RATE | |
|---|---|---|
| | *5 Years* | *12 Years* |
| (millions per cc) | (percent) | (percent) |
| 0.1–1 | 3.9 | 8.7 |
| 1.1–5 | 11.9 | 26.6 |
| 5.1–10 | 22.1 | 34.3 |
| 10.1–15 | 45.0 | 58.5 |
| 15.1–20 | 68.6 | 82.0 |

The pregnancy rate increased as the sperm count increased. Therefore, male infertility is a relative rather than absolute problem. In 1984 Australians Dr. Gordon Baker, Dr. David de Kretser, and Dr. Henry Burger, from Melbourne, made somewhat similar findings when the wife was treated and the husband's sperm count was low. They compiled an elegant graph comparing the pregnancy rate per month among infertile couples with varying sperm counts in the husband and com-

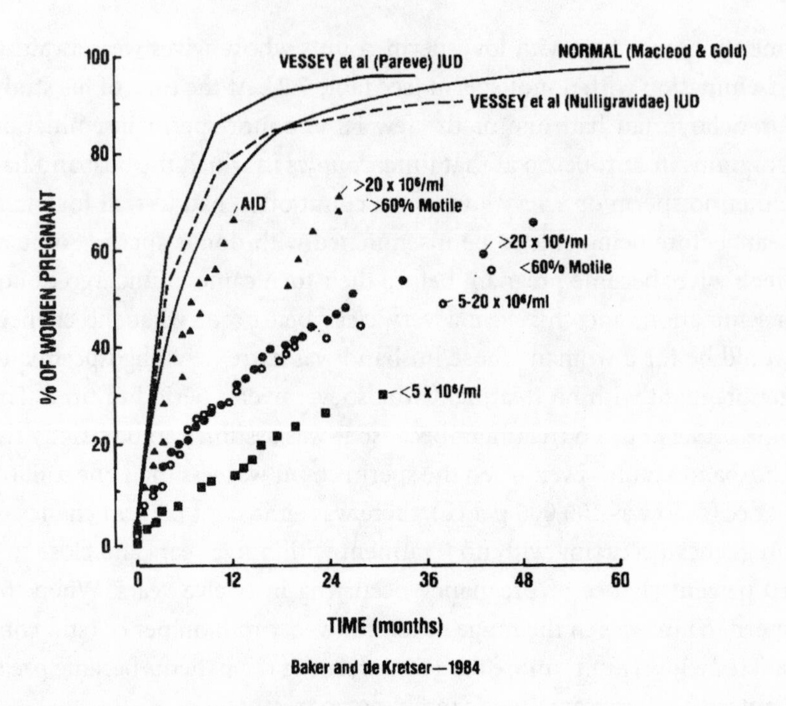


**FIGURE 7.7.** Cumulative and lifetable pregnancy rates.

pared it to the pregnancy rate per month of normal fertile couples (see fig. 7.7).

By a year and a half, normal fertile couples that discontinued contraception had about a 92 percent chance of getting pregnant (Vessey and normal curves). Azoospermic couples undergoing insemination with normal donor sperm (artificial insemination by donor, or AID) had a slightly lower but very similar pregnancy rate to that of normal couples. For infertile couples who had sperm counts of higher than twenty million per cc and greater than 60 percent motility, the pregnancy rate at eighteen months was about 60 percent, considerably less than that of normal couples or couples undergoing donor insemination with normal donor sperm. Couples with greater than twenty million sperm per cc but less than 60 percent motility had a 40 percent chance of pregnancy at eighteen months, and couples with between five and twenty million sperm per cc had a similarly depressed rate of pregnancy of 40 percent at eighteen months. Finally, couples with sperm counts of less than five million per cc had only about a 22 percent chance of pregnancy at a year and a half. Similar studies from Europe showed that pregnancy rate was adversely affected only when sperm counts were below five million per cc. Our thirty-year studies of pregnancy rate in otherwise fertile women whose husbands underwent vasectomy reversal also shows little benefit to having a sperm count greater than five million per cc. A low sperm count does not mean the couple is infertile and can't get pregnant. It just means that it is more difficult for them to get pregnant, particularly if there is a female problem as well.

### *The Hamster Test and Other Wastes of Time and Money*

Scientists have always been fascinated by the fact that fertilization of an egg by sperm is always species specific, meaning that a dog's sperm cannot fertilize a cow's egg, and a human sperm certainly can't fertilize a rat or hamster egg. In the early 1970s, efforts were made to find out what it is that makes it impossible for the sperm of one species to penetrate or fertilize the egg of another species, and this research was used to develop one of the many worthless tests for determining sperm fertilizing capacity. Many patients have spent huge amounts of money on this and other useless male fertility tests.

In nature there are certain types of crossbreeding that work. For example, the domestic bull can mate with a North American buffalo and produce a hybrid called a cattalo, which is a fertile animal that can breed more cattalos. A polar bear will readily mate with a brown bear. Lions will readily mate with tigers, producing an animal called a liger, which is also fertile and can produce more of its kind. The donkey and the horse have perhaps become the most famous crossbred species, resulting in a mule, an animal that carries the stronger attributes of both animals but is sterile and unable to produce more mules. The zebra can also mate with a horse or a donkey, producing a zebhorse, a sort of zebra-stallion that looks like a horse with stripes, or a zebdonkey, which looks like a donkey with stripes. But these animals, like the mule, are sterile and cannot reproduce. Ram sperm seems to successfully fertilize goats, but the resulting embryo invariably dies after the second month of pregnancy. Although very closely related species thus can crossbreed and sometimes produce a new and even fertile species, it is impossible for sperm to fertilize the egg of a distantly related species.

However, if the tough outer layer of the egg (called the zona pellucida) is removed (i.e., the egg is denuded of its outer protective layer), then sperm from any species can penetrate and, therefore, theoretically fertilize the egg of any other species. In fact, sperm from fertile humans can indeed penetrate such a denuded hamster egg. Removing that shell allows the sperm of a human to penetrate the egg of a hamster and initiate what appears to be the very first stages of fertilization. But in truth fertilization cannot possibly occur.

In an effort to improve upon the prognostic limitations of the sperm count, the interesting ability of human sperm to penetrate a denuded hamster egg was turned into the so-called hamster test of sperm function. It was postulated that if a man's sperm can penetrate the denuded hamster egg, then he was supposedly fertile. But instead of clarifying the man's fertility, it turned out to be a huge waste of money, and even had disastrous consequences for gullible patients. It really is worthless, and no credence whatsoever should be placed upon it. The same is true for sperm antibodies and most other andrological tests.

Professor Eberhard Nieschlag from the Max Planck Clinical Research Unit for Reproductive Medicine in Münster, Germany, carefully studied the hamster test in fertile and infertile men, comparing it to information obtained with semen analysis to find out whether the expensive hamster test added any information to what the routine, inexpensive semen analysis could provide. He discovered that although the hamster test correlates with the degree of male fertility, the sperm count also correlates with the degree of male infertility — the hamster test did not yield any additional information. This has been true of all the "new" tests of male infertility that have come and gone over the years.

A case from several years ago demonstrates just how emotionally misleading the shaky information from such tests can be. A thirty-four-year-old couple came to see me after having tried for several years to get pregnant following a vasectomy reversal. They asked that I redo the vasectomy reversal operation because they had been told elsewhere that a negative hamster test showed that the husband's sperm was unable to fertilize. The woman was a busy, hardworking lawyer under great stress who insisted that she was ovulating normally. She felt there was "overwhelming evidence" that the problem was with her husband, and she insisted that I operate on him to make his sperm better. She then explained that she was told by other doctors to consider only insemination with donor sperm because of the negative hamster test. When I suggested that her husband's sperm was okay, she simply got up and stormed out of the office, and her husband dutifully followed. More than a year later, I received an apology from them because she had gotten pregnant with her husband's sperm and delivered a healthy child.

I have no doubt that much of what I say in this chapter, and indeed in this book, will stir some anger and resentment. Most books written on this subject are designed in "handbook" format and take no particular stand on any issue; they just give lists of clinics, tests, and things to do. What I am trying to do in this book is distill all of the conflicting information, the garbage and the quality work, and give to you, the reader, not the confusion and the murky chaos of controversies, but rather the essence of what really works and what doesn't work so that you can avoid the pain and agony this last patient had to endure until her story finally ended happily.

### *Whose Fault Is It, the Husband's or the Wife's?*

If the husband has no sperm at all in the ejaculate (azoospermia), then that is the obvious cause of the couple's infertility. If the wife's tubes are blocked, then that is the obvious cause of the couple's infertility. In such cases, it is easy to say whether it is the male or the female who is "at fault." But these conditions represent only a minority of the millions of couples in this country who are infertile. It used to be said that 40 percent of infertility problems were caused by the male, 40 percent by the female, and 20 percent by a combination of problems in both. The cause of male infertility would then be broken down into such factors as varicocele, infection, obstruction, immunologic, and so on. The female would have a similarly detailed range of diagnoses. However, we now know that a clear diagnosis pinpointing the cause of infertility can only be made in a small number of cases.

In the majority of cases, it is really quite impossible to state for sure whether the husband or the wife is the cause of the problem. Consider, for example, Mr. S., from Texas, who underwent microsurgery to unblock his sperm ducts. One and a half years after surgery, although Mr. S. now had sperm in the ejaculate, the number of sperm was extremely low (only seven hundred thousand per cc), and the wife had still not gotten pregnant. The assumption was that although the microsurgery went beautifully and all the sperm that he was making was reaching the ejaculate, the amount of sperm production was just too low to realistically expect his wife to have much of a chance of getting pregnant. After several more months of agonizing over the dilemma,

Mr. S. and his wife decided to have artificial insemination with donor sperm in Texas. The wife was placed on Clomid to time her irregular ovulation so that they could drive from their small town to the medical center on the day before she was expected to ovulate in order to have the donor insemination. During the first month this was planned, they could not make the trip because of a huge hurricane sweeping the area. They planned to try again the next month. But she didn't get her period, and they figured she was getting so tense and nervous that it was affecting her menstrual cycle. In fact she was pregnant, having conceived through natural intercourse with her husband during that hurricane that kept them from traveling to undergo insemination with donor sperm. Subsequently, this couple has had several more children without any difficulty at all, despite a very low sperm count. In fact, treating the wife with Clomid was all that was necessary for them to have children.

### *The Tragedy of Not Treating the Whole Couple*

The biggest tragedy among couples where "male infertility" is involved is that treatment of the couple is delayed, sometimes for years, while the urologist is going through countless unnecessary tests and futile treatment programs to try to raise the husband's sperm count.

To concentrate strictly on trying to improve the man's sperm count is exactly the wrong way to deal with male-factor infertility in a couple trying to have a baby. The cases in my records over the last thirty years in which patients have gone through unnecessary and ineffective treatment of the husband while completely disregarding the problem of the wife are too numerous to adequately cover. One patient who came to see me had a sperm count of fourteen million per cc, 70 percent excellent motility, and good forward progression and morphology. However, his wife had never had regular periods and had literally never ovulated. Yet her gynecologist told her it was strictly her husband's problem because his sperm count was "low." The gynecologist sent her husband to a urologist who was only too happy to perform a varicocelectomy for a "small" varicocele, which, in truth I am certain was not a varicocele at all. At the time they were seeing me for a second opinion, they had even been advised to have artificial insemination with donor sperm. Yet when we treated her ovulatory problem, she became pregnant quite easily with her husband's sperm without ever having to go through donor sperm insemination.

One of the most shocking cases I've ever seen was a man with ninety million sperm per cc, 85 percent excellent morphology, and progressively forward motility whose wife always had irregular periods lasting forty to sixty days and clearly had never ovulated in her life. Yet the local urologist started the husband on testosterone, telling him that the hormone would improve his fertility. Of course, the testosterone might have made his muscles get bigger (the reason many athletes illegally use it), but it certainly lowered his sperm count drastically. Going off this ridiculous steroid treatment brought his sperm count back up to normal.

Just as tragic is the failure to recognize the male's infertility. Twenty-five years ago, the female partner was always blamed for the couple's infertility. In my previous book, I gave the humorous account of a rather enormous, macho football player who came in to see me with his meek, accepting wife. He looked as if he was going to tear me apart when I told him that his low sperm count could be contributing to their infertility. He leaned forward with a stare of anger and disbelief, saying, "What do you mean, my sperm ain't okay?" After I assured him that his masculinity was not a problem, he calmed down a little bit, but he proceeded to blame his wife for feeding him too much fish and vegetables and not enough meat. He was sure that was the reason for his sperm count problem, which must assuredly be her fault rather than his.

That episode occurred at a time when no one really wanted to take a serious look at the male causes of infertility and always assumed, in the sexist society we lived in then, that it was the female's fault. As you may recall, Anne Boleyn, the mother of Queen Elizabeth I, had her head chopped off by the king because she kept giving birth to only girls. Little did he know that the problem was simply that his Y sperm (which would have led to conception of a boy) never fertilized her eggs — only his X sperm did. It was truly his sperm that were misbehaving, not her eggs.

## The Varicocele Myth

If a man is sent to a urologist because of a low sperm count, he is very likely to receive a diagnosis of varicocele. A varicocele is a varicose vein of the testicle normally found in 15 to 20 percent of all men. That is, 15 to 20 percent of all males on this planet have a varicose vein of the testicle, and it is almost always on the left side. The reason for this is that the testicular vein draining blood back from the testicle on the right side drains directly into the major vein of the body, the vena cava, but on the left side the testicular vein drains into the kidney's vein. This type of anatomy on the left is much more likely to lead to a defect in the valves that normally prevent blood from flowing back down the veins because of the effect of gravity when one stands up. A varicose vein of the testicle is no different from a varicose vein in the leg. When you are lying down, you notice nothing abnormal. However, when you stand up, blood (which would normally be prevented from flowing backward by valves) will fill up and dilate these veins so that they become readily apparent under the skin, even to the naked eye.

The standard urological line is that varicocele is "the commonest cause of male infertility." This is a complete myth. As far back as 1952, an English doctor by the name of Tulloch performed a varicocelectomy operation on a single man with no sperm in the ejaculate, and then reported that within six months he was producing sperm and fathered a child. That single report was picked up with incredible enthusiasm in this country in the late 1960s. It has been alleged that as many as 40 percent of infertile men have a varicocele. In fact, there are some urologists who find a varicocele in almost every infertile male they see. The literature on varicoceles and the operation to repair them for infertility is bewildering in volume and replete with apocryphal success stories.

More than 15 percent of the world's fertile men have a large varicocele and suffer no apparent harm. Why should a problem on the left side cause an underproduction of sperm on both sides? I will never forget a meeting of the American Urological Association in the late 1970s, a time when everyone was gloating over the remarkable success of varicocelectomy in curing male infertility, when Dr. Ruben Gittes got up in front of several thousand urologists and stunned them with a simple statement: "I see no evidence that there is any relationship between the presence of a varicocele and male infertility."

Dr. Gittes was one of the most scientifically disciplined and clinically astute urologists I have ever known. At that time he was a professor of urology at the Peter Bent Brigham Hospital at Harvard and chairman of its urology department. He then became the head of the Scripps Research Institute in San Diego, California. His major interest in urology did not revolve around male infertility, but his brilliance in any urological area he studied was recognized by all. After the momentary shock of his comment, the pro-varicocelectomy forces marshaled their strength and vehemently argued that "years of clinical experience have demonstrated the effect of varicocele on depressing sperm production and the success of varicocelectomy in curing male infertility." As it turns out, they were wrong, and Dr. Gittes was correct.

The enthusiasm for varicocelectomy continued to grow to extremes in the early 1980s. Some urologists in Europe recommended that every postpubertal boy be examined for a varicocele, and if he had one, that it should be operated on at an early age, before it had time to hurt his sperm production. This would mean an automatic operation for at least 15 percent of the world's teenagers. Other urologists recommended that even if a patient did not have a varicocele, the operation to tie off the testicular vein (the same operation one would perform to correct the varicocele) would increase the sperm production of any male with oligospermia, whether or not he had a varicocele. If these studies and claims were to be taken seriously, there would not be enough urological surgeons to do all of these operations. I am sorry to say that may be just how such an outrageous epidemic of varicocele surgery for male infertility got started in the first place.

The fact is, many urologists who treat male infertility depend heavily on varicocelectomy for their income. I used to perform varicocelectomy routinely myself, many years ago. I was fooled by a "scientific" literature that was filled with enthusiasm, and by the intrinsic variation in sperm count from month to month in various patients that led to the false impression that one third of them had an improvement as a result of the operation. However, there have now been hard, scientifically controlled studies performed by nonsurgeon endocrinologists with a special interest in male infertility, but with no strong preexisting need to find varicocelectomy surgery beneficial.

In the late 1970s, Dr. Luis Rodriguez-Rigau, Dr. Keith Smith, and Dr. Emil Steinberger, from the University of Texas in Houston, presented the first large controlled studies that showed absolutely no difference in the pregnancy rate between couples who underwent varicocelectomy and those who did not. Around the same time, Nilsson, from Göteborg, Sweden, reported a similar study in the *British Journal of Urology*, demonstrating no statistically significant improvement in sperm count, motility, or morphology in men with varicoceles who had surgery versus those who did not. More important, the pregnancy rate was even lower in the wives of men who had the operation. In 1984, Dr. Vermuelian, from Ghent, Belgium, also reported no improvement in pregnancy rates in those couples whose husband had a varicocelectomy versus those who did not.

The clincher paper, however, was published in 1985 in the *British Medical Journal* by Dr. Gordon Baker and his group at Prince Henry Hospital in Melbourne, Australia. They did an incredibly detailed study following 651 infertile couples in whom the man had a varicocele. In 283 of those 651 couples, the man underwent a varicocelectomy, and in 368 of the couples, the man did not. There was no improvement in pregnancy rate whatsoever in the couples in which the man had a varicocelectomy, and there was no improvement in the semen analysis either. This finding was further strengthened in 1994 by Dr. Eberhard Nieschlag, from Germany, who showed that in men with varicocele, psychologic counseling resulted in as high a pregnancy rate as having a varicocelectomy. Despite the overwhelming evidence that Dr. Gittes's statement in 1978 challenging the role of varicocele in male infertility was correct, urologists still go on performing varicocelectomies on at least 30 percent or more of men whose wives' gynecologists refer them to a urologist.

Years ago, I saw a patient whose wife was scheduled to undergo a reversal of tubal ligation later in the year. Her husband, trying to do the prudent thing and prevent his wife from going through surgery that might be unnecessary, decided to see a urologist first and make sure that he was fertile. He had a high sperm count with excellent motility. Yet the urologist who saw him insisted that he had to have a varicocelectomy, telling him that he had a large left-sided varicocele and absolutely had to have that surgery done before the wife could undergo the tubal reversal operation. I thought the story sounded strange, so I asked him to make a separate trip to St. Louis before the planned time of the wife's operation. It would have been ridiculous to operate on his varicocele, especially with a sperm count that good, and when I examined him I found he didn't even have a varicocele.

Several years ago, my office received a call from a patient who had read my first book and wanted to know whether the varicocelectomy her husband was scheduled to undergo in two weeks was necessary. It would be months before I would be able to see them for an appointment, but I told her that varicocelectomy usually does not benefit male infertility and that there is certainly never any reason to rush into it. She called two months later, just before she was to have her appointment with me, to inform me that thanks to our advice her husband did not have the varicocelectomy and that she was now pregnant and wouldn't need to see me. Interestingly, if he had undergone the varicocelectomy, the doctor who did it might have claimed that that was the reason she got pregnant.

In December 1993, I saw a lovely thirty-year-old couple who had been trying unsuccessfully for five years to get pregnant. His sperm count five years earlier was ten million per cc with 25 percent motility, and the urologist to whom he was immediately sent performed a bilateral varicocelectomy. Instead of the sperm count going up, as the patient had been promised, it was now down to less than a few thousand. The varicocelectomy had actually compromised the blood supply of the testicle and had virtually sterilized him. In IVF attempts elsewhere, his sperm did not fertilize his wife's eggs, and she failed to get pregnant. Fortunately, we performed ICSI in April 1994; the wife became pregnant and delivered a healthy baby in January 1995. The story ended happily because despite the drastic deterioration in his sperm count caused by the bilateral varicocelectomy, there were a few sperm still available for successful ICSI, and this man now has two children.

A twenty-nine-year-old couple I saw in July 1994 was not quite so fortunate. They had suffered five and a half years of infertility, and his sperm counts had averaged five million per cc with 50 percent motility. He had unfortunately undergone bilateral varicocelectomy in 1991, and thereafter he had absolutely zero sperm. A similar case involved a thirty-five-year-old couple who had a five-year-old child and were now trying for their second one. His sperm count was apparently in the low range (five million per cc, but with excellent motility). When he saw his local urologist he was told he had a bilateral varicocele, and he had a bilateral varicocelectomy performed. When I saw him six months later, he was completely azoospermic and would therefore not be able to have any more children. He had been perfectly fertile before, but his treatment had now made him sterile.

Although a varicocelectomy should be a relatively simple, innocuous operation, it can also be tricky at times because in an effort to get every single vein tied off (which would be necessary to prevent any blood from flowing back into the testicles), a surgeon can accidentally tie off the spermatic artery, which is extremely small and delicate. This destroys the blood supply to the testicle. A clumsy surgeon might even tie off the vas deferens.

Many portions of this book will not win me friends among certain infertility doctors. But on so many of these issues related to "male infertility" enough is enough. Drugs and hormones do not increase sperm count in oligospermic or azoospermic men, and neither does varicocele surgery.

CHAPTER 8

# Sperm Washing, Intrauterine Insemination (IUI), and Ovarian Stimulation

Now that you know what can go wrong in the female and male, and what treatments you are likely to encounter early on, you're ready to learn about more advanced treatments. The usual first step before going to IVF in most infertility clinics is IUI and ovarian stimulation. IUI (intrauterine insemination) simply means putting the sperm (after washing) directly into the uterus via a catheter. Ovarian stimulation means injections of various forms of the hormone FSH to yield greater numbers of follicles to ovulate. These techniques of sperm washing and ovarian hyperstimulation must also be employed with any IVF procedure. Therefore, learning about these techniques is a stepping-stone toward complete understanding of IVF.

## Sperm Washing and IUI

Ironically, semen, the fluid in which the sperm is normally transferred to the female at intercourse, is the worst possible environment for sperm. Sperm in an ejaculated semen specimen not only die rather quickly (anywhere from two to eight hours later), but also cannot undergo the rapid movement necessary to fertilize the egg. Furthermore, semen is, in a sense, a toxic substance. If it is injected in volumes greater than 0.5 cc directly into the female's uterus, it causes violent cramps. Sperm in semen are completely incapable of fertilizing the egg, and semen placed directly into the female anywhere other than the vagina not only interferes with the fertilization process but can actually make the woman quite sick. Therefore, sperm must be separated from the ejaculated semen. That is the essence of "sperm washing."

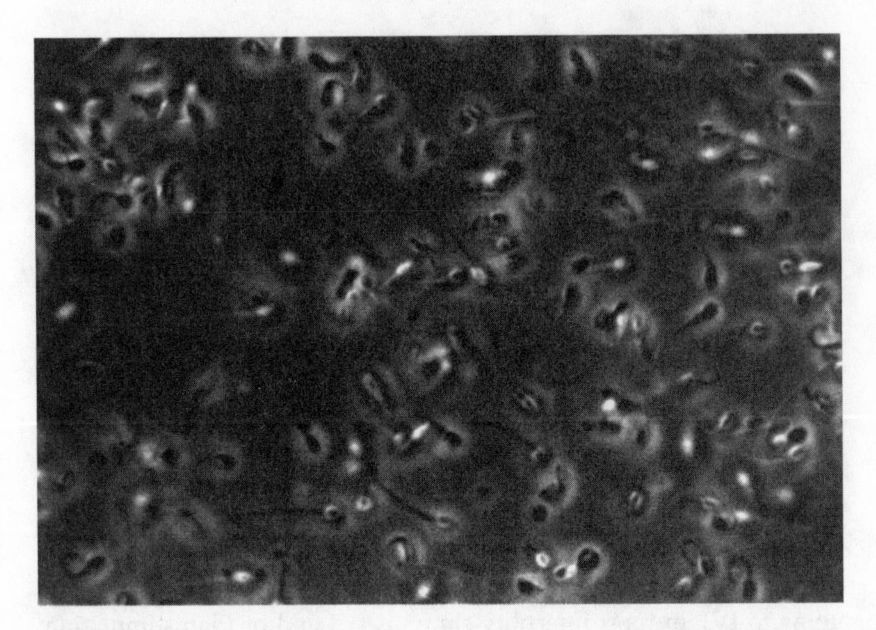

**FIGURE 8.1**

Microscopic view of tremendous increase in the velocity and the force of sperm propulsion after sperm are capacitated in culture fluid.

Simple sperm washing with common laboratory culture media has a dramatic effect on increasing the motility of the sperm (see fig. 8.1). Sperm washing is performed with nutrient fluid, or culture media, that is essentially no different from the media used to nourish the sperm and the egg for IVF. The detailed requirements of these fluids for nourishing sperm, eggs, and embryos will be of more interest in the context of the chapters on IVF.

### *Several Methods of Sperm Washing*

The simplest method of sperm washing is to mix the semen with culture media (in a ratio of three parts media to one part semen) in a test tube and then centrifuge it. By spinning the centrifuge tubes containing this semen–culture media mixture for about five minutes, the sperm all go to the very bottom in what is called a button, a small, dense mass of millions of pure sperm completely separated from the relatively large volume of fluid that they came from (see fig. 8.2). The supernatant is the large volume of sperm-free fluid remaining over the button.

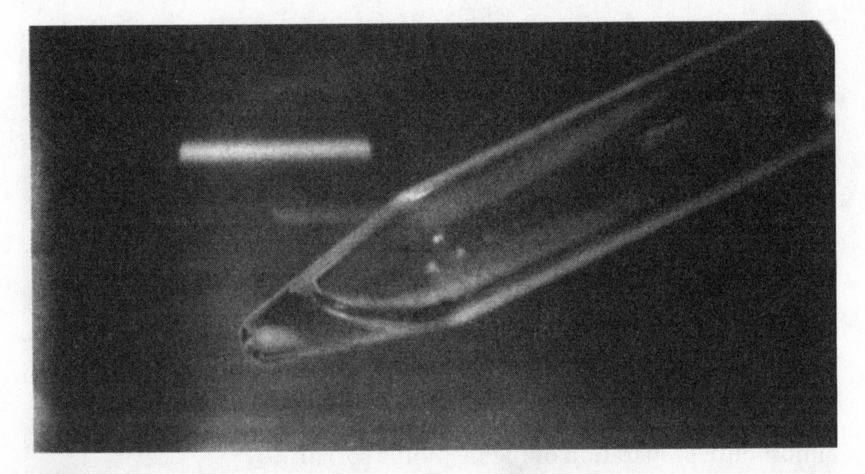

**FIGURE 8.2**

"Button" containing hundreds of millions of sperm at the bottom of the tube after the semen is centrifuged.

This supernatant is then aspirated off of the top with a pipette, leaving the button at the bottom of the test tube intact. Then more culture media is added to the pure sperm and mixed thoroughly. This mixture of sperm and culture media is then spun in the centrifuge once again for five minutes. Once more there is a visible button of pure sperm on the bottom of the centrifuge tube and on top is pure culture media containing the extremely tiny residual amount of semen that had been left in the first button. This supernatant is then pipetted off the top again, and a small amount of fresh culture media is placed once more over the button and thoroughly mixed. The end result of this simple washing technique is that the sperm are completely separated from the semen and now reside in pure culture media.

There are a number of problems with this very simple sperm-washing technique that make it not very suitable for IVF. With this simple technique, the live and dead sperm are not separated, and any white blood cells, bacteria, or debris that were present in the semen will still be present in this washed specimen. Although putting this type of washed sperm specimen in the uterus (using IUI) is routine, putting a lot of dead sperm and white blood cells into a culture dish with the egg, or into the fallopian tube, could interfere with fertilization. For that reason, separating only the most motile and pure sperm from the washed specimen is preferable.

In the swim-up technique, the sperm undergoes a simple wash, but instead of just resuspending the button in fresh media, a small amount of fresh culture media is gently placed on top of the button (usually about 4/100 of a teaspoon). Then the test tube is put in an incubator and kept at a normal body temperature of 37 degrees Celsius or 98.6 degrees Fahrenheit. The most actively motile sperm actually swim up out of this solid mass of millions of sperm from the button into the media that has been overlayed on top of it. The more sluggish or nonmoving sperm, and the white blood cells and debris, are more likely to remain trapped in the button. After the swim-up technique, the overlayed fluid shows very few dead sperm, hardly any debris or white blood cells, and an almost pure preparation of highly motile sperm.

Density gradients have now become more popular than swim-up for separating the most highly motile, fertile sperm from the ejaculate. With this technique several different layers of varying concentrations of isosmotic density gradient are placed on top of each other in a centrifuge tube. It is critical not to allow any mixing of the different layers because sperm separation does not occur simply by virtue of going through the density gradient. Sperm separation occurs as a result of going through the interface between the various density gradient layers.

Sperm is then placed on top of this series of density gradients, and the centrifuge tube is spun for about twenty minutes. During this process, something quite remarkable happens. As the sperm are pushed down through the gradients by centrifugation, poor-quality sperm, as well as white blood cells, debris, and bacteria, are trapped in the upper interfaces. Only the most motile, perfect sperm are able to get all the way down through all three interfaces to the bottom of the centrifuge tube. Then, with a pipette, only the bottom layer is removed, and it is then washed in the routine way and placed in another centrifuge tube with fresh media. At the end of this procedure, extremely hyperactivated, capacitated sperm and very few (if any) poorly motile sperm or debris are left. This method seems to create the purest preparation possible.

You might wonder how this all works. What happens is that the most motile sperm have the greatest ability to penetrate an interface of two different density gradients because the constant movement makes them more likely to break through the surface tension. If you throw a feather into the water, it is likely to float on the surface. However, if the feather had a vibratory mechanism that allowed it to stir up the surface tension of the water, that would make it more likely to sink when tossed into the lake than a feather that simply fell flat on its back and had no motion of its own. That is how density gradients are able to separate out the most highly motile, highly fertile, morphologically normal sperm.

Now that you have learned all about how we wash the sperm, getting it out of the toxic atmosphere of the semen and producing a natural enhancement of the sperm's fertilizing ability by speeding up the process of capacitation, we can discuss how they are put back inside of a woman, or placed in culture with her eggs.

### *Intrauterine Insemination (IUI) of Washed Sperm*

Can the improvement in sperm quality resulting from this washing be used to achieve pregnancy simply by inseminating the sperm back into the vagina or uterus? Well, actually, I think not. The original hope was that by placing washed sperm directly into the uterus (IUI) and bypassing the cervix and cervical mucus barrier, one could accomplish results equivalent to IVF but with obviously much greater simplicity. Because of this allure, virtually every female infertility patient goes through a series of IUIs (whether rightly or wrongly) before she takes the step toward IVF.

The idea behind this approach is very appealing, even though in reality it is not highly effective. It can be performed easily in the office without any surgery, anesthesia, or sedation whatsoever. The patient feels no different than she would when getting a pelvic exam, and a complicated laboratory setup is not necessary. It is logical to expect a higher pregnancy rate because much greater numbers of viable sperm will reach the uterus with this technique than with normal intercourse. That is why it is so popular and so widely used. But in truth, pregnancy rates with this procedure are not great unless accompanied by ovarian stimulation with FSH hormones. Even then the rate is only about 12 percent per cycle. We have found that when combined with ovarian stimulation, sexual intercourse works just as well as IUI, and is much easier emotionally on the couple. However, this is not the usual advice. Many couples go through six to twelve cycles of IUI and ovarian stimulation, and become exhausted emotionally and financially. They would have been better off doing no IUI and, if three cycles of ovarian stimulation with regular sexual intercourse failed, going straight to IVF. It is only the combination of IUI with ovulatory stimulation that seems to result in a respectable 12 percent pregnancy rate per cycle. IUI itself gives no major improvement over intercourse, and it's less fun.

## Ovarian Stimulation with Gonadotropins

Often there is nothing obviously wrong with a woman's ovulation, yet there may still be a problem that could hamper the proper preparation of her eggs for fertilization. Remember from chapter 1 that FSH in the follicular phase and the LH surge that induces ovulation accomplish a lot more than just ovulation. The early FSH stimulation helps the egg grow and form its protective zona pellucida, and then makes the follicle surrounding the egg fill with estrogen-rich fluid; in turn, the estrogen prepares the uterine lining and the cervical mucus for sperm entry. The LH surge then causes the egg to resume meiosis, which reduces the number of chromosomes from forty-six to twenty-three, an absolute genetic necessity before the sperm's twenty-three chromosomes can properly fertilize the egg. Furthermore, the prior FSH stimulation prepares the egg to be genetically competent to respond to the LH surge by resuming meiosis. So a lot more is happening under the stimulation of FSH and LH than just ovulation.

The most effective and powerful method for stimulating your ovary is to use drugs like human menopausal gonadotropin (HMG) and FSH. The reason that these drugs are so effective is that they are purified preparations of FSH (HMG also has a small amount of LH), which directly stimulates the ovary in the early part of the cycle to make better and more follicles. These drugs (FSH and LH) are called gonadotropins because they are the natural pituitary hormones that stimulate the gonads (ovaries and testes). These drugs do not just act indirectly by stimulating the pituitary gland to make more FSH and LH (as Clomid does) — they *are* the FSH and LH. Thus, gonadotropins are more direct and potent than any other treatment utilized for stimulating ovulation. The early FSH stimulation must also be accompanied by a small amount of LH. FSH (with a small amount of LH) only sets the stage for proper ovulation by inducing the formation of good follicles in the first half of the cycle. For ovulation to occur, the woman then needs an injection of a high dose of human chorionic gonadotropin (HCG — the equivalent of LH) when the follicles are mature and ready. Hormonal stimulation is an important key to the success of modern IVF, and there are several different approaches you will need to understand.

### *Lupron (or GnRH Agonist) to Prevent Premature LH Surge*

It is important in the follicular phase of egg maturation that the pituitary does not respond with a premature LH increase. A tiny amount of LH potentiates the early stimulatory effect of FSH, and normally in the early follicular recruitment stage in a normal menstrual cycle, some LH is needed. In the natural fertile state, FSH never exists in the absence of a small amount of LH. But there must not be a large amount of LH released from the pituitary until the follicle is large and ripe. In a normal cycle, the estrogen level goes up toward midcycle and surges to a high level around day twelve or thirteen, and this surge from the mature, large follicle stimulates the pituitary to suddenly release a huge amount of LH, the so-called LH surge. This LH surge causes the mature egg to resume meiosis and the follicle to ovulate twenty-four to forty-eight hours later.

If the LH goes up too early, before the egg is ready, i.e., before it has reached meiotic competence, this results in low pregnancy rates. So LH must not be allowed to go up until the egg is mature and ready for the ovulatory surge. Also, in IVF cycles, care should be taken not to lose the eggs as a result of premature ovulation prior to follicle aspiration. For these reasons, it became popular in the late 1980s to administer Lupron prior to day one of the stimulation cycle to prevent a premature LH release. In fact, this is one of the major reasons for the increase in IVF success rates in the last fifteen years.

Here is how Lupron works. The only reason the pituitary can secrete FSH and LH is that a primitive region of the brain, the hypothalamus, releases a short, brief pulse of GnRH hormone every ninety minutes. A drug like Lupron (or in Europe, buserelin, Lucrin, or Suprefact) is a GnRH agonist, which means it first stimulates and then eventually completely prevents the pituitary from releasing GnRH. When you start taking Lupron, there is a tremendous increase in the pituitary's release of FSH and LH for the first three days. But after five days the pituitary has become down regulated and is completely incapable of releasing any more LH or FSH (except for tiny amounts) until the drug is stopped. Once the drug is stopped, the pituitary eventually begins to function normally again. Thus, if a woman is started on HMG to stimulate ovulation, placing her on Lupron first will completely control the pituitary and prevent a premature LH surge.

Lupron can be administered in either of two fashions, long phase or short phase. With long phase, Lupron is started in the luteal phase of the preceding cycle or for two weeks before beginning HMG or gonadotropin. Long phase means that the Lupron is allowed two weeks to settle down the pituitary to a steadily suppressed LH secretion. If Lupron is given during the luteal phase of the previous cycle, then after about five days the pituitary is down regulated. The woman will have a menstrual period at the end of this luteal phase, and then she can begin HMG anytime thereafter. By the time she starts her first injection of HMG, her pituitary will not be able to release its own FSH or LH, so it won't interfere with the HMG regimen. Many doctors prefer this luteal phase, or long phase, approach because they don't want LH levels to be elevated in the early part of the cycle.

If a doctor wants to reduce the overall amount of HMG that has to be given, or wants to get greater stimulation in a woman who has resistant ovaries, he or she could give Lupron beginning on day three of the cycle (short phase). Two days later the woman would start the HMG or FSH and take advantage of the early stimulatory effect of Lupron on the pituitary. There has been a great deal of debate about which is the best way to administer Lupron, long phase or short phase. However, it is clear from controlled studies that long-phase Lupron with a stable, low LH level prior to beginning HMG or FSH yields the highest pregnancy rates.

### *How Are HMG and FSH (Gonadotropins) Made?*

HMG (as well as HCG) is a natural, not synthetic, hormone. The way in which this drug was discovered is somewhat ironic. HMG means human menopausal gonadotropin. As you get older and go through menopause, your ovaries eventually run out of eggs and shrivel up into very small, atrophied organs that no longer make estrogen. In women who have passed the age of menopause, their pituitary makes enormous amounts of FSH in response to the lack of negative feedback from the ovaries. Since FSH is excreted largely in the urine, the urine of a postmenopausal woman has enormous amounts of FSH (as well as LH) in it. Thus, the urine of postmenopausal women makes for a great fertility drug.

Pergonal was the very first brand of HMG, produced by Serono, originally in Italy. To begin this revolution in infertility treatment, they simply needed to find an efficient way to harvest huge amounts of this FSH-rich urine from postmenopausal women so that it could be processed for extraction of FSH. So they arranged for nunneries to have central processing vats in which all of the postmenopausal nuns would urinate. These postmenopausal nuns were more than excited to donate their services for this enterprise because they knew that it would help hundreds of thousands of infertile women get pregnant. Therefore, in a sense, the Catholic church was crucial to the development of IVF.

Naturally, there is some LH in human menopausal gonadotropin. This can't be avoided because postmenopausal women will have increased LH as well as FSH. The amount of LH, however, is physiologically not very significant. Interestingly, purified FSH is not as reliable itself as standard HMG, which has FSH plus a little bit of LH. Some LH is actually required to stimulate proper follicular development, even in the early phase of the cycle. Pure FSH therefore, in some cases, does not yield as good an ovarian response as old-fashioned HMG. Therefore, many clinics will stimulate a woman with a combination of HMG and pure FSH out of fear that giving pure FSH with no LH in it might not stimulate the ovary quite as well. This is particularly a problem when the woman's own LH level is too low. This is the so-called mixed protocol. A small amount of LH is important in maximizing the effect of FSH.

### *Monitoring HMG or FSH Treatment and Timing When to Give HCG*

HMG or FSH will only mature the eggs and prepare the follicles for HCG. Resumption of genetic preparation of the egg for fertilization, and then ovulation, must be induced at the appropriate time by the injection of HCG (which mimics the LH surge). If the follicles develop too rapidly and the estrogen level climbs out of control, it is a warning that it would be dangerous for this woman to ovulate. As long as she is not given her HCG injection at midcycle, the woman will not develop hyperstimulation syndrome. If she is given HCG when her ovaries are too enlarged, the follicles may be too numerous and produce inordinate amounts of estrogen. The ovulation induced by HCG in such a case could result in severe ovarian hyperstimulation syndrome. (Hyperstimulation syndrome will be explained more fully in a later section.) Thus, if the estrogen level is too high, that is a warning *not* to give HCG. The woman can then be given a month or so to rest, and her ovaries will shrink back to a more normal size. The other problem (unless IVF is being used) is that she will ovulate too many eggs and be in great danger of a high-order multiple pregnancy. Despite severe ovarian enlargement, with more than forty follicles and a sky-high estrogen level, she will not be in danger as long as HCG is not administered.

How does the physician decide when to give HCG? How do we know that the egg is mature enough and is ready for the LH stimulus to cause the resumption of meiosis, and that the follicle is mature enough to proceed with ovulation? When the leading (or biggest) follicles have reached 1.8 centimeters to 2.0 centimeters (four fifths of an inch) in diameter, they have reached the stage of maturity where they are ready for HCG. At this stage, each mature follicle should be releasing about two hundred picograms per milliliter of estrogen. Thus, if there are ten mature follicles in the ovary, the estrogen level at this point should be about two thousand picograms per milliliter. If there are five mature follicles in the ovaries, the estrogen level should be around one thousand picograms per milliliter. So the time to give HCG is judged by the follicular size, and the maturity of the eggs is verified by seeing whether the estrogen is at a high enough level for that number of follicles.

For IVF, more follicles are desired than for routine HMG treatment. We're happy to have ten to twenty eggs for IVF. With just HMG and IUI, it is better to have a smaller number (three would be ideal). Sometimes it is very hard to adequately control the number of follicles achieved in an ovarian stimulation cycle. For that reason, ironically, IVF is actually much simpler and safer than just plain HMG or FSH stimulation using only IUI.

### *Indications and Directions for Using HMG*

The first scientific paper openly advocating the use of HMG therapy in patients with idiopathic infertility (infertility of unknown cause) came from Dr. Alan DeCherney of Yale University in the early 1980s. He openly attempted "empirical HMG therapy" for patients with idiopathic infertility. Most previous studies of HMG tried to come up with some kind of diagnosis of ovulatory failure before. Dr. DeCherney was the first to use it even in patients who had no problem with ovulation. He noted a 12.7 percent pregnancy rate per cycle using HMG in couples with long-term infertility of unknown origin compared to a control group of patients undergoing no treatment who had only a 1 percent pregnancy rate per cycle. DeCherney was thus the first to openly recommend the administration of HMG, or FSH, to couples with infertility of unknown origin with no clear-cut diagnosis of poor ovulation. Infertility doctors no longer had to struggle to try to manufacture a diagnosis of some type of ovulatory defect in these patients.

Why does this work? There is a tremendous amount of preparation the egg must go through during the first half of the cycle in order to be fertilized, and these preparations are aided by an increased level of FSH. Ovarian stimulation is useful in most cases of infertility not caused by tubal blockage because it overrides whatever subtle defect might exist in the whole process of egg maturation and preparation for fertilization. Normally, eight to twelve days of HMG are required before the follicles are ready for HCG. When the largest follicle is 1.8 to 2.1 centimeters in size, the eggs are mature. From thirty-eight to forty-eight hours after HCG, ovulation will occur. Intercourse or IUI should take place one to two days after the HCG injection.

### *Progesterone Injections*

Because ovarian stimulation cycles often exhibit low progesterone production and subsequent loss of pregnancy, progesterone injections must be administered for eight to twelve weeks, beginning two days after HCG. Pregnancy rates are poor without some sort of progesterone supplementation. There are several reasons that progesterone injections are necessary. One is that Lupron, which is used to prevent premature LH release, also inhibits the stimulation of the corpus luteum by LH to make progesterone. This effect can last until the HCG produced by the embryo itself takes over. Furthermore, in IVF cases, emptying the follicles by suction to retrieve the eggs reduces the potential progesterone production from a subsequently deficient corpus luteum. A third reason is that the higher-than-normal estrogen level caused by the ovarian hyperstimulation may require a higher-than-normal complementary progesterone level to allow implantation. Whatever the reason, we know from experience that without progesterone supplementation you are not likely to get pregnant with IVF.

The package insert from the FDA on progesterone may scare you quite unnecessarily because it alleges in big, bold letters a risk of fetal damage from progesterone injections. This is another silly example of political stupidity and foolishness. No physician who specializes in infertility or IVF anywhere in the world feels that this warning is valid. Progesterone is a natural hormone that you normally make during pregnancy to allow the embryo to implant and grow. You would not be taking any synthetic, progesterone-like substances to support the pregnancy, but rather just the same exact progesterone your body would otherwise normally be making. Any pregnancy carries the risk of fetal abnormality, however low, and it would be foolish not to acknowledge such a risk. However, progesterone does not increase that risk. Progesterone is just a natural hormone that your placenta needs to keep the pregnancy alive. The FDA is so burdened by congressionally mandated bureaucracy that unfortunately no intelligent review by the government of any aspect of this field seems possible. So don't let the package insert on progesterone worry you.

### *Using Birth Control Pills for Timing the Cycle*

Sometimes your cycle will come at an inconvenient time for you, your husband, or even your doctor. In order to prevent that, and to "schedule" your cycle rationally, the first day of Lupron or gonadotropin stimulation can be delayed by taking birth control pills during the early follicular phase of the previous cycle. This will "put you on hold" quite safely until it is time to start day one of Lupron or gonadotropin treatment. In fact, this approach, called "programming" your treatment cycle, allows us to schedule the days your husband has to be available many months ahead of time. You're usually likely to require eight to twelve days of gonadotropin. For example, for IVF, we can plan rather precisely when you will have your procedure by scheduling a "target" day (plus or minus two days) and then counting back twenty-eight days to figure out when to start Lupron. On the third day of Lupron, you would stop taking the birth control pills. Two weeks after starting Lupron, you would begin taking the gonadotropin, either HMG or FSH.

Another scheduling approach is simply to "keep you on hold" with Lupron alone (without using birth control pills) and then start the HMG or FSH injections when the timing is appropriate. This works fine if you are already in the luteal phase of an ovulatory cycle. Premature stimulation during the first three days of Lupron causes two different cohorts of eggs to develop asynchronously if the Lupron is not begun either in the luteal phase or while you are still on birth control pills.

Because the initial release of large amounts of LH has occurred during the luteal phase, your ovary would not be prematurely stimulated in the first three days of taking Lupron.

There are several reasons why, in some cases, it is better to accomplish this scheduling, or programming, of your cycle with birth control pills rather than just going right to Lupron. If there has been any excessive endometrial buildup from poor ovulation and subsequent "unopposed" estrogen effect, the progesterone-like action of the birth control pills will guarantee a clean menstrual slough before starting the HMG cycle. Also, taking birth control pills before going on Lupron will more effectively prevent the ovarian cyst formation that occasionally results from the GnRH release during the first few days of Lupron. However, starting Lupron in the luteal phase is often also effective in controlling those first few days of GnRH release.

After you have completed your HCG injection and have ovulated, if you have a period before you are due to get a pregnancy test, you will need to take progesterone. There are some poor progesterone substitutes, such as Crinone and Prometrium, that are being promoted by some drug companies. They must not be used, even though they have been "FDA approved." That just means the drug companies have put a lot of money into lobbying for them. If you do not have adequate progesterone support for your luteal phase, you will bleed early. This will never happen with the use of the proper progesterone. You can only trust the old-fashioned, low-profit "progesterone in oil" in the United States (or Gestone, which is sold only in Europe) or high-dose progesterone suppositories as a distant second choice. The FDA has been not only useless, but quite detrimental to the well-being of infertility patients, and this is just one of the many examples.

### *Comparison of the Different Stimulation Protocols and Drugs*

There have been a variety of approaches to ovarian hyperstimulation that have had differing impacts upon IVF success rates (see tables 8.1 and 8.2). As we have discussed in several previous chapters, the number and quality of eggs that can be retrieved from a stimulation cycle determine what the pregnancy rate will be for any IVF cycle. A good stimulation cycle means a high pregnancy rate, and a poor stimulation cycle means a lower pregnancy rate. There have been many comparison studies, some of which can be very confusing at first glance, between the types of stimulation protocols administered and between the specific types of drugs being used. The drug companies have only added to the confusion because they are motivated purely by profit. I will try to clear up this confusion for you.

As discussed in the last section, in the 1990s some would have recommended that Lupron be started at the same time that the stimulation protocol with HMG or FSH begins. That way, Lupron would stimulate the pituitary during the first three days to release large amounts of FSH and LH, which would be additive to the effect of the administered FSH or HMG. Thus, it was thought that a more powerful stimulation could be achieved with lower, less-expensive doses of HMG or FSH. This was called the "flare protocol." However, comparative studies have shown that pregnancy rates are higher if FSH or HMG is not administered until the Lupron has had enough time (ten to fourteen days) to completely settle down the pituitary so that there is no extra LH secretion. Too much LH in the early follicle-recruitment phase of the cycle results in poorer-quality eggs with lower pregnancy rate. Therefore, even with resistant ovaries, we have found that the long-phase Lupron protocol, even if it requires higher doses of HMG or FSH, gives better results than the short-phase protocol.

### Recombinant FSH Versus Menopausal Gonadotropins

Now that the drug companies can genetically produce pure FSH, with no trace of LH, there is a heated marketing controversy that you will need to understand. Until the late 1990s, the only forms of gonadotropin available for stimulating the ovary were derived from the urine of menopausal women. Since the 1960s, as mentioned earlier, most gonadotropins were obtained from older women, usually nuns in a convent, who urinated into common vats or brought huge jugs of urine to a factory to be processed so that the FSH and LH could be purified. This ultimately led to the production of Pergonal, Humegon, Menogon, and Repronex, different brands of "urinary" gonadotropin that were used for ovarian stimulation. In fact, some of these menopausal gonadotropins would still be the most popular drugs for ovarian stimulation if drug companies had not taken them off the market in their greed to increase profits. Attempts to improve upon them were made in the 1980s and early 1990s by completely removing the LH. This, however, only reduced their potency and was of no clinical benefit.

Two drug-manufacturing giants in this field, Serono and Organon, are now producing pure FSH preparations, not by extracting FSH from the urine of menopausal women, but rather via recombinant DNA technology. This means that genes for producing the FSH are inserted into cell cultures in which they then direct the production, in test tubes, of FSH. This use of genetic technology to produce recombinant gonadotropins rather than menopausal gonadotropins required a large initial investment by the drug companies, but it will pay off because of the cheaper production costs and the easier supply — they no longer have to scour the world for postmenopausal women's urine. More important, they now have an excuse for charging patients even more exorbitant prices.

The drug companies have a clear financial interest in promoting the use of these recombinant gonadotropins. Furthermore, their marketing pitch to physicians is that they are cleaner and purer, with less batch-to-batch variation in dosage effect. However, no physician using both recombinant and menopausal gonadotropins feels there is really any difference in results, except that the older HMG product may possibly be better than the new pure-FSH product. This is owing to the absence of any LH in the new recombinant products. The contention that the newer recombinant-DNA drugs are more effective is just marketing hype designed to increase profit margin.

However, there is one advantage of the recombinant FSH (brand names of Gonal-F and Follistim) that to a few patients may be worth the tremendously increased cost. The recombinant FSH can be given via a subcutaneous injection rather than an intramuscular injection (SubQ versus IM) with no pain. In fact, the menopausal gonadotropins like HMG can be given SubQ also, but that would cause some irritation and discomfort. That is why they are usually given IM. The advantage of a SubQ injection is that the needle is extremely tiny and short, the injection is just under the skin, and there really is no pain with it. Despite the increased cost of what is already an outrageously expensive drug (three thousand to four thousand dollars per cycle), many patients prefer the recombinant FSH. However, others do not mind the minor irritation of SubQ injection with HMG.

There is one severe disadvantage to using pure FSH. A very small amount of LH is necessary for FSH to have its full effect, as we have seen before. For most patients, there is enough secretion of their own LH (even while taking Lupron) to allow the administered FSH to provide good stimulation of the ovary. However, in many cases, the woman's endogenous LH level is so low that pure FSH alone gives only a meager response. A small number of women who have been on Lupron down regulation for several weeks have LH levels below 1.0 milliIu/ml. At this low level of endogenous LH, the stimulatory effects of FSH are quite diminished. Thus, the old-fashioned, discontinued menopausal gonadotropins were more forgiving in that their small amount of LH content was of great benefit.

The major HMG preparations have been taken off the market by the big drug companies in an effort to force physicians to use their more expensive products. The HMG preparations that remain on the market have some use in adding to administration of recombinant FSH in that they supply this small amount of LH. However, they also have a large amount of HCG added in to correct this LH effect (fully approved by the unvigilant eye of the FDA). This HCG component in the remaining generic HCG preparations has a much longer half-life than LH, and therefore can accumulate over the course of a stimulation cycle, reaching levels as high a ten to twelve international units per milliliter, three times higher than the desired LH level for the follicular phase of ovarian stimulation. Therefore, you now must go through what we call mixed stimulation protocols involving the newer recombinant gonadotropins, Gonal-F or Follistim, along with much lower doses of an HMG, such as Repronex, Menogon, or Lepori, all at the same time. Physicians can solve the problems created by drug company profiteering, but it is the drug companies that benefit most from these newer, more expensive products.

## Step-Up and Step-Down Protocols

The next aspect of administering your ovarian stimulation cycle is whether to go with the step-up or the step-down protocol. With the step-up protocol, you are started on a very low dose of FSH, such as one or two ampules. You then begin monitoring your estrogen levels and ultrasound visualization of your ovaries. After four or five days, if this monitoring reveals a low response, without much of an estrogen rise or without any observable follicles developing, then the dosage of HMG or FSH is increased. You are then monitored every other day for estrogen and by ultrasound, and your dosage is increased or maintained according to whether there appears to be an adequate follicular response with an adequate estrogen level and an adequate number of follicles developing.

This so-called step-up protocol is not as successful as the step-down protocol.

The step-down protocol is based on the concept that all of the follicles you recruited to mature with FSH were actually recruited during the first five days. If you remember from chapter 3, after seventy days of prior development, the antral follicles have reached the stage where they are finally sensitive to FSH stimulation during a brief five-day window, develop into maturing, ovulatory follicles only under the early influence of FSH, which sensitizes the follicles more and more to lower levels of FSH as the days progress toward ovulation. Thus, it makes physiological sense to start out with a high dose of FSH rather than a low dose. This will allow the most effective, and the most normal, early recruitment of follicles.

If it turns out that this initial high dose is too high for you (and there is no way to know until you actually undergo ovarian stimulation), then it can be reduced on day five, in plenty of time to avoid hyperstimulation. In fact, if you have a good initial response to a high enough, early dose of FSH, your follicles will be sensitized enough to FSH (just as in a normal ovulatory cycle) that decreasing amounts of FSH in subsequent days will in no way hinder egg development or quality.

Let's review tables 8.1 and 8.2. With the step-down protocol, instead of starting the patient on a modest dose of one or two ampules per day of HMG, we started her on six ampules per day. After four days of HMG, on day five, her monitoring showed an E2 (estrogen) level that was high for day five, and she had nine follicles measuring at least one centimeter. But there were seventeen follicles that were less than one centimeter, which possibly would have led to twenty-five eggs, too many for a safe IVF cycle. Thus, we lowered her dose to three ampules of HMG per day. Her estrogen rose, and her follicles developed in a smooth and even fashion. By day eleven, after ten full days of HMG stimulation, she had fourteen mature size follicles (71.5 centimeters). Fourteen eggs were retrieved, eleven were fertilized, and three good-quality embryos were transferred. She became pregnant and delivered a healthy singleton baby. We'll get into the details of IVF in the subsequent chapters, but the point here is that ovulation stimulation beginning with a high dose that can be lowered then according to the estrogen and ultrasound response gives much higher pregnancy rates and better embryo quality than starting with a low dose, getting inadequate early recruitment, and then trying to catch up with that inadequate recruitment with subsequent increases in the dose.

### *Mini-Dose Lupron*

For older women who are at the end of their biological clock with very few eggs the mini-dose Lupron protocol may sometimes be suggested. However, despite the enthusiasm registered by some doctors, it has the same problems as short-phase Lupron protocols, and there is no evidence that it improves the pregnancy rates in this poor category of patients. Mini-dose Lupron means that you go through the short-phase Lupron protocol but use a much lower dose than the usual 0.2 milliliters (1 milligram). You might use one fourth to one tenth of that dose. Theoretically, this might give a more vigorous response to ovarian stimulation with HMG or FSH because it would suppress the pituitary gland's secretion of FSH and LH less vigorously. In other words, mini-dose Lupron is another version of short-phase Lupron, but with a lower dose, which will cause your pituitary gland to continue to release FSH and LH over a longer period of time during your stimulation.

Although I don't think mini-dose Lupron works any better for women with poor ovaries, you need to understand how it works. This will help you decide whether to use Lupron in your stimulation cycle, or go to one of the newer GnRH antagonist drugs. Lupron is a GnRH agonist, meaning it stimulates the pituitary gland, just like your own GnRH would, to release large amounts of FSH and LH. GnRH agonists like Lupron are actually acting just like your own GnRH, except that your own GnRH disappears immediately after its secretion and, therefore, has a very short-lived effect of just a matter of minutes. A GnRH agonist, like Lupron, lasts for as long as a day, and therefore, the pituitary gets no rest whatsoever from its continuous, forced secretion of FSH and LH. Normally, the pituitary only secretes a modest amount of LH and never tires of secreting it. However, with a GnRH agonist like Lupron, which is not metabolized immediately like your own GnRH would be, the effect lasts for a whole day, and the pituitary responds by releasing huge amounts of LH and FSH.

After three to six days of releasing this large amount of FSH and LH, the pituitary is actually depleted, literally drained of its LH and FSH reserves. That is called down regulation. Continuing to take Lupron over the course of two weeks forces the pituitary gland to push out whatever little FSH and LH is left, and prevents it from building up reserves as it normally would under the natural influence of pulsatile rather than continuous GnRH secretion. After the first five days of stimulation of LH release by the pituitary, LH then becomes depleted.

If the continuous endogenous secretion of LH is too high, it cannot have a normal or beneficial effect on recruiting pre-antral and antral follicles. When you take injections of HMG (which contains both FSH and LH), the FSH stays around for a full day and has a beneficial effect on recruiting follicles, but the LH goes down within hours, mimicking more closely the limited LH exposure that your ovaries should have in the follicular phase of your cycle. However, relying on your pituitary to secrete large amounts of LH via GnRH agonist creates a continuous early elevation of LH, which is detrimental to the developing eggs.

### *GnRH Antagonist Protocols*

Since 2001, a different kind of GnRH drug has become available to prevent premature ovulation and control ovarian stimulation. This is the so-called GnRH antagonist. The GnRH antagonist has the opposite effect of GnRH agonists like Lupron. Instead of simulating the effect of GnRH on the pituitary and causing a massive outflow of FSH and LH so that the pituitary eventually becomes depleted, the GnRH antagonist actually blocks the release of FSH and LH from the pituitary by interfering with the effect of your brain's own GnRH secretion on the pituitary. Thus, the antagonist causes your pituitary FSH and LH secretion to drop instantly, instead of in three to six days. An advantage of using the antagonist rather than Lupron is that you do not have to be on Lupron injections for two weeks to down regulate the pituitary gland before commencing with ovarian stimulation.

There are three disadvantages of using the antagonist. First is that the antagonist is so expensive that despite having to be on it for one quarter of the time you would have to be on the agonist, it still winds up costing more. It certainly doesn't cost any more to produce the antagonist than it does to produce the agonist. The drug companies have simply designed another way to dramatically increase their profits at the expense of infertility patients. The second disadvantage of using the antagonist is that it drops the LH level so low (usually much lower than Lupron does) that it lowers the ovarian response to stimulation. A third disadvantage is that if you forget to take the antagonist on a particular

TABLE 8.1

## Ovarian Stimulation Summary: Step-Up

| DATE | CYCLE DAY | # | FOLLICLE SIZES Right ovary | FOLLICLE SIZES Left ovary | # | E2 LEVEL | LH LEVEL | UTERINE LINING | MEDICATION PER SJS GnRH, GONADOTROPIN, HCG |
|---|---|---|---|---|---|---|---|---|---|
| 2/21/03 | Day 3 of of prev cycle | | | | | | | | Begin birth control pills |
| 3/11/03 | | | | | | | | | Begin Lupron |
| 3/14/03 | | | | | | | | | Stop birth control pills |
| 3/17/03 | | | 15<1 cm | 1.1, 10<1 cm | | | | | |
| 3/18/03 | | | Normal bleeding began after stopping birth control pills | | | | | | |
| 3/25/03 | 1 | | | | | | | | Gonadotropin 150 iu |
| 3/26/03 | 2 | | | | | | | | Gonadotropin 150 iu |
| 3/27/03 | 3 | | | | | | | | Gonadotropin 150 iu |
| 3/28/03 | 4 | | | | | | | | Gonadotropin 150 iu |
| 3/29/03 | 5 | 0 | 0>1 cm | 0>1 cm | 0 | 87 | 3.7 | 5 mm | Gonadotropin 450 iu |
| 3/30/03 | 6 | | | | | | | | Gonadotropin 450 iu |
| 3/31/03 | 7 | 3 | 1.2, 1.1, 1.1 | 1.6, 1.0 | 2 | 457 | 3.0 | 8 mm | Gonadotropin 450 iu |
| 4/1/03 | 8 | | | | | | | | Gonadotropin 450 iu |
| 4/2/03 | 9 | 7 | 1.5, 1.4, 1.3, 1.2, 1.2, 1.1, 1.1 | 1.6, 1.3, 1.2 | 3 | 1200 | 2.9 | 1 cm | Gonadotropin 450 iu |
| 4/3/03 | 10 | | | | | | | | Gonadotropin 450 iu |
| 4/4/03 | 11 | 8 | 2.0, 1.9, 1.9, 1.6, 1.6, 1.3, 1.3, 1.1 | 1.8, 1.5, 1.3, 1.2, 1.0 | 5 | 2463 | 2.5 | 1.2 cm | Gonadotropin 450 iu |
| 4/5/03 | 12 | | | | | | | | Last day for Lupron HCG 10,000 units |

TABLE 8.2

## Ovarian Stimulation Summary: Step-Down

| DATE | CYCLE DAY | # | FOLLICLE SIZES RIGHT OVARY | LEFT OVARY | # | E2 LEVEL | LH LEVEL | UTERINE LINING | MEDICATION PER SJS GnRH, GONADOTROPIN, HCG |
|---|---|---|---|---|---|---|---|---|---|
| 1/20/03 | Day 3 of prev cycle | | | | | | | | Begin birth control pills |
| 2/6/03 | | | | | | | | | Begin Lupron |
| 2/7/03 | | | 9<1 cm | 10<1 cm | | | | | |
| 2/9/03 | | | | | | | | | Stop birth control pills |
| 2-12-03 | | | Normal bleeding began after stopping birth control pills | | | | | | |
| 2/20/03 | 1 | | | | | | | | Gonadotropin 450 iu |
| 2/21/03 | 2 | | | | | | | | Gonadotropin 450 iu |
| 2/22/03 | 3 | | | | | | | | Gonadotropin 450 iu |
| 2/23/03 | 4 | | | | | | | | Gonadotropin 450 iu |
| 2/24/03 | 5 | 3 | 1.6, 1.1, 1.0, 9<1 cm | 1.7, 1.4, 1.3, 1.1, 1.0, 1.0, 8<1 cm | 6 | 585 | 3.0 | 1 cm | Gonadotropin 225 iu |
| 2/25/03 | 6 | | | | | | | | Gonadotropin 225 iu |
| 2/26/03 | 7 | 7 | 1.8, 1.5, 1.2, 1.2, 1.1, 1.1, 1.1, 6<1 cm | 1.7, 1.5, 1.4, 1.4, 1.3, 1.0, 1.0, 1.0, 4<1 cm | 8 | 1489 | 3.1 | 1.1 cm | Gonadotropin 225 iu |
| 2/27/03 | 8 | | | | | | | | Gonadotropin 225 iu |
| 2/28/03 | 9 | 10 | 1.8, 1.6, 1.6, 1.5, 1.5, 1.4, 1.3, 1.1, 1.1, 1.1 | 2.0, 1.9, 1.7, 1.6, 1.4, 1.3, 1.2, 1.1, 1.1, 1.1, 1.1 | 11 | 2354 | 2.7 | 1.2 cm | Gonadotropin 225 iu |
| 3/1/03 | 10 | | | | | | | | Gonadotropin 225 iu |
| 3/2/03 | 11 | 10 | 2.0, 1.9, 1.8, 1.8, 1.7, 1.7, 1.6, 1.5, 1.3, 1.3 | 2.2, 2.1, 1.9, 1.8, 1.6, 1.5, 1.3, 1.3, 1.3, 1.3, 1.3 | 11 | 3205 | 2.4 | 1.2 cm | Last day for Lupron HCG 10,000 units |

day, you could get an immediate LH surge and a premature ovulation, ruining your cycle. If you forget to take Lupron, the effect is lingering because the pituitary has been depleted of its store of FSH and LH, and it would therefore take several days to a week for that store to be replenished. Thus, forgetting Lupron for a single day is much more forgiving than forgetting the antagonist.

As I have said, one of the disadvantages of the antagonist is too much suppression of LH. This can be solved by not starting the antagonist injections until the stimulation cycle has been well established, and your leading follicle has reached 1.3 or 1.4 centimeters in diameter. Remember, once follicles have become over one centimeter in size, they are sensitized to FSH (and to LH). They are all capable of becoming dominant follicles and require very little continuing boost to keep on developing properly, just a modest amount of FSH or LH. Therefore, by withholding the antagonist until your follicle size reaches about 1.3 centimeters, you still prevent premature ovulation but do not interfere with follicle development.

So is there any real advantage to using the GnRH antagonist rather than the agonist in the stimulation protocol? Well, actually, the advantages are minor, but it is possible that this would be the ideal way to stimulate a marginal ovary with poor ovarian reserve in an older patient. You would essentially have no pituitary suppression until you needed it, and your eggs would not be poisoned by the rapid, early stimulation with LH, which would occur with short-phase Lupron. Furthermore, you don't have to have a prior two weeks of medication to down regulate your pituitary before beginning your stimulation cycle. The disadvantage of the antagonist protocol is simply that you have to be looked at and monitored more closely in order to prevent the risk of inadvertent, premature LH surge and premature ovulation. In addition, the sudden drop in LH during stimulation may be detrimental. Overall, I am not convinced that these new drugs like pure FSH or GnRH antagonist are any improvement over older drugs like HMG or Lupron, and they may have some distinct drawbacks.

### *Ovarian Stimulation for Timed Intercourse or IUI Versus Ovarian Stimulation for IVF*

There are contradictory objectives in ovarian stimulation for IUI (or timed intercourse) versus stimulation for IVF. Let me explain.

The most dreaded complication of infertility treatment is multiple pregnancy. Most women have no problem with twins, and in fact, some infertile women look forward to twins. However, triplets represent a very difficult pregnancy. In the hands of a good high-risk obstetrician, most triplet pregnancies in our region do well. Nonetheless, we try to avoid triplets as much as possible because of the increased risk of attempting to carry such a pregnancy. The risks are not only medical, but also social, in that the relationship between couples is stretched to the extreme by having three kids all at one time. Quadruplets and higher numbers are medical tragedies. Even though we read about successful cases in the media, they are, for the most part, very dangerous and dreaded.

You may have read with enthusiasm all of the media hoopla and excitement about the birth of septuplets (seven siblings) in Iowa. This was lauded in the media as some kind of great medical success. In truth, it was tragic. Most of the septuplets have some sort of medical or developmental problem, despite a huge team of medical specialists and an extraordinary outpouring of financial help from the public. In fact, the mother was not really an infertile woman at all, but a woman in her twenties who had already had a child and was eager to have more children. Her doctor placed her on gonadotropin injections for ovarian stimulation, and this woman who was quite fertile anyway wound up conceiving with seven embryos.

This is the type of problem that can be avoided with IVF because you can select the number of embryos to place back into the woman's uterus and freeze the extras. With simple ovarian stimulation, followed by either IUI or timed intercourse, you really have no control over the number of embryos that can implant in the uterus other than to make sure you have no more than three follicles developing. The inherent problem with ovarian hyperstimulation not accompanied by IVF is that you have to use minimal doses of gonadotropin to create minimal hyperstimulation so as not to run the risk of high-order multiple pregnancy. But with minimal stimulation, you dramatically reduce the chances for pregnancy. That is precisely why I do not recommend continuing with cycle after cycle of ovarian stimulation but rather proceeding more directly to IVF. With IVF, you can stimulate the ovaries strongly enough to obtain between ten and twenty eggs, and then simply select two or three embryos to replace; if there are more embryos that are viable, those can be frozen for a later date.

Therefore, for simple ovarian hyperstimulation, it is better to start with the step-up protocol, beginning with very low doses. For IVF, it is better to employ the step-down protocol, beginning with much higher doses. With the step-down protocol, as mentioned before, you can reduce the dose after the initial recruitment phase if monitoring shows that it is too high. If the dose had been low in the initial recruitment phase, you would have gotten smaller numbers of eggs, and this is not ideal for IVF. However, the step-up approach is the only safe way to stimulate the ovary if it is not accompanied by an IVF procedure.

### *Hyperstimulation Syndrome*

When gonadotropin was first available (in the 1960s), doctors did not know about the importance of monitoring daily estrogen levels, and ultrasound wasn't available. There was a high incidence of multiple births, serious hyperstimulation syndrome, and even a few deaths. With modern daily monitoring of blood estrogen levels, ultrasound evaluation of the follicles, and appropriate modification of dosage, these dangerous complications should not be a problem. However, 1 percent of women undergoing gonadotropin therapy will get some degree of hyperstimulation syndrome despite the most careful monitoring. This unlikely complication should not scare you away from ovarian stimulation, because nowadays we are quite well equipped to handle this condition.

Hyperstimulation syndrome occurs when you ovulate from a large number of follicles, causing a huge amount of estrogen-rich fluid to be poured directly out of the enlarged and fragile ovaries into the abdominal cavity. This estrogen then coats the peritoneal surface of the abdominal cavity and causes it to become very permeable to fluid leakage, allowing fluid to accumulate inside the abdomen. You then become dehydrated, and your abdomen swells. You get light-headed as a result of relatively low blood pressure, and you may even get dizzy because of decreased blood volume. Furthermore, you might feel some shortness of breath because all this fluid is pushing up against your diaphragm. At one time, this was a very dangerous condition because it was not fully understood. With modern monitoring, severe hyperstimulation syndrome is very unusual, but it can still occur.

In the past, doctors would treat this condition by withholding fluids, under the mistaken impression that this would somehow prevent the abdominal cavity from filling with so much fluid. That notion was incorrect and dangerous. The problem is that the blood volume that is lost has to be replaced with intravenous fluid. Something also has to be done to eliminate the continued irritation of the lining of the abdomen by this estrogen-rich fluid.

We now know that by putting a small paracentesis catheter into the abdomen and draining all of this fluid, the patient is made much more comfortable and can breathe more easily. By getting rid of this estrogen irritation, fluid leakage into the abdomen slows down dramatically. At the same time, fluids can be taken liberally to overcome the dehydration. Thus, even in these unusual cases of severe hyperstimulation syndrome, knowledgeable treatment prevents any dangerous outcome.

Many women will have mild degrees of hyperstimulation syndrome with a little bit of lower abdominal swelling and discomfort. This does not require hospitalization, only a little bed rest at home. It is only the rare, *severe* cases that require hospitalization. But with the proper, simple treatment, the woman just has to wait it out while her ovaries recover over a few days to a week. During that time, she will need to be on IVs and peritoneal fluid drainage, but she should be quite comfortable.

There is one very good side to having this occasional complication. The worst cases of hyperstimulation syndrome occur when a woman becomes pregnant. This is because her placenta is making HCG and stimulating the ovaries to continue to pour out large amounts of estrogen-rich fluid. So although it is a very unpleasant side effect to endure, hyperstimulation syndrome often means good news. Eventually the symptoms resolve, the patient feels fine, and she is happy to be pregnant.

### *No Increased Risk of Ovarian Cancer*

In January 1993, the FDA asked fertility-drug makers to change labels to "acknowledge a potential link between the drugs and ovarian cancer." This irresponsible announcement from the FDA followed a fairly irresponsible publication that suggested that women who had taken fertility drugs have a higher risk of developing ovarian cancer. The study claimed that women in the 1960s and 1970s who were infertile (and were therefore placed on Clomid or Pergonal to stimulate ovulation) had a higher risk of developing cancer of the ovary than fertile women. This erroneous conclusion scared women into thinking that Clomid and Pergonal increased the risk of ovarian cancer. This claim has now been put to rest.

The truth is that it has been known for years that infertility increases the risk of ovarian cancer, and having several children dramatically decreases that risk. Infertility also increases the risk of uterine cancer and even breast cancer. Infertile women who get pregnant after being treated with Clomid or Pergonal have no greater risk of ovarian cancer, or any other cancer, than a normal population. It was only women who failed to get pregnant who had this increased risk. Using these drugs *does not increase* the risk of ovarian cancer. Infertility increases that risk, and if these drugs overcome your infertility and help you get pregnant, then they will have decreased rather than increased your risk of getting ovarian cancer.

Furthermore, a detailed National Institutes of Health (NIH) study that has been ongoing for more than a decade now has demonstrated no increase in cases of ovarian cancer in women whose infertility was treated by IVF.

### *Multiple Births and Selective Reduction*

With any infertility treatment designed to stimulate ovulation, there is a risk of multiple births. Twins create obstetrical problems, but the couple is usually happy with such an outcome. Triplets are very risky but are manageable with extensive and expensive modern obstetrics and pediatric care. Quadruplets or quintuplets are an extremely dangerous complication. The likelihood of such multiple births is low, but if it occurs, it can be a disaster. The odds are that many such children will die or be severely retarded, and the mother runs a much greater risk of danger to her life and health as well. Any couple entering treatment for infertility must be aware of this risk, however small it may be.

The doctor can keep the risk of multiple births low by not administering HCG if the woman has a huge number of follicles. However, it should be understood that going to a GIFT or IVF procedure reduces the risk of multiple pregnancies because although the doctor obtains the eggs from every follicle, the doctor puts back only the number that he or she thinks would safely give the best chance of pregnancy. Therefore, IVF should dramatically reduce the risk of multiple pregnancy caused by ovarian stimulation.

Another option, which every couple must think about carefully and decide on ahead of time, is selective reduction. With modern ultrasound techniques, the embryonic sac can be detected as early as three to five weeks after fertilization. The ultrasonographer can very easily insert a needle and terminate any dangerous extra sacs. To some, such a procedure might carry a moral or ethical problem, and each couple will have to decide whether they will take advantage of this modern option that could convert the potential tragedy of quintuplets into the joy of healthy twins. Most religious leaders who have pondered this problem have decided that since selective reduction salvages the lives of at least two of the fetuses, and reduces dramatically the obstetric risks to the mother, it is ethically justifiable. But it is emotionally difficult, and to some it may still be morally repugnant. Selective reduction is certainly not ethically or medically acceptable if too many eggs or embryos are routinely replaced, or if it occurs frequently. It is only medically acceptable if there is just the occasional case (perhaps 1 percent or less) where too many embryos unexpectedly implant. Nonetheless, every couple must decide beforehand whether it is psychologically or morally acceptable to them. If it is not, then they should not have more than two or at most three embryos replaced. But if selective reduction is an acceptable moral option for them, then in cases of an older woman, or one with poor embryo quality, replacing more than two or three embryos would improve the chances of pregnancy.

### *Subsequent Pregnancies Without Treatment*

Problems with a woman's hormonal cycle that were corrected with gonadotropin stimulation sometimes remain corrected for subsequent cycles. Once the ovary gets stimulated properly, it may continue to respond normally to the body's own FSH. The most remarkable example of this in our practice was a woman in her early thirties who had been trying to get pregnant for eight years. When we put her through an HMG stimulation cycle for IVF, we found that all of her follicles were completely empty and devoid of eggs. We tried again in a second cycle, this time using very large doses of HMG.

We were finally able to get five good eggs from her ovaries after the fourth cycle of treatment. Three of those five eggs fertilized in vitro with her husband's sperm, but unfortunately, she did not get pregnant during that cycle. We were all very sad because so much effort had gone into those four cycles of massive gonadotropin therapy. But she became pregnant on her own the very next month. This is a dramatic example of gonadotropin stimulation correcting an ovarian problem (of which we have a very poor understanding).

Of course, this does not happen in the majority of cases. Most couples need to come back and go through ovarian stimulation and IVF again to get pregnant. But the fact that some couples have a permanent correction of their problem indicates that there are some mysteries about ovarian function that we still don't understand.

CHAPTER 9

# IVF (In Vitro Fertilization)

On a Tuesday evening, July 25, 1978, at 11:47 p.m., the world's first human test-tube baby was born. Louise Brown was a beautiful, normal, five-pound, twelve-ounce girl with blond hair and blue eyes. Dr. Robert Edwards and Dr. Patrick Steptoe, in a little clinic near Manchester, England, were responsible for this giant step forward into the "brave new world." Dr. Edwards's first statement upon seeing the child was, "The last time I saw the baby it was just eight cells in a test tube. It was beautiful then and it is still beautiful now." The child's mother, Leslie Brown, and father, John Brown, had been married for nine years and were unable to have children. The problem was that Leslie's tubes were so badly destroyed by scars and inflammation that surgery could not help her. Her ovaries and her uterus were normal, however, and all that was required was to take an egg from her ovary, mix it with her husband's sperm in a test tube, and then transfer the three-day-old embryo into her womb to grow for the next nine months into a full-term baby.

This achievement was the culmination of twelve years of painstaking research by the two doctors. Their experiments had involved an incredibly complicated variety of techniques, which had to be tested over and over again in animals before being tried in humans. Determining the composition of the fluid in which the sperm and egg were to be bathed, figuring out the best time to remove and then implant the egg, and establishing how to monitor the hormone levels of the mother prior to the retrieval of the egg all required years of patient effort. Their work was not funded by the medical hierarchy, and even after their first successful result, they were ridiculed because it was so difficult at first to make it happen again. Drs. Steptoe and Edwards courageously ushered in a new era, making it possible today for virtually any couple to have a baby.

As with all other advances relating to reproduction — no matter what politicians, theologians, and medical critics may think — test-tube fertilization has been widely accepted by the public. IVF is now the dominant form of therapy for childless couples. Research in this area was severely retarded in the United States because in the 1970s, under the Carter administration, federal support for research into IVF was halted for fear that IVF was unethical. Therefore, most of our early knowledge in this field had to be imported from Europe and Australia. The U.S. government refused to recognize IVF, and the first IVF clinic in America (in Norfolk, Virginia), which was completely privately funded, had to go through tremendous obstacles to get permission to open. Political activists protested IVF because they felt it "tampered with nature." But infertile couples continued to support this developing field despite no government research funding whatsoever. Now, because of privately funded improvements, IVF is the most successful treatment available for infertility today.

I wrote in a series of predictions in my first book in 1981:

> Now that we have already stepped over into that brave new world, think of the other possibilities. What if a woman has had a hysterectomy? She has no uterus at all, but does have normal ovaries and a fertile husband. It would now be possible to remove one of her eggs through the laparoscope, fertilize it in a culture dish with her husband's sperm, and then implant this new embryo into another woman, who could act as a "surrogate" mother. Then when the baby is delivered nine months later, it could be turned over to the mother who originally provided the egg. From the opposite point of view, what if a woman had a perfectly normal uterus and a fertile husband, but her ovaries were incapable of producing eggs? An egg could be extracted from a donor through the laparoscope, fertilized with her husband's sperm, and then implanted into her own uterus.

Now such treatment is commonplace and can be done in a nonoperative setting. Almost 5 percent of all children born in Europe today are the result of IVF. Most important, for all types of infertility, not just the dramatic ones described above, the success rate is so good with this technology that most infertile couples are more likely than ever to achieve their dream.

## Improvement in IVF Pregnancy Rates

All IVF-type procedures are referred to in general as ART, or assisted reproductive technology. When Steptoe and Edwards first reported on IVF, the pregnancy rate per cycle was no more than 2 percent. This made it simply an exotic procedure, too expensive for most, that was not likely to result in very many happy couples. Even in the mid-1980s, the pregnancy rate per cycle (meaning the couple took home a baby) was still only about 8 percent. An occasional program boasted 15 percent. So although IVF was an exciting new horizon for infertility treatment, it remained a curiosity for most patients, and indeed, in the eyes of most fertility specialists, it took a backseat to plodding, conventional treatments. What led to the sensational popularity of ART and the rapid establishment of IVF clinics was the improvement in pregnancy rates as a result of a variety of technical modifications.

With classic IVF, sperm and eggs were mixed in a culture dish and put in an incubator, where the eggs were allowed to fertilize. Two days later, the fertilized egg, or embryo, was replaced in the woman's uterus (see fig. 9.1). Fertilization in a petri dish was not a problem. The frustrating stumbling block to the wider success of IVF was not in getting fertilization to occur, but rather in getting the transferred embryo to implant in the uterus and result in a pregnancy. Hundreds of thousands of fertilizations were accomplished in IVF laboratories around the world in the 1980s, but when those precious embryos were replaced in the uterus, only a small percentage of them were able to implant and become babies. We now understand this dilemma much better and have dramatically increased pregnancy rates.

Gamete intrafallopian transfer (GIFT) was the first attempt to solve the implantation problem. With GIFT, everything proceeded the same way as with classic IVF except that sperm and eggs were placed directly into the fallopian tube (rather than in a laboratory culture dish) and allowed to fertilize there, so that the fallopian tube would then move the embryo down into the uterus at the appropriate time via natural processes. It had been questioned then whether embryos could get the same nutrition in a laboratory petri dish that they would receive in the fallopian tube. If this fear were well founded, then certainly the best place for the embryo from the very beginning of its inception would be the fallopian tube. Remarkably, the pregnancy rate with GIFT in the 1980s was dramatically better (35 to 40 percent) than that of conventional IVF.

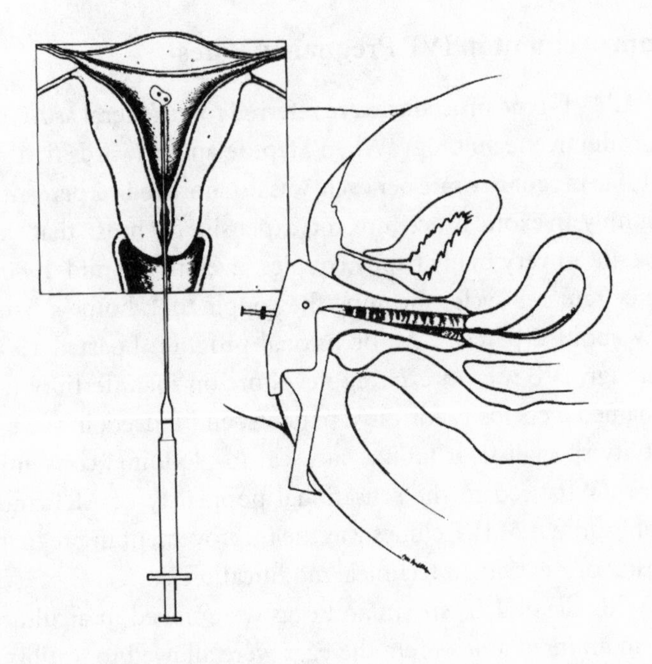

**FIGURE 9.1**

**In classic IVF, fertilized eggs, or embryos, are placed without surgery directly into the uterus, and the fallopian tubes are not involved.**

That was the original rationale for GIFT's rise to popularity in the mid-1980s and early 1990s. The obvious problems with GIFT were that (1) there was no way to ensure that fertilization had occurred or to evaluate embryo quality, and (2) it required a surgical procedure. There were two reasons that GIFT resulted in dramatically higher pregnancy rates, and those two reasons are now utilized to make IVF pregnancy rates almost equivalent: (1) the embryo's nutritional requirements for the first three days (while in the tube) are different from those over the next three days (in the uterus), and (2) the slightest irritation of the uterus by a catheter works just like a contraceptive IUD, and prevents implantation.

One of the remaining advantages of GIFT is that Catholic couples can follow the papal injunction against IVF. The Catholic church still fully approves of GIFT because the papacy prefers that fertilization of the egg take place inside the body rather than in a petri dish. A variation of GIFT, called ZIFT (zygote intrafallopian transfer), was devised to solve the problem of not knowing whether the eggs fertilized. With ZIFT, the eggs are first fertilized in a petri dish; the resultant embryos are then transferred two days later into the fallopian tube. However, today, IVF pregnancy rates are so much improved that GIFT and ZIFT are only occasionally preferable.

IVF pregnancy rates per treatment cycle are now averaging 50 percent in good centers, and if you are relatively young and have a high ovarian reserve, pregnancy rates of over 65 percent per treatment cycle are routine in the best centers. With older patients, pregnancy rates are lower. It is obvious that overall pregnancy rates are much higher now than they were in the mideighties, when the average pregnancy rate for IVF was 8 percent and when the very best programs boasted pregnancy rates of only 15 percent. Despite taking on many low-prognosis cases, our center's overall pregnancy rate for women under thirty-eight years of age, whether favorable or unfavorable cases, is 55 percent per cycle. For the rest of this chapter, I would like to explain how IVF has been improved over the last five to fifteen years so that you will have enough information to determine where you should go for help.

### *Ovarian Stimulation Protocols and Egg Retrieval*

IVF can be divided into three phases. First is the use of drugs for ovarian stimulation to obtain mature eggs, along with the ultrasound-guided retrieval of those eggs at exactly the right time. Second are the IVF laboratory techniques for manipulating and culturing eggs and embryos, as well as freezing extra embryos. Third is the technique for transferring those embryos back into the uterus with minimal irritation so that they will have the best possible chance of implanting.

The first and primary step is to obtain good-quality eggs. As I discussed in the previous chapter, it is clear that a larger dose of gonadotropin should be given during the first five days because that is when egg recruitment truly begins. After those first five days, the follicles that have been recruited are already sensitized to FSH, so the actual dose of FSH is not that important in making sure good-quality eggs are obtained. Therefore, if on your first day of monitoring, after four or five days of gonadotropin, your estrogen level has gone very high, or you have too large a recruitment of follicles, the dose can be reduced until the lead follicles become mature over the next four to six days. This so-called step-down protocol has worked much better than starting with an initial low dose of gonadotropin and then having to increase it later (step-up).

Another major factor in obtaining good-quality eggs is prevention of an early LH surge and premature ovulation. The introduction of

Lupron to prevent this LH surge and to allow "controlled" ovarian hyperstimulation, combined with the step-down protocol, caused an immediate improvement in pregnancy rates in the late 1980s. Good programs now prefer a long-phase Lupron protocol, which ensures that the pituitary is not secreting too much LH during the early recruitment phase, when gonadotropin stimulation begins.

A new avenue of stimulation that accomplishes results similar to that of long-phase Lupron is simply to avoid Lupron altogether, begin stimulation with gonadotropin only, and then watch the follicle size closely so that a GnRH antagonist (brand names Cetrotide and Antagon) can be administered before the follicles get too big, to prevent a premature LH surge and premature ovulation. Using a GnRH antagonist accomplishes the same result as long-phase Lupron. All of these successful stimulation protocols are based on the same overriding principle: Make sure there is a small amount of LH and a maximal administration of FSH during the first five recruitment days of the stimulation cycle, and continue to stimulate the ovary (without fear of premature LH surge and ovulation) until the follicles are fully mature.

Transvaginal ultrasound-guided needle aspiration for egg retrieval has been perfected for quite some time. However, it is clear that in the last decade, anesthesiologists have become much more skilled at so-called conscious sedation. There are some programs that use a general anesthetic to put the patient completely to sleep for egg retrieval. There are other programs that administer no sedation other than the standard premedication injection. Neither of those approaches is as comfortable for the patient as conscious sedation with a board-certified anesthesiologist or anesthetist. With conscious sedation, the patient is as awake as she wants to be, and she can watch the ultrasound screen to actually see her follicle aspiration if she cares to. The patient has an IV in place, and if she feels the slightest discomfort (which is highly variable from patient to patient), the anesthetist or anesthesiologist who is sitting right next to her can administer exactly the right amount of sedation (usually propofol or Versed) she needs to be comfortable. With this conscious sedation approach, the woman does not feel drugged and can leave the hospital with her husband very soon after the procedure with no uncomfortable side effects such as nausea, vomiting, or grogginess. The whole experience, therefore, becomes much more pleasant and less anxiety provoking.

### *Egg and Embryo Culturing Techniques*

The details of laboratory IVF techniques and embryo culturing will be covered in the next chapter. This chapter will provide a simple overview of what improvements have been made in these areas — improvements every good IVF program should be employing — to give the very highest pregnancy rates.

In the old days, we used to prepare all of our own culture media. Culture media is simply the fluid in which the eggs and the sperm are maintained in the laboratory and in which the fertilized eggs and subsequent embryos can best develop and grow. Therefore, the culture media must include the purest water, usually triple distilled, without any trace ingredients whatsoever that could be toxic to the embryo. Added to this water is a proper mix of sugar, electrolytes and salts, amino acids, and proteins that best mimic the natural conditions the embryos and eggs would find in the fallopian tubes and uterus. Such media was available for tissue culture long before there was IVF. However, labs that were involved in the time-consuming chore of mixing their own media were so distracted from their primary work, IVF embryo culture, that quality control was a real problem. So perhaps the most important advance in IVF culture media is the fact that almost any good IVF program now purchases their media from competitive distributors, companies that are devoted to rigorously controlling their media batch production. Furthermore, any good IVF program today is under unprecedented regulation and oversight by the Society for Assisted Reproductive Technology (SART), the College of American Pathologists (CAP), and the Centers for Disease Control (CDC). Although this regulation is not very useful per se, it sets up an administrative reminder that the good laboratories are very happy to follow — to keep meticulous records of results and quality-control testing of the media.

In the same respect, most good laboratories are now paying very close attention to air quality. We had observed in the early 1990s that whenever there was driveway construction outside the hospital, or wallpapering or remodeling going on anywhere within the vicinity of the operating room or laboratory area, our pregnancy rates plummeted. Therefore, we are meticulous about knowing the schedule of any kind of construction or driveway work going on within the entire vicinity of the hospital and do not schedule IVF cycles during such times. More important, however, we have state-of-the-art air-filtration systems, both in our laboratory and within each incubator. Any potentially toxic element that could be in the atmosphere is filtered out so that the air quality in which we work and in which the embryos are cultured is guaranteed to be pure.

The formulation of ingredients in the culture media now is more carefully in sync with the actual needs of the eggs and the embryos during each day of development. This improvement in tailoring the media specifically to the day of development is called sequential media. Again, the details of the media will be covered in the next chapter, but the key breakthrough in embryo culture in this new millennium is that the early embryo, during the first three days of development, requires no glucose whatsoever for its energy metabolism and, in fact, prefers an energy source called pyruvate. Reducing or eliminating the glucose from the media by putting it in a very low concentration of 0.5 millimole per liter, at most, makes it more consistent with the fluid in which the embryo is normally bathed in the fallopian tube during its first three days. It is only after day three, the eight-cell stage of the embryo, that further development is benefited by having a high concentration of glucose (up to as high as 6.1 millimoles per liter) as well as an increase in pyruvate (instead of 0.33, an entire 1.0 millimole per liter). In addition, after the eight-cell stage, the embryo requires a whole variety of amino acids and vitamins that do not really help in the first three days of development. This modern understanding of the embryo's metabolic requirements in culture has allowed us to mimic more closely the environment found in nature. It has not only improved our routine IVF pregnancy rates, but has even allowed us to culture embryos to days five or six, giving us time to make a genetic analysis of the embryos (which will be discussed in a later chapter).

The next area of improvement in laboratory technique is an awareness of how important it is for all environmental conditions of the cultured embryo to remain constant. A little droplet of media containing an embryo can evaporate, change temperature, and even "go flat" (an analogy to what happens to a glass of Coca-Cola if allowed to stand out for a while before drinking). Just taking the petri dish containing the embryo out of the incubator to look at it under the microscope can result in a drop in the temperature, some evaporation (and, therefore, change in concentration of ingredients), and a release of carbon dioxide

($CO_2$) (which is what happens to a carbonated beverage when it goes flat), changing the acidity dramatically. Good laboratories are much more attentive now to the possibility of such changes and guard against them in several ways.

Every single microscope and every single tabletop upon which the petri dish is placed temporarily (either to view it or to manipulate the embryo) has a heating block with a digitally controlled temperature of 37 degrees centrigrade (98.6 degrees Fahrenheit). The temperature must be kept at this exact, constant level, the temperature at which your body would normally maintain the embryo. Particularly for the egg, any minute drop in temperature can damage its chromosomal spindle apparatus. Furthermore, nowadays, almost any good laboratory will culture the embryos in individual microdroplets with a pure oil overlay. Test tubes are virtually never used anymore, and open petri dishes are unacceptable. The pure oil overlay, which requires some extra work, keeps the temperature more constant and prevents the slightest evaporation even during the short periods of time that the embryos are out of the incubator.

Even the opening and closing of the incubator door can allow carbon dioxide and heat to escape, and it might take a few minutes for the incubator's automatic temperature and $CO_2$ injection systems to return to normal settings. Thus, to prevent too much opening or closing of the incubator door, small desktop incubators are positioned right by the microscope so that several embryos at a time can be looked at or manipulated while kept at a constant temperature, pH, and humidity. In fact, good laboratories will not even take the embryos out to monitor their development on relatively unimportant days, such as day two or day four. They will only be viewed the day after aspiration to check for normal fertilization, and just prior to transfer on day three, or day five.

Incredibly close attention must be paid to the acidity of the media, which can change within seconds. Let me explain. When a bottle of Coca-Cola is opened up, you begin to see bubbles come out of the solution. These are carbon dioxide bubbles that are released from the solution when the bottle is opened and the pressure is reduced. This carbon dioxide dissolved in fluid forms carbonic acid, a very weak acid that provides the twang in the taste. As the carbon dioxide evaporates and bubbles away from the open bottle of Coca-Cola, the acid content of the Coca-Cola begins to go down. Once the $CO_2$ evaporates from the fluid, what is left in the place of carbonic acid ($H_2CO_3$) is simply water ($H_2O$).

The reason this is important for all cell culture, whether embryos or any other cells, is that bicarbonate ($HCO_3$) is absolutely critical for all cellular metabolism. The Krebs cycle is the chemical system that allows every cell in our body to utilize oxygen to create energy. The Krebs cycle is completely dependent on the presence of bicarbonate. Thus, no cell can survive in culture media without bicarbonate ($HCO_3$). However, this bicarbonate will always be evaporating as $CO_2$. In our bodies, we manage this complex system by breathing off $CO_2$ via our lungs. If we did not breathe off this $CO_2$, our bodies would become too acidic. For cell culture in petri dishes, this mechanism doesn't work. Thus, for more than fifty years, biologists have been careful to make sure that the media (which contains the bicarbonate necessary for cell development) is kept in an atmosphere of 5 percent carbon dioxide ($CO_2$). It is this 5 percent concentration of $CO_2$ in the incubator that keeps the acidity (or the pH) of the culture media constant. When the petri dish is removed from the incubator and is in the atmosphere of the laboratory (which contains very little $CO_2$), $CO_2$ evaporates from the media rapidly, and although you don't even notice it, the alkalinity of the media is rising above neutral as the $CO_2$ invisibly evaporates. This will quickly and silently kill the egg or the embryo, or any other cell in culture.

There are three ways to prevent this surreptitious and rapid rise in alkalinity of the media. The first is to maintain exactly the right percentage of $CO_2$ in the incubator that will allow the pH to stay just below the neutral 7.4. Thus, if the embryos are taken out of the incubator for a few moments, the pH might rise slightly, up to the neutral 7.4, but will still remain in a safe range. The second way is to always use oil overlays, which will retard the $CO_2$ from evaporating. An oil overlay gives you an extra ten or fifteen minutes with which to manipulate the embryos. The third way is to make use of desktop incubators, through which 5 percent $CO_2$ is always flowing, whenever the embryos are out of the main incubator. Finally, for prolonged periods of manipulation, which might be as long as a half an hour, the eggs or embryos are placed into a culture media that contains very little bicarbonate, and has a different type of acid-based pH buffer, called Hepes. Embryos should not be cultured in this nonbicarbonate-containing Hepes-buffered media for longer than an hour, because the embryos, over the long haul, will always need bicarbonate for their metabolism. However, for short periods of time, up to an hour, a Hepes buffer allows one to work with the embryos, whether injecting sperm, doing an embryo biopsy, or performing any other type of manipulation, with no fear that there will be a change in pH. So, the next time you drink a glass of flat cola or any other carbonated beverage, you will understand the importance in an IVF laboratory of rigidly maintaining the pH (acidity) of the media at a constant, normal biological level.

### *Intracytoplasmic Sperm Injection (ICSI)*

One of the biggest problems with IVF throughout the 1980s and in the early 1990s was "failure of fertilization." This was most commonly a problem in couples where the men had very low sperm counts or poor sperm motility or morphology. However, it was also a problem with a small number of cases in which there was no apparent defect in the sperm count. The most frustrating aspect of IVF in these early days was failure of the sperm to fertilize the egg. This was solved in 1992 and 1993 in Brussels, in collaboration with our microsurgery team from St. Louis. The procedure developed is frequently referred to as ICSI or, for the severest sperm defects, TESE-ICSI. This simply means that instead of allowing the sperm to fertilize eggs on their own within a microdroplet in a petri dish, individual sperm are selected in a microscopic pipette, which is completely invisible to the naked eye, and are injected directly into the egg. (ICSI will be discussed in detail in chapter 11.)

We are now performing ICSI so flawlessly that we are no longer afraid of harming the eggs at all and are quite willing to perform it for every single case of IVF, not just those cases in which there is known male infertility. By doing this we can be sure that any problem the sperm might have in fertilizing the egg, whether obvious or not, will be routinely overcome as a standard part of the IVF procedure. Some might be afraid that ICSI is a risk that should only be taken with clear-cut cases of male infertility. But very careful studies in both Brussels and St. Louis have demonstrated that ICSI represents no increased risk, but by using ICSI for all cases, failed fertilization of normal eggs is a virtually nonexistent problem. In our program, there is no extra charge or fee for ICSI because we feel that it is a routine part of good IVF procedure.

### *Longer Culturing*

In the early days of IVF the embryos would routinely be transferred back to the patient, either to the uterus or the fallopian tube, as soon as possible, usually on day two, when they are normally two to four cells.

The thinking was that the sooner the embryos got back into the patient, the safer they would be because of fears about the inadequacy of laboratory culture methods. It is now routine to transfer the embryos back to the woman on day three, when they normally should be at somewhere between six and eight cells. The major advantage of transferring embryos to the uterus on day three is that of "embryo selection." Day-three embryos more clearly indicate by their appearance whether they are likely to go on to become normal pregnancies than day-two embryos. On day two the embryo may very well be only two cells, and therefore appear to be slow in developing, yet by day three it could be a normal eight-cell embryo with a high prognosis. On the other hand, an embryo on day two could appear to be at a properly developing four-cell stage, yet it may arrest at that stage, never to develop into a proper eight-cell embryo on day three.

Our laboratory culture conditions are so precise now that we have no problem keeping the embryos in culture in the laboratory for up to five days. There are those who have argued since the late 1990s in favor of routinely culturing the embryos to day five. By this so-called test of extra culturing, the better embryos could more easily be selected as those that continue to develop to the day five blastocyst stage. However, most laboratories choose embryos on day three to transfer, freeze the healthy-appearing embryos on day three, and only culture on to day five those embryos they are not sure will develop. Pregnancy rates are clearly not improved by day-five transfer as opposed to day-three transfer, whereas pregnancy rates were dramatically improved by switching from day-two transfer to day-three transfer. The few IVF programs that routinely culture to day five and report good results are selecting out only those patients with a very high ovarian reserve and very good-quality embryos on day three. For more difficult cases, even the enthusiasts for blastocyst culture will transfer at day three rather than day five.

### *Assisted Hatching*

The embryo normally sits around in the uterus making no effort to implant until around day six. Until day six, the embryo keeps growing within its very tough zona pellucida (outer shell). But on day five or six, that zona pellucida begins to thin out, and the embryo eventually hatches, just like a chicken out of an eggshell. At this moment of hatching, the embryo, now called a blastocyst, implants into the uterine lin-

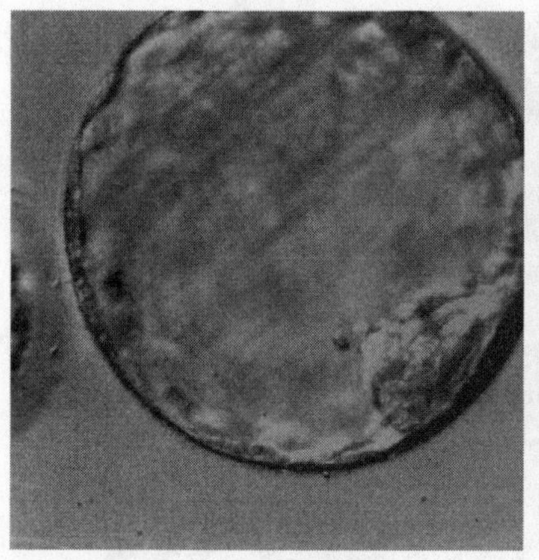

**FIGURE 9.2.** Day five: blastocyst.

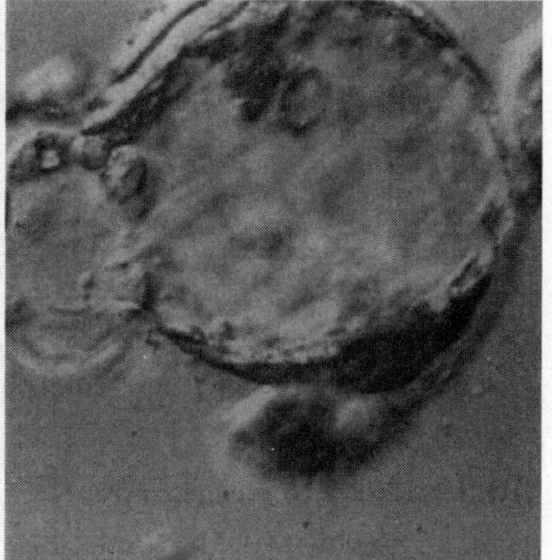

**FIGURE 9.3.** Day six: hatching blastocyst.

ing, the endometrium. It is then, around day seven after fertilization, that pregnancy actually occurs, and this free-floating ball of cells finally becomes a part of the mother.

In figures 9.2 and 9.3 you can see the process whereby the day-five, blastocyst-stage embryo has thinned its outer zona pellucida completely and then begins to hatch. The embryo at this stage, between day five and day seven, simply has to escape from that thick outer wall that up until now protected it much like the shell of a bird's egg. However, the great deal of energy expended by the embryo during this natural hatching process can result in lower pregnancy rates. That is why we routinely perform assisted hatching on all of our embryos just before we transfer them on day three.

Figures 9.4 through 9.7 demonstrate what assisted hatching accomplishes. You can readily perceive how important this could be for improving pregnancy rates. In figure 9.4 you see an embryo on day six — the zona pellucida has thinned out so much that the embryo is just beginning to break through a leak in that thinned-out shell. Natural hatching is just beginning to occur.

With assisted hatching on day three, just prior to transferring the embryo into the woman's uterus, a small slit is made in the outer shell. It can be done mechanically with a microscopic needle, chemically with an acid Tyrode's solution directed only at this one spot, or with a microscopic laser. Each of these three methods creates an opening in the zona pellucida so that the embryo can hatch three days later without using its energy to thin out the outer shell.

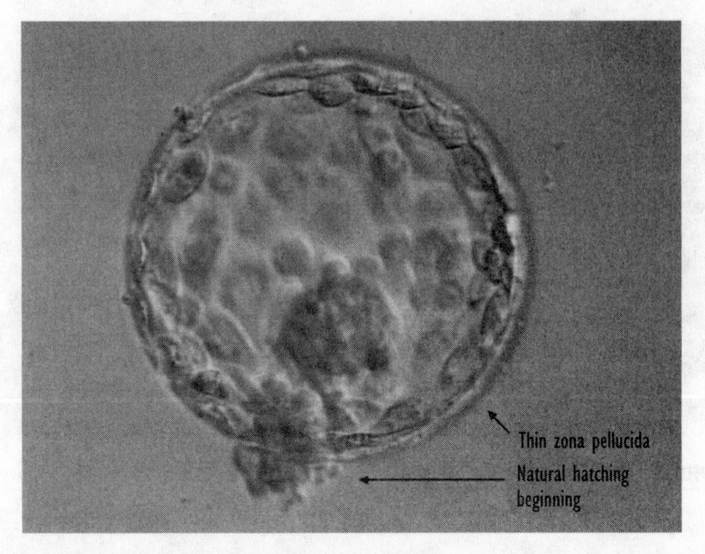


FIGURE 9.4. Naturally hatching blastocyst.

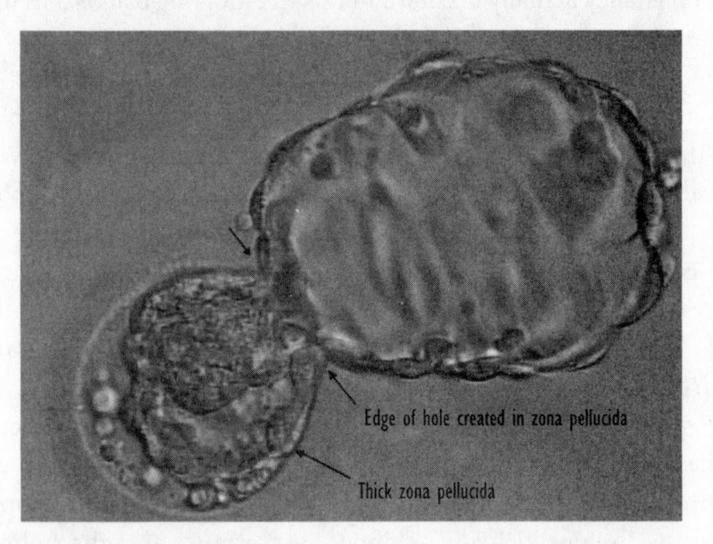


FIGURE 9.5. Assisted hatching: first stage.

Figure 9.5 demonstrates the beginning of the blastocyst hatching from an embryo that underwent assisted hatching several days earlier. Note that the zona pellucida is still thick and has not been thinned out by the embryo's own energy. Rather, you can see the embryo starting to escape from its shell via the opening that was made three days earlier. Figure 9.6 shows the embryo almost completely hatched from the zona

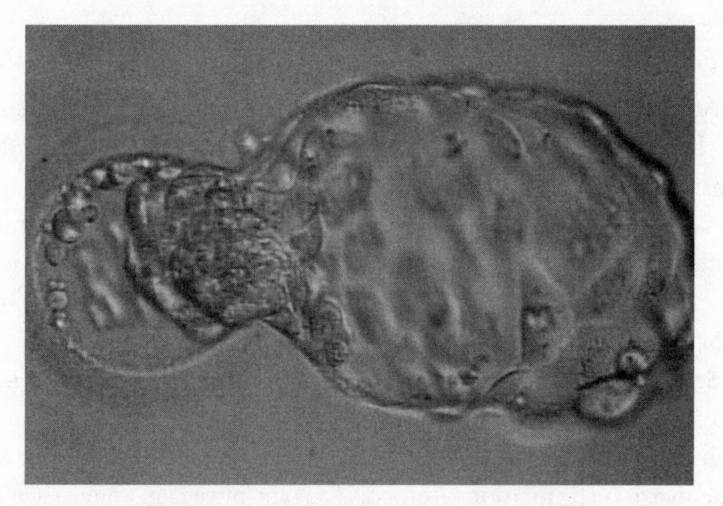

**FIGURE 9.6.** Assisted hatching: second stage.

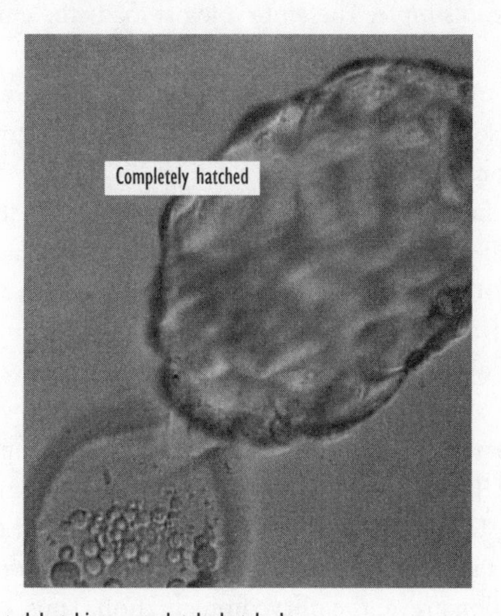


**FIGURE 9.7.** Assisted hatching: completely hatched.

pellucida. Figure 9.7 exhibits the completely hatched blastocyst free of its constraining zona pellucida, and ready to implant into the uterine wall. These figures demonstrate lucidly the tremendous benefit of routinely making an opening in the zona pellucida prior to embryo transfer so that when the embryo is ready to implant it doesn't have any difficulty escaping from its confines.

### *Embryo Transfer*

After all of the work that the patient, her physicians, and the laboratory have put into reaching the point when the embryos are ready to be transferred back to the woman, it is tragic how little attention many physicians pay to doing this transfer correctly. In fact, of all the improvements that have increased IVF pregnancy rates, the most important reason may be that closer attention is being paid to the technique of embryo transfer into the woman's uterus.

Several centers have discreetly kept track of differences in pregnancy rate related to different physicians performing the embryo transfer. With the same laboratory, the same population of patients, and the same ovarian stimulation protocols, certain physicians have very high pregnancy rates, and others have very low pregnancy rates. The transfer process seems so simple. The embryologist loads the embryos under a microscope into a little catheter, and the physician simply places that catheter into the woman's uterus through her cervix and injects the embryos. Yet some physicians consistently have very good results and some very poor results.

If there is any uterine irritation whatsoever during the transfer, the chance that an embryo will implant is much reduced. This is easy to understand if you think about the simplest contraceptive method of all, i.e., the IUD (intrauterine device). The mere placement of a painless, nonobtrusive object (which is what an IUD is) of any kind into the uterus is a safe and effective contraceptive with a very low failure rate. In fact, if a woman has had intercourse while not on a contraceptive, she can have an IUD put into her uterus the very next day, and she will not get pregnant. Despite some claims to the contrary, the way an IUD works is that it sets up the most minor, painless irritation in the uterus, and this irritation prevents embryo implantation. Thus, any irritation to the uterus caused by an embryo transfer would act temporarily like an IUD and prevent implantation.

In addition to the physician's gentle technique, the next most important feature to embryo transfer is to use an extremely soft "wet noodle" type of catheter. The slightest stiffness in the catheter (which makes it much easier to insert) will be irritative to the uterus. We prefer the Wallace catheter because it is so incredibly soft and also has a microscopically machined tip, which prevents the inadvertent leakage of any fluid until the moment of injection. The difficulty with the Wallace catheter (which is an old device), and what kept it from being popular for so many years, is that it is not as easy to place through the cervical canal as any of the stiffer catheters, which were most popular in the eighties and nineties. The Wallace catheter is so soft that it will not go in unless the cervix is completely relaxed, and the physician must have a very, very fine fingertip touch to maneuver it. There is an outer stiff sheath that can be used to place the catheter initially into the opening of the cervix, but that stiff sheath must never be placed into the uterus itself because of the irritation that it would cause. Many physicians are tempted to do this in what they find to be a "difficult" transfer, but that is always a mistake. Always. Whether it appears to be a difficult transfer or not, the physician must be patient and quiet, not in a hurry and not nervous, until he or she can eventually slowly guide the soft "wet noodle" inner catheter into the uterus.

The patient must also be quiet and relaxed. This is very seldom recognized by the physician and is very often poorly handled in large, commercial-style IVF programs. The patient's cervix is a sphincter, which is designed to keep everything but sperm from getting in and, during pregnancy, to hold the baby within. In fact, a weak cervix (called incompetent) is a common cause of miscarriage between the fourteenth and twentieth week of pregnancy. Thus, it is important to recognize that this cervix, the muscular canal that leads into the uterus, is a sphincter just like your rectal or bladder sphincter. This sphincter is under the unconscious but powerful control of your emotions. If you are anxious, tense, or the atmosphere is emotionally stressful, your cervix is very likely to contract, making the embryo transfer more difficult.

A difficult embryo transfer is never caused by cervical stenosis, i.e., some sort of intrinsic blockage in your cervix. If you had such a problem your menstrual bleeding could never get out, and that would be a deadly situation. It is a complete misconception on the part of many physicians that a difficult transfer is related to the cervical anatomy. Certainly there could be more or less of a curve in the cervix, which might require a certain amount of delicacy on the physician's part. However, the single most important factor in making the transfer delicate and easy is the patient's ability to relax. I have explained some of the relaxation techniques we teach to our patients in chapter 6.

## Improving IVF Results When There Is Tubal Disease

For women with diseased fallopian tubes, an IVF transfer of the embryos directly into the uterus gives a lower pregnancy rate than IVF in patients with normal tubes. There are several possible reasons for this reduction in pregnancy rate in women with poor-quality fallopian tubes. One is that damaged tubes may leak toxic substances into the uterus, which can hurt the embryos before they can implant. Another explanation is that when the embryos are placed in the uterus, they will often migrate back into the fallopian tubes for several days before once again returning to the uterus on day five, prior to implantation. If the tubes are diseased, the embryos will not get proper nurturing in the fallopian tube and, indeed, may never be transmitted back into the uterus. Therefore, many centers are now recommending, in an effort to improve pregnancy rates with IVF in women with diseased fallopian tubes, that these fallopian tubes actually be removed via laparoscopy prior to the IVF procedure. Thus, if the tubes are not good enough to contribute to the pregnancy, they can be bypassed completely.

## Rationale for Doing IVF Sooner in All Cases of Infertility

In a sense, the majority of infertile patients have nothing wrong with them. But even when there is a specific diagnosis, IVF will generally have a higher success rate than conventional treatment. By bypassing all of the normal reproductive processes, it is possible to achieve high pregnancy rates despite not knowing what the problem is. No matter what the apparent cause of infertility, even poor sperm or diseased fallopian tubes, some form of ART is the best chance for getting pregnant (with a few exceptions like vasectomy reversal or tubal ligation reversal).

The monthly pregnancy rate with IVF is so good that it always saddens me to see a couple that has been through years and years of costly and often painful conventional treatment just give up when they are confronted with the amount of money and effort they will have to now put into a single IVF cycle. The hassle of daily tests and shots can be overwhelming after they have already gone through years and years of failed treatment. IVF should be an exciting adventure rather than an ordeal at the end of a long, dark tunnel.

My views on this started with a patient I treated many years ago. She was a nurse who counseled couples on the scientific use of rhythm methods of birth control. She obviously knew her cycle inside and out, and was extremely knowledgeable. Her menstrual cycle was that perfect model chart that you see in the textbooks, with a temperature rise on day fourteen, a drop on day twenty-eight with menstruation, and perfect, regular cycles — she could predict almost to the hour when she expected to start her next period. In fact, all of her studies and her husband's tests were completely normal. Yet even with proper timing of intercourse, making sure they never missed the day or two before she ovulated, for many, many years, they still had not gotten pregnant.

She did not want to go through any of the preliminary treatments like IUI, Parlodel, Clomid, or even HMG plus IUI. She asked point-blank for IVF. I explained to her that this was not our usual pattern and that we would rather put off doing IVF until she had gone through many cycles of HMG and IUI and had had at least several years of conventional therapy. She told me that this was baloney, that she understood everything that was involved, that she had looked at the statistics, and that she did not want to mess around with less-effective remedies just to appease the doctor's sense of guilt. She was a strong feminist and told me exactly what she wanted to have done. I agreed; after the first cycle with IVF, she became pregnant with twins, and we were all quite delighted.

This woman avoided years and years of Clomid plus IUI, Parlodel, laparoscopic surgery for minimal lesion endometriosis, and months and months of HMG plus IUI. She explained to me that if she had to go through all of these other treatments without a pregnancy, she would lose her zeal for pursuing treatment any further. That's why she wanted to go right for the IVF procedure, which carried the highest yield immediately. As it turns out, she was right.

On the other hand, this same woman had a friend she referred to us who had been through three years of Clomid, hysterosalpingograms, and laparoscopic surgery, and nine cycles of HMG and IUI, and she and her husband were fed up. It is understandable that she had been placed on so many cycles of HMG plus IUI, because of an initial diagnosis of irregular menstrual cycles and poor ovulation. Her husband's sperm count was normal, and everything else about her was normal. Yet despite the "reasonableness" of putting her on all of these cycles of ovulatory stimulation, the couple was so exhausted that when she saw us and the option of IVF was presented she had heard all she really wanted to and wasn't going to go through any more. She was emotionally and financially at the end of her rope. The right approach would have been to dispense much earlier with preliminaries and go right for the highest-yield procedure.

Most of the aggravation and expense the patient goes through in an IVF cycle involves the stimulation and monitoring of the ovaries. By the time the patient has been through her Lupron, HMG or FSH, and HCG, along with daily ultrasound and blood estrogen tests, she has already done all of the work. The IVF procedure itself is relatively effortless compared to all of the injections, which are no different than what she would also have to go through for conventional treatment.

Another reason for going to IVF sooner is that with so many infertile couples in their thirties who want to have a child, both the husband and the wife have very responsible positions, and it is often hard to find the time to go through an entire treatment cycle of any kind, without interruption for business trips, meetings, and so forth. Why not give them the best possibility for pregnancy resulting from the ovarian stimulation? It may seem radical to suggest this, but with this kind of couple, why not go to IVF right away and dispense with the prerequisite of many conventional cycles of unsuccessful ovarian stimulation? (For a sample summary chart of a complete IVF cycle, see figure 9.8.)

Patient wants embryo freezing: yes / no / undecided

**month/year** **SART #** ________

___ Cycles of GIFT ___ Cycles of ICSI/IVF

___ Cycles of FET/IVF ___ Cycles of ICSI/ZIFT

___ Cycles of FET/ZIFT ___ Cycles of IVF

Patient Name: ____________ Age: ___ FSH: ________

Ultrasound to be perfomed on: ________

Day 1 of menses: ________ Birth control pills began: ________

| Day of Week | Date | Cycle Day | Follicle Sizes | | | | E2 Level | LH Level | FSH Level | Uterine Lining | Medication per SJS | Pt. Rcvd. Instructions | |
|---|---|---|---|---|---|---|---|---|---|---|---|---|---|
| | | | # | Right Ovary | Left Ovary | # | | | | | Lup/HMG/HCG Amt. | Date | Initials |
| | | | | | | | | | | | Birth control pills begin. | | |
| | | | | | | | | | | | **Daily Lupron injections begins.**<br>**Last day of birth control pills.** | | |
| | | 1<br>2 | | | | | | | | | Gonadotropins begin | | |
| | | 3<br>4 | | | | | | | | | | | |
| | | 5 | | | | | | | | | | | |
| | | 6 | | | | | | | | | | | |
| | | 7 | | | | | | | | | | | |
| | | 8 | | | | | | | | | | | |
| | | 9 | | | | | | | | | | | |
| | | 10 | | | | | | | | | | | |
| | | 11 | | | | | | | | | | | |
| | | 12 | | | | | | | | | | | |
| | | 13 | | | | | | | | | | | |
| | | 14 | | | | | | | | | | | |
| | | 15 | | | | | | | | | | | |
| | | 16 | | | | | | | | | | | |

Pregnancy test results:

Date/Time Semen Collected:

Pre-Wash Motile Sperm Count:

Post-Wash Motile Sperm Count:

| Sperm Frozen This Cycle: yes / no | Sperm Type: ejac / test / epid |
|---|---|
| # straws: ___ / freeze #: ______ | Sperm Source: partner / donor |

Type of transfer: IVF or ZIFT

Ultrasound findings:

Embryo transfer notes:

Plan per SJS if no pregnancy this cycle:

Ob/Gyn:

| U/S date: | |
|---|---|
| # fetal sacs: | |
| # fetal HB: | |
| Misc. date: | |
| Deliv. date: | |
| # boys born: | |
| # girls born: | |

Rcpt #: ____________

Dbase Entry: STL___M/T___

Sperm Wash Tech: Volume:

Motility:

Motility:

| Egg/Embryo/Blastocyst/ Cryopreservation Info: | # eggs/ embryos | Egg/Emb Quality |
|---|---|---|
| # eggs retrieved | _____ | |
| # eggs inseminated/ICSI | _____ | |
| # eggs fertilized | _____ | |
| # eggs/emb transferred | _____ | |
| overall embryo quality | good / fair / poor | |
| **Existing # Froz D2, D3, Blast** | _____ | |
| # Froz Today D2, D3, Blast | _____ | |
| # D2, D3, Blast Thawed Today | _____ | |
| # Froz Emb/Blast Transferred | _____ | |
| **# Froz Emb/Blast Remaining** | _____ | |

| Freeze list |
|---|
| / |
| BMI = |
| IOV date/time: |
| |
| Sel Red/ Cryo: |
| / |
| ART Cons. Signed |
| yes / no |
| "Y" Chromosome |
| date drawn / results |
| / |
| Karyotyping |
| date drawn / results |
| |

**FIGURE 9.8.** ART summary chart.

CHAPTER 10

# Step-by-Step Details of Your IVF Cycle

Now that you have a general overview of what assisted reproductive technology (ART) offers, and how it is performed with a realistic view of results, I'll try to explain in greater detail what each of the steps of these procedures entails. I suggest that IVF not be viewed as a horrendous ordeal, but rather as an exciting adventure during which you can thrill to the view of your own eggs developing on the television screen of an ultrasound monitor, following every step of the procedure with the same excitement that I look forward to with each patient.

As a former athletics coach of young children, I know how badly they want to win each game, and how seriously disturbing a loss or a failure can be. But I always remind the kids to take each game one at a time. You may not get pregnant in any given cycle, but with the technologies that are available today — IVF, ICSI, egg donation, PGD, or even having someone else carry your genetic baby for you, virtually everyone is able to have a baby. Persistence and keeping an open mind to technology in even the most difficult cases will usually pay off sooner or later.

In a CBS documentary in the 1990s a couple was filmed who had gone through eight previous IVF attempts without a pregnancy. They were still trying, for their ninth time, when many would have given up and might have viewed such an optimistic persistence with bitterness. But that couple did finally get pregnant on their ninth try. The chance of pregnancy per cycle stays just as good (as long as you do not have a diminished reserve of good-quality eggs), even after as many as six or seven previous cycles in which no pregnancy occurred.

I often notice my nurses wince when they hear me sincerely tell patients, "This is the most romantic possible way to get pregnant." Rather than just the casual result of an impulsive toss in the bed, an IVF pregnancy is a truly treasured event. The children arising from such parental efforts tend to be, if anything, more emotionally sound and intellectually alert than their peers, probably because they are so appreciated by their parents. Thus, I hope you will go through the rest of this chapter with the same thrill that I have about witnessing the miracle of fertilization and conception.

## Obtaining the Eggs

In the very early days of IVF, the eggs were always obtained via laparoscopy. This meant that IVF required a surgical procedure to get the eggs, and then the embryos were replaced several days later nonsurgically into the uterus. With the advent of transvaginal ultrasound and transvaginal-guided needle aspiration of the eggs in the late 1980s, all that changed (see figs. 10.1 and 10.2). IVF today is a completely nonsurgical outpatient procedure. The same ultrasound used to monitor ovarian stimulation is used for egg retrieval. The echoes created by the tip of the needle can be seen clearly on the ultrasound machine. Placing the ultrasound probe directly against the ovaries through the vaginal wall, the needle can be inserted right into the follicle. You can actually see the needle puncture the follicle, and as gentle suction is applied, you can see the follicle empty completely.

The egg is not contained in the fluid of the follicle. Rather, the egg sits on a stalk attached to the follicular wall. Thus, the egg is almost never located in the first part of the fluid to come through the needle into the

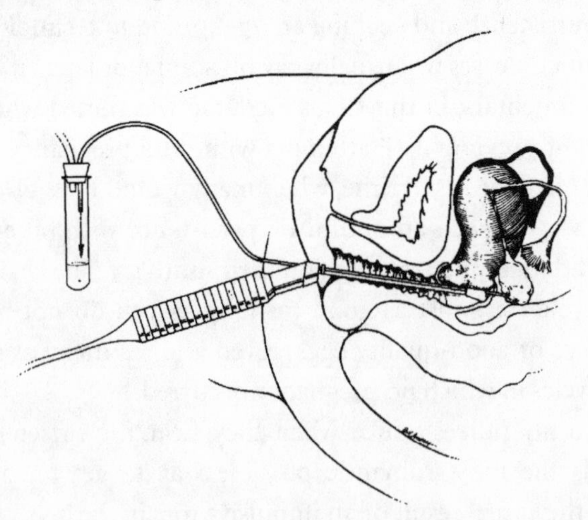

**FIGURE 10.1.** Placement of the ultrasound probe for transvaginal needle aspiration of eggs.

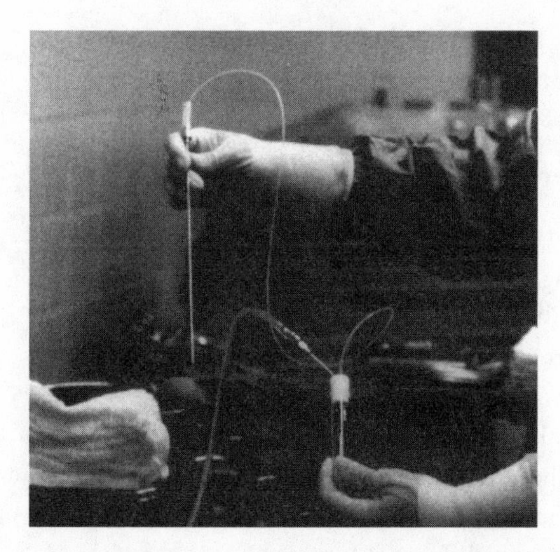

**FIGURE 10.2.** Suction trap and tubing for collecting the eggs.

suction trap. As the follicle wall becomes completely collapsed, the egg gets drawn into the needle only at that point and literally gets pulled off the stalk (see fig. 10.3). The needle is then inserted into the follicle closest to the first one that was punctured. The fluid from the next follicle washes the egg through the needle and tubing into the suction-trap test tube. As this second follicle collapses around the needle, its egg also gets drawn up into the needle. The fluid that is aspirated will either be clear yellow or somewhat bloody. If the fluid is very bloody, it means that this follicle was already aspirated, and is refilling with blood. This is no different from what normally occurs with ovulation. If the fluid is dark brown, it means

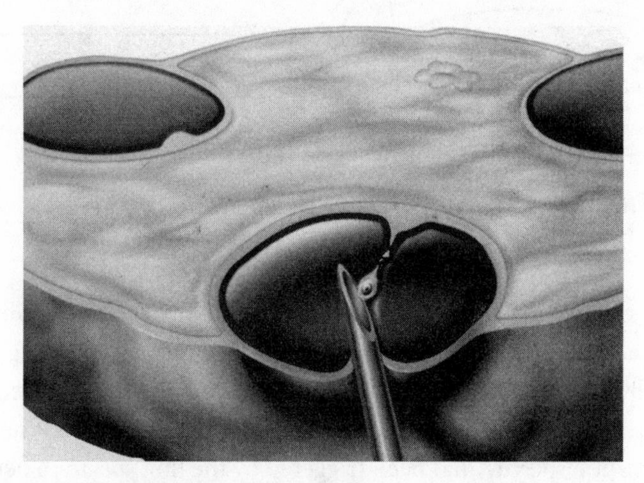

**FIGURE 10.3.** Egg aspiration from an ovarian follicle.

that the follicle was actually an endometrioma, a big cyst of the ovary containing endometriosis tissue. It does not affect pregnancy rate.

## Preparation of the Sperm

Sperm preparation for IVF is no different from what was described in chapter 8 on sperm washing. The husband provides a specimen about two hours before the projected time of the procedure. That allows sufficient time for the sperm to be properly washed, separated, and capacitated.

Just exactly how many sperm should be placed in culture with the egg? As you know, a normal male will ejaculate anywhere from one hundred to three hundred million sperm into the vagina, but only about ten thousand sperm ever make it to the fallopian tube. In the past, about one hundred thousand to one million motile sperm have been placed in a one-cc culture dish or test tube with the eggs for IVF. Today, most good IVF programs culture each egg individually in tiny (thirty thousandths of a cc) microdroplets (see fig. 10.4) with only about three thousand motile sperm placed into each microdroplet.

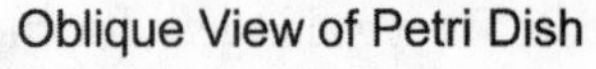


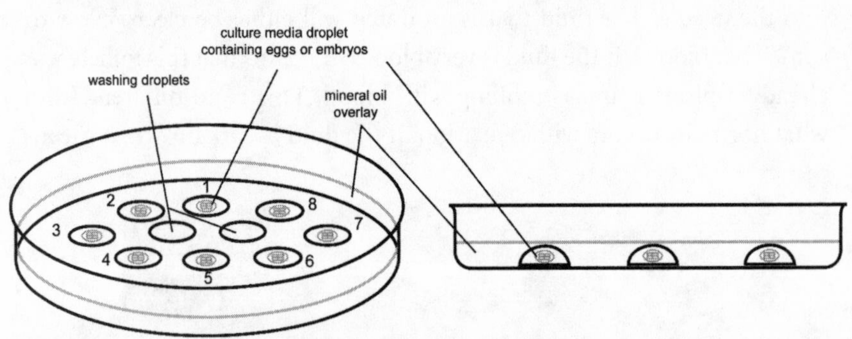


**FIGURE 10.4.** Petri dish setup for IVF culture in microdroplets.

You might ask why we don't put in five million or ten million sperm, just to increase even further the egg-sperm interaction. If the egg is completely overwhelmed by too many sperm, there is a risk that when one of the sperm fertilizes the egg, another sperm will get in before the normal "block to polyspermy" has been triggered by the first sperm to penetrate. In fact, we know that in any conventional IVF procedure, about 5 percent of the eggs will exhibit polyspermy, meaning they have been fertilized by more than one sperm, and will not develop. Polyspermy occurs in a certain percentage of the eggs and is usually caused by an inherent defect in the ability to harden the zona after the first sperm penetrates. Nonetheless, it can also occur if the egg is overwhelmed by millions of sperm (instead of just a few) in the microdroplet.

In the past, if sperm quality was extremely poor with very low motility, it would be common to put many more sperm than three thousand in contact with the egg, to increase the chance for fertilization. Because of ICSI, however, such an approach is now outmoded, and in such cases a single sperm is injected into each egg. I will discuss ICSI in more detail in the next chapter.

## Culture Techniques for Egg and Sperm

### *Culture Media*

Culture media is a fluid that contains the necessary ingredients for proper cell growth outside of the body. A pure, nontoxic culture media with constant acidity, temperature, and no evaporation is critical if the egg, and eventually the embryo, is to survive in the laboratory culture dish or test tube. The egg, sperm, and embryo must reside for the next two to five days in the same type of fluid they would find if they were in the fallopian tube or the uterus.

There are basically two categories of media: bicarbonate-buffered and air-buffered. A buffer is an ingredient that keeps the acidity of the media constant. Acidity is reflected by the pH. The higher the pH, the more alkaline the fluid: the lower the pH, the more acidic the fluid. The pH of all of our bodily fluids and in our cells is 7.4. This is a biological constant. When the acidity, or pH, of the fluid gets above 7.5, most cells, and particularly eggs, will die. When the pH gets below 7.2, the cell will die. The buffer in the media is what keeps this pH at a constant level and prevents its fluctuation. The reason this is necessary is that as a cell metabolizes, it releases acids, and the buffer is the ingredient that absorbs these changes in acidity and keeps the pH constant.

Life would be much easier in the IVF laboratory if all we had to use was air-buffered media, which means the pH stays constant in ordinary room air. The problem with air-buffered media is that the cells can only function in such media for limited periods of time. You cannot expect a cell or embryo to live for hours and days in air-buffered media. They need bicarbonate (baking soda) to live. That is why we have to use bicarbonate-buffered media for all of our culture work, and can only resort to the convenience of air-buffered media for short periods of time in which we are grading, manipulating, or otherwise handling the eggs or embryos outside of the incubator.

### *$CO_2$ Incubator*

You have to put the bicarbonate-buffered culture media into an incubator designed to maintain a constant concentration of 5 percent carbon dioxide ($CO_2$) in the atmosphere. With this 5 percent concentration in the atmosphere, carbon dioxide, which would otherwise evaporate from the culture media, is prevented from doing so. If your incubator isn't functioning properly and has a concentration of 10 percent carbon dioxide, the culture media will be too acidic (pH less than 7.2), and the egg will die. If the concentration of carbon dioxide in the incubator is only 2 percent, the media will become too alkaline (pH over 7.5), and the egg will die. Therefore, you must have an incubator that maintains a constant atmosphere of 5 percent carbon dioxide. There are some media formulations that require somewhat higher or lower concentrations of $CO_2$ in the atmosphere to maintain the proper pH. That is why we take nothing for granted, and meticulously check pH every day. If the pH of the media is not right at 7.3, we adjust the $CO_2$ concentration in the incubator.

But what happens when we open and close the door of the incubator to take culture dishes out to transfer the embryos? The more the door is opened and closed, the more $CO_2$ leaks out. Therefore, without our even being aware of it, the pH of the media can go up, and the egg can quietly and unobtrusively die. Keeping the $CO_2$ in the atmosphere constant and the pH in the 7.3 to 7.4 range remains one of the major issues of quality control for IVF embryo culturing. For that reason, we do not open and close the large incubator door frequently, and we keep the eggs or embryos in a smaller desktop incubator while we are working with them.

### *Culture Dishes and Test Tubes Designed to Keep pH Constant When out of the Incubator*

Now that we have the problem of maintaining constant pH in the incubator solved, what do we do when we absolutely have to take the culture dishes out into room air for brief periods of time? How much time are we allowed before we have to either transfer the egg or embryos to an air-buffered media or get them back into the $CO_2$ environment of the incubator? Unfortunately, with most culture dishes, that period of time is only a couple of minutes at most.

Typical culture dishes have a broad surface area that allows one to visualize easily the egg or embryo under the microscope. You simply put the culture dish on the stage of the microscope, and the embryo comes right into view and can be manipulated quite easily. That is the advantage of these common, broad-based culture dishes. However, the $CO_2$ evaporation is so rapid that within several minutes the pH will go way too high and the egg will die.

On the other hand, if the eggs or embryos are kept in a small test tube, which has a much narrower area for evaporation, the pH of the media can stay constant in air for fifteen minutes or longer because of the reduced surface area for $CO_2$ evaporation. The problem with these test tubes is that it is very difficult to visualize the egg or embryo under the microscope in a test tube, and it is technically very demanding to remove these embryos from the test tube without the possibility of losing them.

Therefore, the common solution for minimizing $CO_2$ loss and pH changes while the culture fluid is out of the incubator is an oil overlay. With this technique, very small microdroplets of culture media are placed on the bottom of a broad-based culture dish, and purified mineral oil or paraffin oil is laid over this droplet. With this approach you can take the culture dish out of the incubator for periods as long as ten minutes without a serious risk that the pH will go up. Of course, there is some $CO_2$ evaporation even through the oil, but it is slowed down tremendously. Using this method, we can keep the pH stable for a limited period of time while the embryo is out of the incubator, while guaranteeing the proper pH while it is in the incubator. In a good IVF lab today, all culturing should be done in this way, i.e., in microdroplets with an oil overlay (see fig. 10.4).

This oil overlay cannot be a casual substitute for carefully keeping track of how long the embryos are out of the incubator. The $CO_2$ still evaporates out through the oil overlay, just more slowly than if there were no overlay. If you were to keep the petri dish out of the incubator for ten minutes (the maximum allowed), return it to the incubator for an hour, and then take it out again for ten more minutes, it would be as though it were out for a total of twenty minutes. The pH would go too high, and the embryos would die. This is because it takes much, much longer for the $CO_2$ in the atmosphere to be absorbed into the media than for the $CO_2$ in the media to evaporate. Therefore, the total amount of time the embryos are out of the 5 percent $CO_2$ environment of the incubator is additive in its destructive effect.

### *Osmolality of Media*

The osmolality of a fluid is the number of dissolved molecules in a given volume. All body fluids and cells have an osmolality of about 280. If the osmolality of the fluid around the cell is too high, then water leaks out of the cell into the surrounding fluid by osmosis and the cell shrinks.

If the osmolality of the fluid is too low, fluid will enter the cell by osmosis, cause it to swell, and certainly kill it. When vigorously active, motile sperm are placed in fluid of low osmolality, they die instantly. The effect is quite dramatic and visible. When embryos are placed in fluid with low osmolality, they also swell and die.

While the culture media is sitting in a warm incubator over a period of time, the osmolality of the fluid might go up as evaporation of water occurs. Protection against this is afforded by creating a 98 percent humidity saturation in the incubator.

### *Temperature*

Our normal body temperature is 98.6 degrees Fahrenheit, or 37 degrees Celsius. Without this constant temperature, our normal biological processes simply would not proceed. The incubator maintains a constant temperature of 37 degrees Celsius for this reason. How sensitive is the egg, or the sperm, to changes in temperature? Actually, when the temperature goes down, the sperm movement slows down, but there is no major effect on the sperm's viability. When the temperature goes back up again, the sperm once again become vigorous. However, with the egg, when the temperature goes down even a little, its chromosome spindle is seriously damaged, and a chromosomally viable embryo cannot develop. The egg and embryo must be at 37 degrees Celsius in order to develop properly.

What if the temperature goes above 37 degrees Celsius? A slight elevation of the temperature above 37 degrees Celsius can also be very damaging to the egg. You won't notice what happened. The egg simply will not fertilize because it died from overheating. If the temperature in the incubator goes much over 98.6 degrees Fahrenheit, the eggs quite literally get poached.

### *Protein*

The ingredient in culture media not frequently mentioned is protein. Very few IVF centers would risk trying to culture eggs or embryos without some type of protein added. The amount and type of protein, however, vary considerably and may not really make a significant difference. Previously, the simplest approach was to draw the patient's blood the day before the procedure, separate off the serum from the red blood cells, and add some of her serum to the culture media, usually in a concentration of 10 percent. However, fear of transmitting any infectious agent has halted that practice. Today, commercially prepared protein supplements, carefully sterilized, are added to all media (six grams per 100 milliliters). These supplements include the major proteins found in your blood, i.e., albumin, alpha and beta globulins, and gamma globulin. The role of these proteins in cell culture is not clear, but at the very least they are necessary to lubricate the eggs and embryos so that they don't stick to the glass of the petri dish or the pipette.

### *Sequential Culture Media*

At different stages in the egg's development and during the first five or six days of the embryo's development there are different nutritional needs. For many years it was considered impossible to culture embryos for more than three days, and to culture more than even two days was risky. In the late 1990s, however, Dr. David Gardner, from Australia, and Dr. Rusty Poole, from Texas, discovered that the fluid from the human fallopian tube contains very little, if any, glucose, and that the embryo needs very little if any of this sugar for its development during the first three days of life. For the next three days, however, the embryos need a high concentration of glucose. Therefore, the sugar that is necessary to maintain rapid fetal growth is actually harmful to the embryo during the first three days, and is only needed after that time. The next finding was that the embryos actually need very few ingredients at all in the media during the first three days. Out of these studies developed what is now commonly referred to as sequential culture media. Table 10.1 lists the ingredients of the typical, simple culture media required for the first three days, and table 10.2 lists those in a typical, very complex culture media designed for the next three days of the embryo's development.

**TABLE 10.1**

**Culture Medium (Fourteen Components): First Three Days (until Eight-Cell Stage)**

| COMPONENT | FORMULATION mM |
|---|---|
| Glucose | 0.5 |
| NaCl | 102.6 |
| KCl | 2.50 |
| $MgSO_4$ | 0.20 |
| $CaCl_2$ | 1.70 |
| $NaHCO_3$ | 25.0 |
| Na pyruvate | 0.33 |
| Na lactate | 20.77 |
| Alanyl-glutamine | 0.50 |
| Taurine | 0.05 |
| Na citrate | 0.15 mg/L |
| EDTA | 10 μ M |
| Phenol Red | 0.005 g/L |
| Gentamicin | 10 μg/mL |

**TABLE 10.2**

**Culture Medium (Thirty-three Components): Days Three to Five (Eight-Cell Stage until Blastocyst Stage)**

| COMPONENT | mM |
|---|---|
| **Energy** | |
| Glucose | 3.0 |
| Sodium pyruvate | 0.2 |
| Sodium chloride | 101.5 |
| Potassium chloride | 2.5 |
| Potassium phosphate | 0.35 |
| Calcium chloride | 1.7 |
| Magnesium sulfate | 0.2 |

| | |
|---|---|
| Sodium bicarbonate | 25.0 |
| Phenol Red | .005 gm/L |
| Gentamicin sulfate | 10 μg/mL |
| Sodium citrate | 1.0 |
| Sodium lactate | 20 |
| **Amino Acids** | |
| Alanine | 0.05 |
| Alanyl-glutamine | 1.0 |
| Arginine | 0.3 |
| Asparagine | 0.05 |
| Aspartic acid | 0.05 |
| Cysteine | 0.05 |
| Glutamic acid | 0.05 |
| Glycine | 0.05 |
| Histidine | 0.1 |
| Isoleucine | 0.2 |
| Leucine | 0.2 |
| Lysine | 0.2 |
| Methionine | 0.05 |
| Phenylalanine | 0.1 |
| Proline | 0.05 |
| Serine | 0.05 |
| Taurine | 0.05 |
| Threonine | 0.2 |
| Tryptophan | 0.02 |
| Tyrosine | 0.1 |
| Valine | 0.2 |

Thus, the first three days of the embryo's life require an extremely simple media that just provides a constant pH, protein, and basic electrolytes, with little sugar and very few, if any, amino acids. But after the morning of day three, when the embryo has reached eight cells, a much "higher octane" media is needed to fuel the rapid growth of the developing blastocyst, to aid hatching out of the zona pellucida, and to allow implantation into the uterus to become a pregnancy. In fig. 10.5 you see several embryos that have been cultured beyond the simple ball of eight cells on day three into the day-five blastocyst, with the inner cell mass as shown and the outer trophectoderm as shown. The outer trophectoderm will become the placenta of the pregnancy, and the inner cell mass

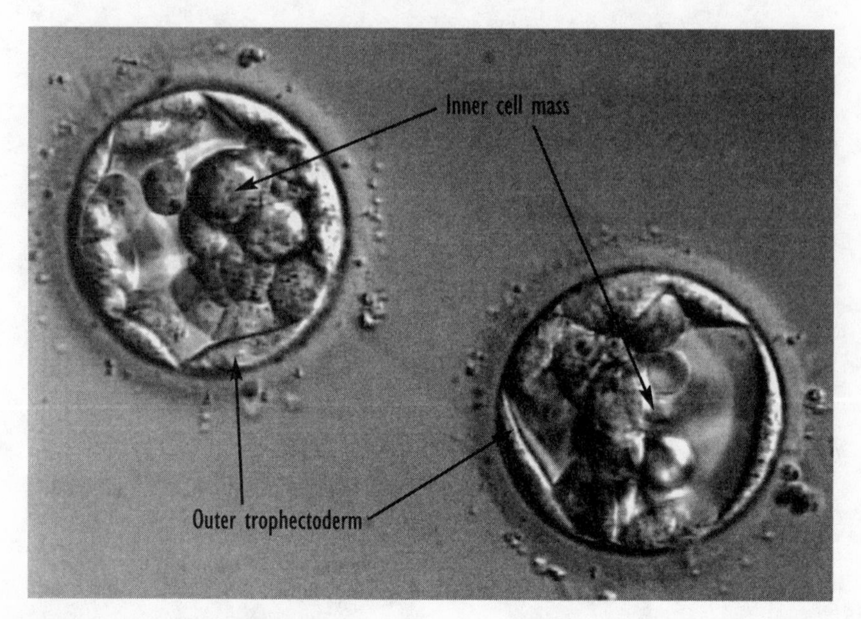


**FIGURE 10.5.** Day-five blastocysts.

will become the fetus proper. This complex development to day five or day six in vitro has only been made possible by closely mimicking, in the culture media, the sequential and varying requirements of the early embryo for growth and development.

This concept of sequential media is currently being challenged by a different global kind of media called KSOM, a complex media designed by a trial-and-error approach, which provides whatever the embryo needs at any time and is not related to its changing metabolic requirements. Whichever approach is used, sequential or global, modern embryo culture media is able to support life safely in the test tube for five to six days.

## Egg Handling After Retrieval from the Ovary

The test tube containing the follicular fluid is immediately brought to the laboratory worktable, which preferably is directly connected to the operating room. The contents of the test tube are immediately emptied into a large petri dish. This petri dish is then scanned under the microscope to find the egg. The egg is an incredibly serene, beautiful object in contrast to the millions of frantically moving sperm, only one of which will be able to fertilize the egg. When I'm looking at the egg I get a wonderful feeling knowing that I am looking at something that might someday grow up and be able to write a poem. Sperm are very impersonal because any one of the millions of them might be the one to get into the egg. But the egg is something truly personal and exciting to look at.

The human egg is actually visible to the naked eye because of the sticky, gooey cumulus mass that surrounds it. A bare egg could never be picked up by the fallopian tube, so nature has provided this gooey mass, which cradles it and allows it to be grabbed by the cilia of the fallopian tube. Because of this, you can almost always find the egg in the petri dish before even looking through the microscope. The egg is then picked up under microscopic control, with a small pipette, and placed in a droplet of culture media.

The egg is also surrounded by corona cells, which are closely attached to the outside of the zona pellucida shell. As the egg matures in the follicle under the stimulus of FSH and estrogen, and prepares for the LH trigger, the egg grows from 20 microns to 140 microns in size, and the densely packed granulosa cells surrounding it begin to spread out circumferentially in a fan-shaped pattern, like the spokes of a bicycle wheel. In fact, looking at a mature egg with a completely developed corona often reminds reproductive scientists of stylized drawings of the

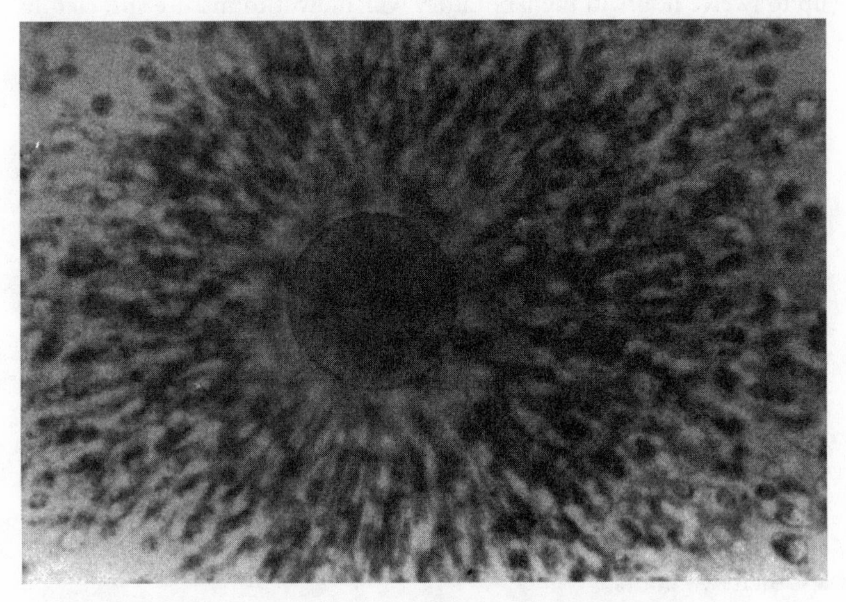

**FIGURE 10.6.** Sunburst appearance of a mature egg ready for fertilization.

sun (see fig. 10.6). When you look at the sun, there is a center orb of brilliant light surrounded by flashes and streaks of hot gases extending and trailing off circumferentially outward from the sun's surface. That is the reason these granulosa cells in a mature egg are referred to as the corona radiata.

The granulosa cells and the cumulus mass are critical for pregnancy. The egg cannot possibly develop into a viable embryo without the nourishment provided by these granulosa cells and cumulus mass before the LH surge has induced it to resume meiosis. If the corona is widely dispersed and spread out in a beautiful fan-shaped pattern, that means that the cell is very mature and very likely to be fertilizable, particularly if the cytoplasm is clear and not clumpy or dark; such an egg would be graded as very high quality. Looking carefully at such an egg, one would almost always find a first polar body, indicating that the egg has received the LH trigger and is genetically ready for fertilization. However, in practice, the first polar body is not often looked for (except when doing ICSI) because it may be difficult to find under an ordinary dissecting microscope.

If the corona is tightly packed against the zona pellucida, without very much spreading out, then the egg is very immature and definitely not ready for fertilization. It most likely will not have undergone a first polar body extrusion. Sometimes culturing such an egg for a period of up to twelve hours in the laboratory will allow it to mature sufficiently to extrude its first polar body in vitro, and therefore become able to be fertilized.

## Culturing the Sperm and Eggs, and Embryo Transfer

The patient leaves the operating room shortly after egg aspiration and goes home with virtually no pain at all. The sperm are then placed into culture dishes (or test tubes) containing the eggs. It used to be thought that a certain period of time was required for the egg to mature in culture, and also for the sperm to capacitate before this insemination procedure could be performed. With modern stimulation protocols, as discussed earlier in this section, one really doesn't have to go through this long period of waiting. The sperm that have already been washed, and therefore capacitated, can be placed in culture with the eggs within less than two hours.

The eggs should be checked somewhere between thirteen and eighteen hours after insemination to see if pronuclei have formed and if the second polar body has been extruded. These signs would indicate that the egg has fertilized and that it will most likely undergo cleavage into an embryo. At this point, the egg may be fertilized, but it is not yet really a new individual. The chromosomes have not truly met and united into a new cell. It has not undergone the process of syngamy, in which the two pronuclei seem to miraculously move toward the center and become one. Usually, this occurs sometime after eighteen hours. Three days after the initial egg retrieval and insemination procedure, the embryos should be ready for transfer back to the patient.

After two days, the embryos will normally have two to four cells. In three days, the embryos should be five to eight cells. Seven- to eight-cell embryos on day three have a better chance of becoming a pregnancy than five- to six-cell embryos (see fig. 10.7). Each one of these cells in a cleaving embryo is called a blastomere. The quality of the embryo is judged by several factors: (1) how many blastomeres are present, indicating the rapidity of embryo cleavage, (2) equal size of blastomeres, (3) the presence of a single nucleus in each blastomere, and (4) the relative absence of loose cellular fragments. Embryo quality and how well it can predict successful pregnancy will be discussed in more detail later in this chapter.

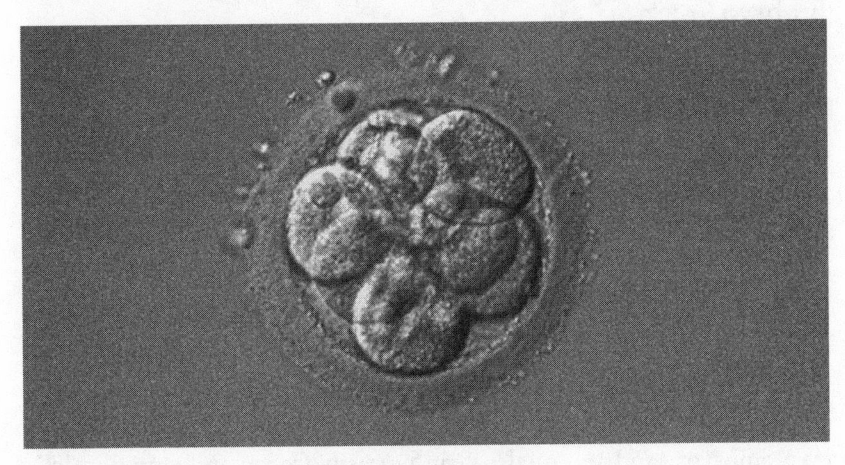

**FIGURE 10.7.** Normal, good-quality eight-cell embryo.

The physician must distinguish between a good embryo, with healthy-looking, rapidly cleaving blastomeres, and a poor embryo, with unequal size or multinucleated blastomeres and greater than 30 percent fragmentation. The healthy-looking embryos are loaded into a catheter in a low volume of fluid (about one hundredth of a teaspoon) to transfer either to the woman's uterus (IVF) or to her fallopian tube (ZIFT).

Finally, the physician is ready to transfer the embryo via a tiny catheter through the cervix into the uterus, or surgically into the fallopian tube. An impeccable study from Finland in 2002 of almost five thousand IVF cycles compared pregnancy results to the ease or difficulty of the embryo-transfer technique. The findings were astounding. Transfers that were considered difficult had a 60 percent lower pregnancy rate than those that were considered easy. If the doctor pays attention to my advice in chapter 6, and is patient and gentle, almost all embryo transfers should be easy.

The ball of cells being transferred is no larger than that original tiny egg (about 1/250 of an inch in diameter) and is no longer surrounded by a sticky, gooey cumulus mass. It is just a tiny, fragile little ball that even in a small culture dish looks like a mere speck in the universe. Although the egg looks very impressive with all of its outer vestments of corona radiata and sticky cumulus, it is hard to believe that this tiny mass of cleaving cells called an embryo can ever become a human being.

## Embryo Freezing

When many embryos are obtained with an IVF cycle, obviously they cannot all be placed back into the woman. If the embryos are of good quality, and the woman is less than thirty-eight years old, it is usually safe to transfer only two or three. Transferring more would create too big a risk of quadruplets or quintuplets, or even greater. Some infertile couples will yield many eggs in a stimulation cycle and many embryos. It would be foolish and unethical to waste these extras after the best-looking two or three embryos have been replaced. It is for that reason that embryo freezing was developed.

Eggs, until recently, could not be frozen without killing them. However, embryos (and sperm also) can be easily frozen and stored indefinitely in liquid nitrogen tanks for future replacement into the uterus. In order to understand how we can actually hold this form of human life on call for future use without killing it, you need to understand why freezing normally kills a cell or an organ.

Lowering the temperature to –196 degrees Celsius does not poison any metabolic processes. It just stops everything. One would not, therefore, logically expect freezing to harm the body at all. The only reason that freezing kills relates to a peculiar property of water (the cells in our body are more than 70 percent water). When the temperature reaches freezing, water crystallizes instead of just turning solid. We all know that ice cubes do not sink. The reason is that when water freezes, unlike most other liquids, it actually expands and forms a crystalline structure of much greater volume. If you put an enclosed bottle of water in a freezer, the water, by virtue of freezing, will burst the bottle. Thus, when cells are frozen, they die only because the formation of ice crystals inside them expands and damages the inside of the cell.

The cell must be protected in two ways: (1) by getting as much water out of it as possible, and (2) by getting a cryoprotectant (literally an antifreeze solution) into it to prevent formation of ice crystals. One reason that eggs cannot easily be frozen without killing them but embryos can is that the outer cell membrane of the egg is not very permeable, and it is harder to get water out of it and cryoprotectant into it. The other reason is that the mature egg is in the process of chromosome separation (meiosis) on a delicate spindle that is easily damaged by the slightest temperature drop, or by ice-crystal formation. Most of the cells of an eight-cell embryo (most of the time) are not in the process of chromosome division, and so the spindle is no problem. The reason that a sperm is relatively easy to freeze is that it is one of the few cells in the body that has hardly any water in it. A sperm head is just solid DNA with virtually no cytoplasm. There is hardly any ice-crystal formation to worry about.

The method for freezing the extra embryos is relatively simple. We place the embryos into a solution containing propanediol (the antifreeze) and sucrose (a sugar that stays outside the cell and "pulls" water out osmotically). The embryos in this solution are then aspirated into a tiny plastic freezing straw, and the ends are hermetically sealed. The straw is very carefully labeled and placed into a programmed freezing machine (see fig. 10.8). The temperature is then slowly reduced at a tightly controlled rate. Once it is just below freezing (–8 degrees Celsius), ice-crystal formation outside the egg membrane is induced in a controlled fashion via a process called seeding. Then the temperature continues to be slowly reduced to about –30 to –40 degrees Celsius. After that, the straw is immediately plunged into the liquid-nitrogen storage container.

The reason for the slow, carefully controlled freezing rate is that it

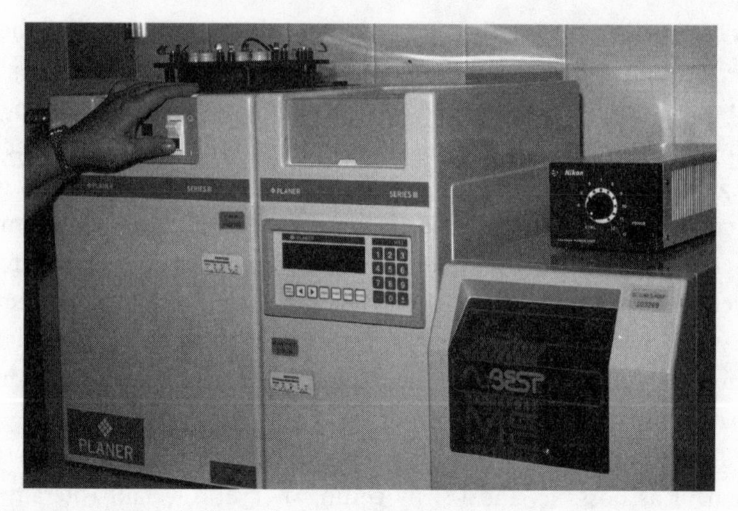


**FIGURE 10.8.** Computerized controlled-rate embryo-freezing apparatus.

allows ice crystals to form first on the outside of the cell. This increases the osmolality outside the cell, thereby drawing more and more water out of it. Ideally, once the solution in the straw crystallizes, there is virtually no water left inside the embryo. All the ice crystals are left on the outside.

When thawing the embryos (at a future date) for putting them back into the patient, a similarly rigorous, gradual approach must be used, or they will die from what is called osmotic shock. These dehydrated little embryos would swell and burst if just placed back into the body's normal osmotic environment. They must first be put into successively less-diluted solutions of sucrose to gradually get all the antifreeze solution (propanediol) out and to put small amounts of water back into the cell. Finally, the embryos are fully restored, alive, and ready to start a new life.

Not all embryos survive this freezing and thawing process, no matter how carefully it is performed. However, it is usually the least-healthy embryos (which would have been least likely to result in a pregnancy anyway) that fail to survive the freezing process. That is why most programs freeze only the embryos that are completely normal-looking. The others are left in culture to see if they can continue to develop. If they do, they are then frozen several days later. If they don't, then it means they never could have made it anyway. With a methodical, careful approach to both freezing and thawing, frozen-embryo pregnancy rates are very high.

The purpose of freezing embryos is not to tamper with or destroy life. If there are more embryos available than can be *safely* put back into the patient at one time, then freezing the extras for later is a way of maximizing their chance of eventually becoming a baby.

## Embryo Quality and Embryo Selection

Even in fertile couples, the majority of human embryos are abnormal and incapable of resulting in a viable pregnancy. That is why it is customary to replace more than one embryo in order to have a high pregnancy rate with IVF. If there were some way we could tell for sure which of the many embryos derived from an IVF cycle were the normal ones that would result in a baby, then one or two embryos could be replaced at a time. The danger of transferring more than two embryos in any given cycle is the risk that the woman might have triplets, quadruplets, or, even worse than that, quintuplets or sextuplets. For that reason, most physicians will transfer just the two or three best-quality embryos and freeze any excess embryos that appear to be viable. Obviously, nonviable, arrested embryos are discarded. The problem is in trying to decide which potentially viable embryos are the "best" ones, i.e., the ones that are most likely to result in a viable pregnancy.

Four characteristics of an embryo's appearance that can be observed readily under the microscope are used to try to make this embryo selection: (1) the number of cells at day two and day three, (2) the percentage of the embryo volume that consists of fragments rather than true cells, (3) the relative equality or inequality of the size of the cells in the embryo, and (4) the presence of more than one nucleus in any or all of the cells of the embryo. Since these are four different characteristics of the embryo, which may vary in combination in any given embryo, there are many different types of embryos. Furthermore, because each embryo in a cohort of, say, ten embryos might have a different appearance, it has been very difficult to pinpoint exactly which embryos will result in the highest probability of pregnancy. Sometimes, very poor-appearing embryos result in a multiple pregnancy, particularly in young women. Sometimes, almost perfect-appearing embryos result in no pregnancy, especially in an older woman. However, despite these limitations in attempting to grade embryos, the overall impression of embryo quality based on these four characteristics, when combined with the woman's age and the number of eggs (ovarian reserve), gives a relatively good prediction of pregnancy rate, and can be used to minimize the number of embryos transferred.

At first, an infertile couple might be pleased by the prospect of triplets or quadruplets, and they are almost always happy about the prospect of twins. However, once they are aware of the increased difficulties of such a pregnancy, and the risk to the offspring, they realize they are much better off having a singleton or at most a twin birth.

Figure 10.9 summarizes pregnancy rate in relation to the age of the wife and her ovarian reserve when using poor-quality embryos and when using good-quality embryos (based on the four characteristics listed previously). Regardless of age or the number of eggs, pregnancy rate is approximately twice as high in cycles where there are good-quality embryos versus when there are poor-quality embryos. With poor-quality embryos, the pregnancy rate is only 23 percent, and with good-quality embryos, the pregnancy rate ranges from 44 to 57 percent. In women over forty, the pregnancy rate is much lower even with good-quality embryos, and that is because the type of chromosomal error associated with older eggs does not result in any decrease in the apparent quality of the embryos. Aneuploid chromosomal errors typical of the aging egg result in perfectly normal-appearing embryos. However, for younger women, these appearance-related selection criteria are usually valid.

**FIGURE 10.9**

**Embryo Quality and Pregnancy Rate in Relation to Age and Ovarian Reserve**

| | <10 EGGS EMBRYO QUALITY | | ≥10 EGGS EMBRYO QUALITY | |
|---|---|---|---|---|
| Age | Poor | Good | Poor | Good |
| **<30** | **30%** | **50%** | **37%** | **60%** |
| **30–35** | **24%** | **44%** | **26%** | **57%** |
| **36–40** | **21%** | **43%** | **17%** | **52%** |
| **Overall** | **23%** | **44%** | **26%** | **57%** |

Simply looking at the percent of the embryo that is fragmented (without paying attention to the other three criteria) gives a relatively good prediction of embryo quality. Researchers in Brussels demonstrated years ago that when there is greater than 35 percent fragmentation in the embryos, there is only a 15 percent pregnancy rate, but when the embryos have less than 25 percent fragmentation, there is a 50 percent pregnancy rate. When the embryos have only 5 percent fragmentation, there is a 62 percent pregnancy rate. They also showed that when there is less than 20 percent fragmentation, 16 percent of the embryos implant and become babies, and when there is greater than 20 percent fragmentation, only 5 percent of the embryos implant and become babies. However, there are so many different variables of these four aspects of embryo morphology all mixed up in different embryos in a given IVF cycle, that it is impossible to make predictions any more accurate than this with embryo grading.

Figure 10.10 is an illustration of what good-quality and poor-quality embryos look like on days two and three of embryo development. Any good IVF lab should be routinely evaluating embryos in this way before selecting which ones to transfer. You'll note from the figure that on day two the ideal embryo would have four cells, each cell would be equal in size, there would be little or no fragmentation, and there would be a single nucleus observable in each cell. On day three the ideal-quality embryo would be eight cells, have equal-size cells, have little or no fragmentation, and, again, there would be a single nucleus observable in each cell. Contrast that to the poor embryos on day two and day three. The poor-quality embryo depicted here on day two is composed of only three cells, and one of those cells has two nuclei rather than one. Notice that the cells are not of equal size and that 35 percent of the actual volume of the embryo is composed of small fragments of cells rather than true cells. On day three the poor-quality embryo depicted has six cells rather than eight, the cells are of unequal size, and more than 35 percent of the embryo's volume is filled with fragments rather than true cells. In two of the cells there is a double nucleus, even though the other cells have a single nucleus. There are a wide variety of combinations of defects in these four different characteristics of embryos on days two and three, but this figure gives you an excellent idea of how to judge overall embryo quality. The best-appearing embryos are the ones most likely to result in a pregnancy.

The reason that the number of cells in an embryo found on either day two or day three is an important criterion is that it reflects the speed of embryo development. Generally, the more rapidly developing the embryo, the healthier it is, and the more likely it will result in a preg-

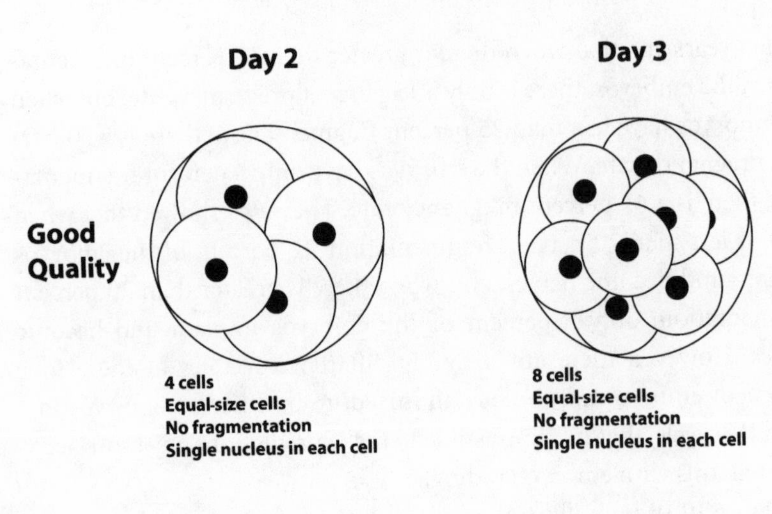


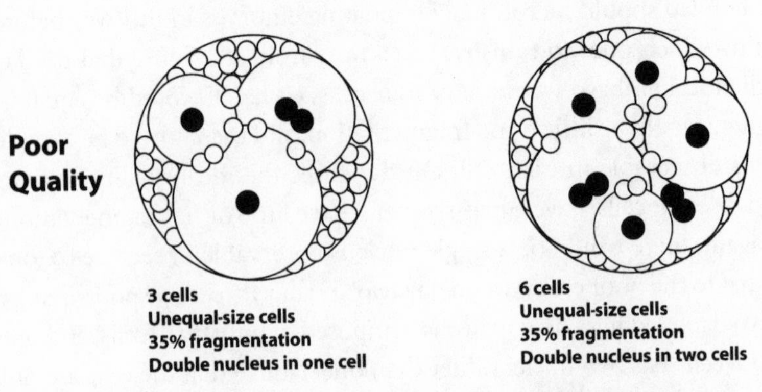


**FIGURE 10.10.** Good-quality versus poor-quality embryos on day two and day three.

nancy. Embryos that are only four cells on day three can certainly result in a pregnancy, but the pregnancy rate is much lower than that of embryos that have eight cells on day three. In a similar fashion, embryos that are only two cells on day two can certainly result in pregnancy, but these more slowly developing embryos are less likely to result in a pregnancy than embryos that already have four cells on day two. On the other hand, embryos that have ten or more cells on day three are also less likely to result in a pregnancy, because even though they are developing rapidly, they have failed to undergo (at the proper time) a process known as compaction.

Compaction means that once the embryo has reached this eight-cell stage, the individual cells of the embryo, all of which are totipotential up until that time, must begin to "talk to each other." The clearly defined cell membranes must begin to "melt" and stick to one another. This process of compaction, during which the cells amalgamate into what looks like a blob rather than individual, distinct cells, must occur right at or just after this eight-cell stage. If cells continue to develop and this compaction does not occur, then the embryo cannot develop any further. If you see eight cells that are beginning to lose the distinctness of their outlines and merge together on the morning of day three, this early compaction is an excellent indication of the embryos most likely to result in a baby.

There are a few centers that embrace blastocyst culture, culturing embryos to day five in order to make (in their opinion) a better selection of embryos likely to lead to a birth. However, the vast majority of good IVF centers prefer to make transfers on day three based on the criteria depicted in figure 10.10. Still, blastocyst culture has very important benefits. When there has been a preimplantation embryo biopsy on day three, the results for those embryos are often unknown until day five, and for that purpose, culturing the embryo to blastocyst is very important. Also, if an occasional young woman has too many embryos on day three, culturing to blastocyst may aid somewhat in selecting which ones are the best to transfer. Blastocyst culture is also beneficial in cases where the best embryos are transferred on day three but the remaining ones are not clearly nonviable, but just of poor quality. After several more days in culture, the vast majority of those embryos will arrest and demonstrate that they were not able to develop into an offspring, just as it was determined on the day-three evaluation. However, an occasional such embryo may develop to blastocyst, and in that case it can be frozen on day five. Thus, blastocyst culture is a way to make sure that no embryo is discarded that might have any chance whatsoever of being viable.

## How Many Embryos Should Be Transferred?

The question remains, how many embryos should be transferred? Transferring a larger number of embryos gives a higher pregnancy rate but also increases the risk of dangerous multiple pregnancy. First, you should understand something that is often confused in the layperson's mind. The majority of these dangerous triplet and quadruplet pregnancies are not coming from IVF. In IVF we have control over how many embryos are transferred. Although the decision-making is often difficult, the incidence of high-order, dangerous multiple pregnancies is much lower with IVF than with simple administration of standard fertility drugs.

Although it makes sense that pregnancy rates for IVF are higher when more embryos are transferred, U.S. statistics from the CDC would, at first glance, seem to contradict that notion. In the CDC report, transferring a single embryo in women under thirty-five resulted in a 30 percent pregnancy rate, and transferring two embryos in women under thirty-five resulted in a 50 percent pregnancy rate. However, transferring more than two embryos resulted in no increase in pregnancy rate, and even appeared to result in a lower pregnancy rate. For older women and women with a low ovarian reserve, the CDC results show a 10 percent pregnancy rate when only one embryo is transferred and a 35 percent pregnancy rate when two embryos were transferred. Once again, transferring more than two embryos did not result in any increase in pregnancy rate but, in fact, resulted in a lower pregnancy rate. How can that make sense?

The reason is that women who have had more than two embryos transferred are more likely to have had poor-quality embryos. In this retrospective report from the CDC, there is no awareness of the embryo quality because this is not reported to the CDC. This is the problem with any conclusions derived from any retrospective rather than prospective study. In fact, if you look at the CDC data, the incidence of triplets is not significantly increased whether you put back three embryos, four embryos, five embryos, or even more than five embryos. No matter how many embryos you put back, the incidence of triplets or more is approximately 6 percent. That would make no sense if not for the fact that clinics are only replacing large numbers of embryos when the embryo quality is poor or the wife is older and has a low ovarian reserve. If, in poor-prognosis cases such as this, clinics were putting back only one or two embryos, the pregnancy rate would most likely be disastrously low.

Once again, clarity on this issue of how many embryos to transfer and the effect on pregnancy rate, as well as the risk of multiple births, is more clearly identified in prospective studies from Europe. The group from Copenhagen strictly limited their study to those cases in which all

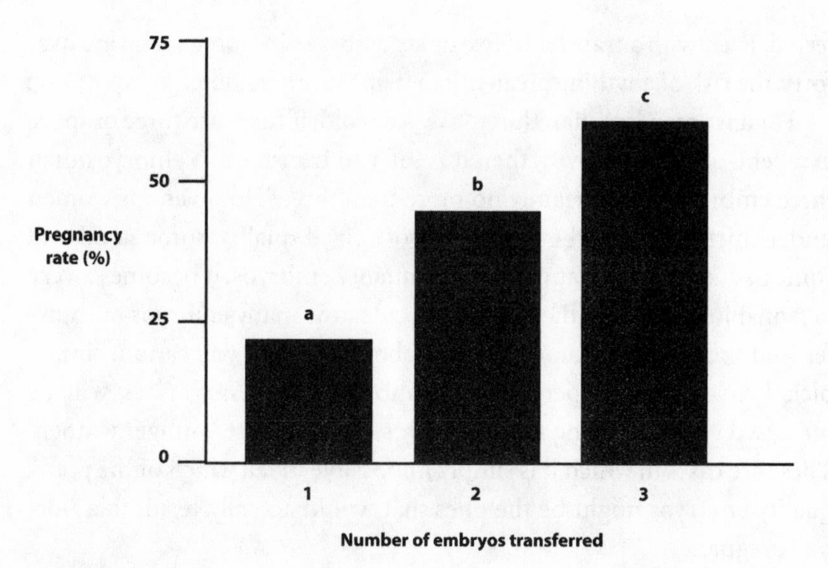


**FIGURE 10.11**

Pregnancy rates in relation to number of transferred embryos when embryos are of equal quality (Copenhagen Study).

embryos had identical quality. This enormously difficult study required many IVF cycles, but the result is very clear (see fig. 10.11). When one embryo is transferred, there is a 24 percent pregnancy rate; when two embryos are transferred, there is a 40 percent pregnancy rate, and when three embryos are transferred, there is a 60 percent pregnancy rate. Thus, there is a clear increase in pregnancy rate related to increasing the number of embryos transferred, so long as all the embryos are of the same quality. It is when embryos are of differing quality that physicians must make judgments about when it would be better to transfer more embryos in an effort to provide an adequate pregnancy rate in women who otherwise might not do as well.

So, what is the right approach for you to take? If you are over thirty-seven years old, and embryo quality is not the best, it is wise to be aggressive in deciding how many embryos to replace. This is not the politically correct thing to suggest, because everyone is extremely concerned about not increasing the incidence of multiple pregnancies. However, the risk of multiple pregnancy in women who are over thirty-seven and who have anything but the best-quality embryos is extremely low, even when three, four, or five embryos are replaced. In fact, for women forty or older, it makes very little sense to restrict the number of embryos that are transferred. Even with a transfer of five or six embryos in women who are over forty, the risk of anything greater than twins is very remote.

For a woman less than thirty-five years old, if there are three or more excellent-quality embryos, then it is safer to transfer two embryos than three embryos, and certainly no more than three. However, for women under thirty-five who have embryos of mixed quality, some good and some bad, or maybe many mediocre-quality embryos, it becomes a very personal judgment on their part to decide how many embryos to transfer, and they must be knowledgeable about it. When you cannot simply pick two or three superb-quality embryos, pregnancy rates will be increased by transferring more embryos, even in these younger women. These are cases in which it is simply impossible to tell which of the poor-quality embryos might be the ones that would actually result in a normal pregnancy.

However, more than three embryos should never be transferred in women who would not be willing to undergo a selective reduction procedure if the guess is wrong and too many embryos implant. The risk of that is extremely low if proper, judicious judgment is applied. Yet couples must think about it ahead of time. Despite there being an extremely low risk of triplets or more in such cases, it is simply too dangerous to risk transferring more than three unless the couple would be willing to undergo selective reduction if more than two or three embryos implanted.

## Selective Reduction

By seven weeks of fetal gestation (that means three weeks after your positive pregnancy test, five weeks after your embryo transfer, or literally seven weeks from the start of your ovarian stimulation with FSH or HMG), simple ultrasound will reveal how many embryos have successfully implanted. Of course, 75 percent of the time this will be a singleton pregnancy, which is really the most favorable outcome. In 22 percent of cases it will be a twin pregnancy, and most couples are quite happy even though twins present more of an obstetric problem. However, 3 percent of the time (unless you are in a program where only two embryos are transferred), you will see viable triplets, and that is a problem. In a program that transfers more than three embryos in carefully selected cases, there will be an occasional (less than 1 percent) risk of quadruplets, and that is an extremely serious problem. These triplet, quadruplet, or quintuplet pregnancies, which should be very rare, can be ameliorated via selective reduction. This concept will be an anathema to many couples, and even bringing it up might be explosive. But if there is more than a triplet pregnancy, selective reduction is the only truly safe alternative to give the pregnancy the best chance of success.

The risk of losing a triplet pregnancy is about 15 percent. Furthermore, if a triplet pregnancy delivers prior to thirty-two weeks, or when the babies are less than three pounds, there is a higher risk of developmental abnormalities despite all the best pediatric attention. Our particular experience with triplets in the hands of our high-risk obstetricians actually yields a better success rate than that. With proper bed rest for the entire second half of the triplet pregnancy, appropriate tocolytic drugs, and meticulous and close obstetric monitoring, we have not seen such terrible results with triplets. Nonetheless, on a national and international basis, triplet pregnancies (in addition to the increased cost to the health system) have dramatically higher risks than twins or singletons. There is a 15 percent chance of losing a triplet pregnancy. If one of the triplet embryos is removed, usually at eleven weeks' gestation, the risk of losing that pregnancy goes from 15 percent down to less than 5 percent. Thus, even though our few triplets have done well, in view of nationwide statistics, reducing a triplet pregnancy to a twin pregnancy makes it more than three times safer for that pregnancy to continue.

With multiple pregnancies greater than three, i.e., quadruplets, quintuplets, and sextuplets, the chance of such a pregnancy surviving is very low, and the chance of the offspring doing well is also extremely low. In fact, quadruplet pregnancies and higher are an absolute medical disaster. It is for that reason that selective reduction has to be considered before any IVF cycle in which more than two or three embryos might be replaced, and the couple has to be sure of what they would and would not be willing to do if too many embryos implanted. The risk of pregnancy loss goes from 25 percent to 7 percent if quadruplets are reduced to twins, and from 50 percent to 11 percent if quintuplets are reduced to twins. Although the IVF program should never transfer more than three embryos if there is any risk of more than three implanting, there will be occasional miscalculations. When that happens, the only safe alternative is selective reduction.

If a couple must resort to selective reduction, and this should be rare, it is best that they go to the one or two most experienced people in the country or in their region at handling such cases. The world's leading authority on selective reduction is Dr. Mark Evans, who used to be at Wayne State University, in Detroit, and who is now at Columbia University, in New York City. Couples who know that their personal or religious values would not allow them to do a selective reduction should never have more than two (or at the very most three) embryos transferred, no matter how poor the quality of the embryos and no matter what the age of the wife. For those very rare couples who find that too many embryos have implanted, here is the approach I recommend.

As soon as you find out you have a multiple pregnancy (at seven weeks' gestation) call and make an appointment to see the leading expert in your region. At exactly eleven weeks of gestation, that is eleven weeks after you began your gonadotropin injections, seven weeks after you got your positive pregnancy test, or four weeks after you did your seven-week ultrasound and found out that you had a multiple pregnancy, you would have a chorionic villus sampling (CVS) procedure. CVS is a fairly routine procedure for women over thirty-five who want to know if their pregnancy is normal. The very next day, analysis of the cells retrieved from this routine CVS will tell you which, if any, of the embryos are chromosomally abnormal. With that information, the physician can remove the abnormal sacs, leaving only the normal ones. In the event that all four or five sacs represent normal embryos, he would still reduce that pregnancy to twins via ultrasound-guided needle injection based only on which sacs were in the safest position. The procedure is actually painless, although emotionally wrenching. But if you have this rare complication of quadruplets or greater, it would be necessary in order to protect the lives of the other embryos. Therefore, you must think about this carefully before deciding how many embryos to have transferred and how many to have frozen.

CHAPTER 11

# ICSI — the Long-Sought Solution to Male Infertility

Four million American couples suffer from infertility, and in almost half of those cases, the problem involves the male. In about 20 percent of these cases, the husband's sperm will not fertilize the wife's eggs via conventional IVF. In about 2 percent of these cases, there is no sperm whatsoever, that is, azoospermia. Before 1992, this had been the major, insurmountable problem in IVF. The development of intracytoplasmic sperm injection (ICSI) provided the solution to that problem.

In the autumn of 1995, the magazine of the IVF World Congress in Vienna stated:

> In April of this year, the American Dr. Sherman Silber, from St. Louis, reported his collaborative work in male factor infertility with the Brussels' group of Dr. Andre Van Steirteghem and Dr. Paul Devroey. To a startled audience at a main auditorium in Vienna, he summarized their results and stated that there are now very few sterile men who cannot father their own genetic children. By September of 1995, the number of groups corroborating Dr. Silber's findings had grown exponentially.

With the ICSI technique developed in Brussels, and sperm-retrieval techniques developed in St. Louis, a man does not have to be fertile to be able to father his own child; indeed, he needs only a few scant sperm. With ICSI, each egg is individually injected with a single sperm under a microscope using delicate microscopic tools (see fig. 11.1). If the sperm quality is poor, that does not mean there is any problem with the DNA content. The only problem is with the delivery system for getting that man's DNA into the woman's egg. The most pitifully miserable, slow-moving sperm, even sperm with abnormal shapes, have normal DNA,

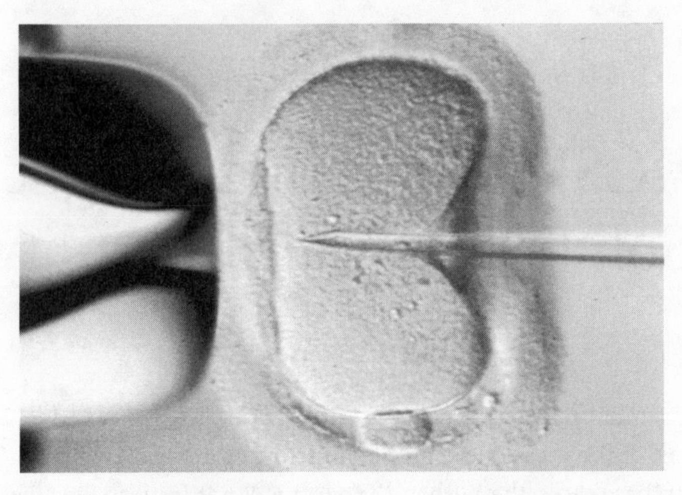

**FIGURE 11.1.** ICSI: injection of sperm into an egg.

and if they are injected into the woman's eggs, they yield a pregnancy rate not very different from IVF in couples whose husbands have completely normal, fertile sperm (see figures 11.2a through 11.2d). In addition, more than a decade of follow-up study indicates that ICSI is safe.

Imagine how tiny the microsurgical detail has to be to inject a sperm safely into a human egg. The diameter of the egg is about 140 microns (6/1,000 of an inch). The sperm head is approximately 4 microns wide by 6 microns long (approximately 1/5,000 of an inch). Can you imagine picking up a sperm (with a diameter of 1/5,000 of an inch) in an injection pipette (a glass needle that has been specially drawn out with computerized glass-pullers), which has a diameter of about 1/4,000 of an inch, and injecting it into the egg, which has a diameter of 6/1,000 of an inch? All of these delicate maneuvers must be performed in a culture dish overlayed with oil under a microscope (making sure that the temperature, osmolality, and acidity that would normally exist inside the body are maintained).

## How the ICSI Technique Was Invented

In 1991, in a modest laboratory in Brussels, Belgium, the first breakthrough in ICSI was made. For years we had been afraid to inject sperm directly into the substance of the egg because we were certain that this would simply destroy the egg. We also had feared that these infertile

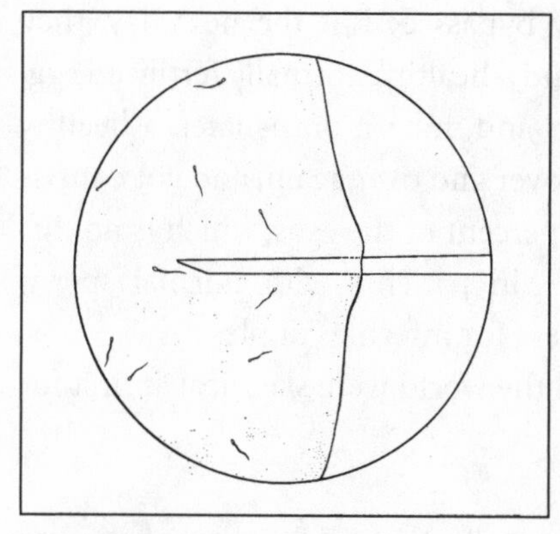

**FIGURE 11.2A.** Picking up a weak, infertile sperm using a micropipette.

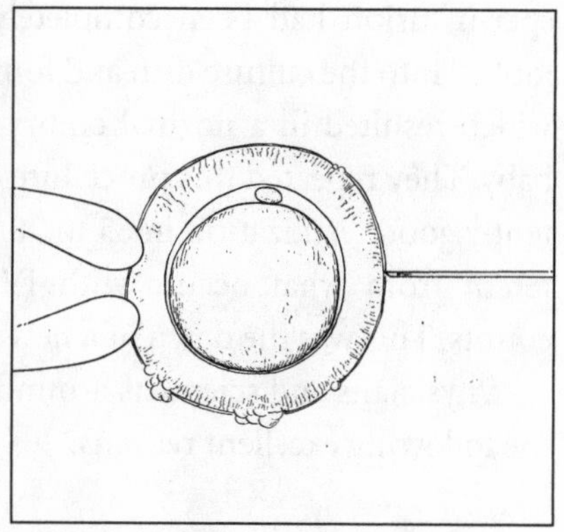

**FIGURE 11.2B.** Preparing to inject the sperm into the egg.

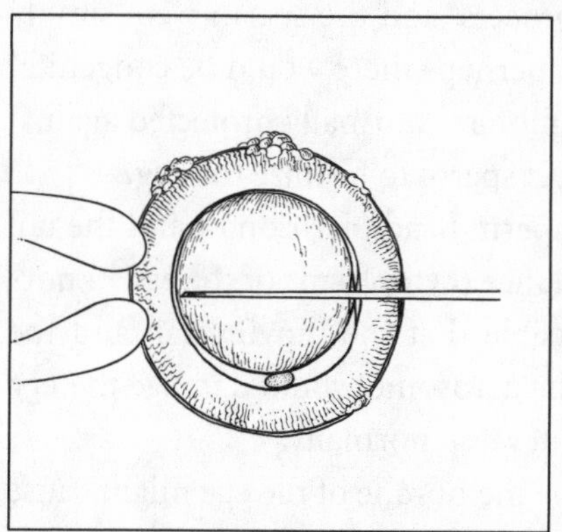

**FIGURE 11.2C.** The sperm being injected through the micropipette into the egg.

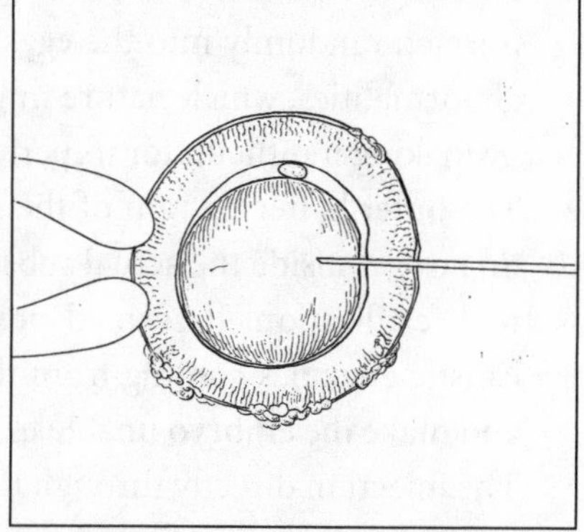

**FIGURE 11.2D.** Removing the micropipette. The egg has been fertilized by the otherwise infertile sperm.

sperm just were not any good and that no matter what mechanical help they might be given, they would still not result in fertilization, normal pregnancy, or delivery of a normal baby. We discovered how wrong we were completely by accident.

In April of 1991, two of Dr. Andre Van Steirteghem's young assistants (Dr. Gianpiero Palermo and Hubert Joris) accidentally punctured the membrane of a patient's egg (which they were trying to avoid doing) and injected the sperm directly into the egg instead of just into the space underneath the outer shell. They were sure that this would result in a destroyed egg and no fertilization, because the natural processes of egg-sperm fusion had been completely bypassed. But the next day, they looked into the culture dish and found a healthy, normally fertilized egg, which resulted in a normal embryo and, nine months later, a healthy baby. They repeated this procedure over and over again, and got consistently good fertilization in 65 to 70 percent of the eggs, which is no different from what occurs with IVF in patients with normal sperm counts. This was the dawn of a new era for infertile couples.

Physicians and scientists around the world were skeptical at first for the following excellent reasons:

- If the sperm couldn't fertilize naturally, that might mean they were abnormal and that abnormal babies would develop, or that the embryos would not develop completely into a normal pregnancy.
- Since there was no "selection" process, and the sperm were simply injected randomly into the eggs, perhaps there would be congenital abnormalities, which nature might have normally protected against by making it difficult for imperfect sperm to fertilize the egg.
- The outer battering ram of the sperm head (acrosome) and the tail do not get inside the actual substance (cytoplasm) of the egg in normal fertilization. It seemed possible that the moving tail and the caustic enzymes coming from the acrosome would damage the egg and make the embryo unable to develop normally.
- The injection directly through the membrane of the egg might cause damage to the egg.

So an international meeting of the world's leading authorities in IVF was urgently needed.

## The Meeting in Adelaide

In November 1992, a small group of scientists from around the world met in Adelaide, Australia, at the request of Dr. Colin Matthews. In this relatively remote outpost of the world, Dr. Matthews directed one of the most scientifically advanced IVF programs anywhere, and recognizing the importance of quickly studying and deciding upon the safety of the Brussels technique, he organized this elite group of fellow infertility researchers to convene in Adelaide and determine the answers to lingering questions. As the very soft-spoken and modest Dr. Van

Steirteghem quietly presented his results, the room was silent with the recognition that a new era was taking place in biological science.

It was astounding to see Dr. Van Steirteghem present demonstration after demonstration of cases in which the male had so few sperm that no one could ever have imagined fertilization would be possible. Rates of normal fertilization, embryo development, and pregnancy were reported to be no different from IVF in couples with normal male fertility. Using ICSI, 70 percent of the eggs fertilized, 80 percent of those fertilized eggs cleaved into normal embryos, and 35 percent of patients in each IVF cycle (who never before could have gotten pregnant) delivered healthy babies. Patients with ridiculously low sperm counts, which in the past meant complete sterility, could now have children. Dr. Van Steirteghem astonished the group further by reporting that neither poor motility nor poor morphology made any difference. The genes that control sperm shape, size, number, and motility appeared to have nothing to do with the genes necessary to produce normal, healthy offspring.

My St. Louis clinic's history of collaboration in microsurgery with the Brussels group now intensified. From November 1992 until the present, we have maintained a continual Brussels–St. Louis shuttle through which ideas are exchanged and developed for the purpose of eventually eliminating all male infertility. By the end of the century, more than one hundred thousand babies had been born from otherwise sterile fathers as a result of this technique, and they are growing up normal and healthy. I will give more detail on that in the next chapter.

## Types of Patients Who Need ICSI

Let me describe a few of the first ICSI patients to demonstrate the incredible impact that ICSI has had for infertile males.

A rural couple in 1993 had never dreamed they would ever be able to have children, because the husband had had mumps as a teenager, which had affected both testicles, and he apparently had no sperm in the ejaculate. As long as they had been married, they had assumed (as explained by many doctors) that there was no chance of getting pregnant. So when they came to see us in St. Louis, they were completely cynical about this new ICSI procedure. At first, the ejaculate did appear to have no sperm whatsoever, but after a careful search, we found seven sperm. Just seven sperm! This was more than enough to inject into the wife's four eggs.

The husband was astonished two days later to see normal embryos on the videoscreen being implanted in his wife's uterus, and nine months later he was a father.

A very healthy couple who had traveled around the world for eleven years seeking the best fertility treatment possible, had undergone more than fifteen IVF procedures with failure of fertilization (because of the husband's very weak sperm). By the time the ICSI technique became available, they had spent more than half a million dollars for therapies that couldn't possibly work because his sperm were so poor. Yet his wife finally became pregnant with his sperm in their first IVF cycle using ICSI in St. Louis.

We recently celebrated the bar mitzvah of the child of a man who had been born with undescended testicles, which were producing "no sperm." We operated on him to see if we could find a few sperm hiding somewhere inside his deficient testicles, but what we found instead was cancer. Luckily, this cancer was at an early stage and was curable, so we removed it. However, in a different region of this testicle (where there was no cancer), we found a few sperm, and we injected them into his wife's eggs. She became pregnant and delivered a normal, healthy baby who is now a healthy teenager.

We are also now celebrating the graduation of the child of a patient who had been diagnosed with Hodgkin's lymphoma (a cancer of the lymph glands) and had been treated with radiation and chemotherapy ten years earlier, resulting in complete destruction of sperm production in his testicles. His oncologist felt that he was cured of the cancer but was irreversibly sterile. Nonetheless, when we operated to search through his testicles, we found a few sperm and were able to use them for successful injection into his wife's eggs, with the result of a normal pregnancy.

These are just a few examples of early cases in which couples who had given up all hope of ever having a child of their own had their unrealistic prayers answered with the ICSI technique. About the only thing that seems to stand in the way of most couples with male infertility having children is, in truth, the biological clock of the wife. This is a complete turnaround from the early 1990s, when it was felt that most female infertility problems were treatable, and that male infertility was the untreatable stumbling block.

## Are All Types of Male Infertility Equally Treatable with ICSI?

No matter what the cause of the male infertility, ICSI bypasses the problem successfully. Whether the man has a normal sperm count, a very low sperm count, or only a rare sperm in his ejaculate (because of deficient or poor-quality sperm production), the results are the same. If he has zero sperm in his ejaculate and a doctor has to surgically remove sperm from his vas deferens, his epididymis, or his testicle, the results are the same (with the occasional exception). No matter what the source or origin of the sperm, whether the patient has normal sperm production or deficient sperm production, whether he's suffering from a previous case of mumps in the testicle, has had chemotherapy that disrupts sperm production, or has undescended testicles, as long as a few sperm can be found, there is a good chance for pregnancy.

Many cases of poor sperm production are caused by identifiable genetic problems in the man. The problem can be congenital absence of the vas deferens caused by a mutation on the cystic fibrosis gene, it can be a chromosomal aberration that is readily detectable in a routine chromosome analysis, or it can be a much more subtle defect in a specific area of the X or Y chromosome that is responsible for sperm production. Even in these cases with a clear genetic origin, the children have all been normal physically, chromosomally, and genetically, except that the inherent fertility defect of the father will in some cases be transmitted to the offspring. For the most part, parents do not appear to be concerned about this possibility, because they figure correctly that if their infertility problem could be solved, then any potential infertility problem in their son or grandson would be equally solvable, perhaps less expensively and more simply, twenty-five years from now. I will discuss all of this in more detail in later chapters.

### *The Role of the Egg in Normal Fertilization*

During ovarian stimulation (in preparation for egg retrieval), when the follicles are forming, the eggs grow from about 15 microns in diameter to 140 microns in diameter. The zona pellucida forms, but genetic preparation for fertilization has not yet occurred. Once HCG is given (the equivalent of the LH surge), the nucleus (germinal vesicle) of the egg begins meiosis, in which the total chromosome number of the egg is reduced from forty-six to twenty-three. The twenty-three chromosomes

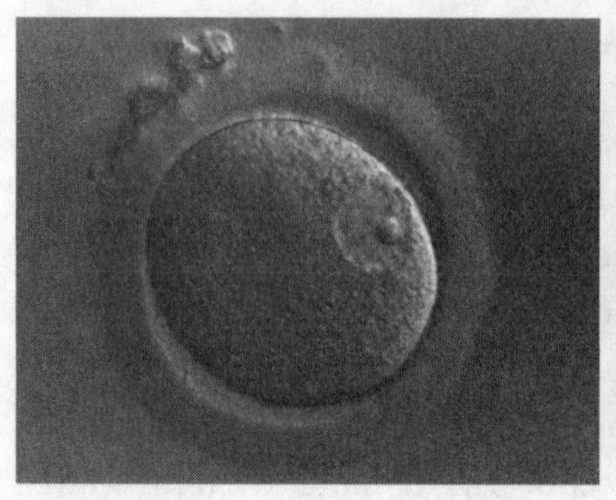

**FIGURE 11.3**
An immature germinal vesicle (GV) egg with intact nucleus containing forty-six chromosomes.

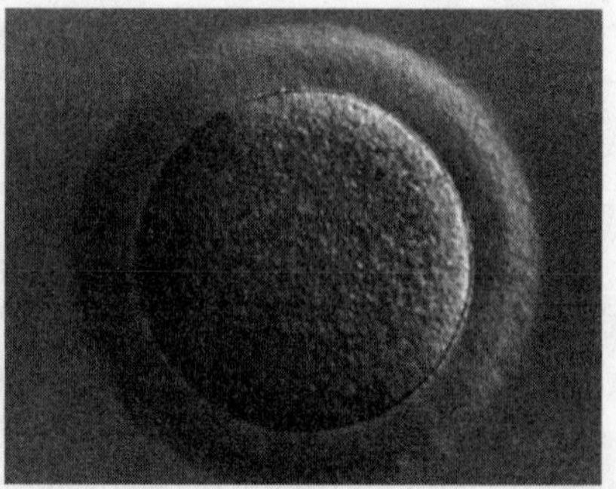

**FIGURE 11.4**
M-I (metaphase-I) egg in the process of maturing, but not ready yet for fertilization.

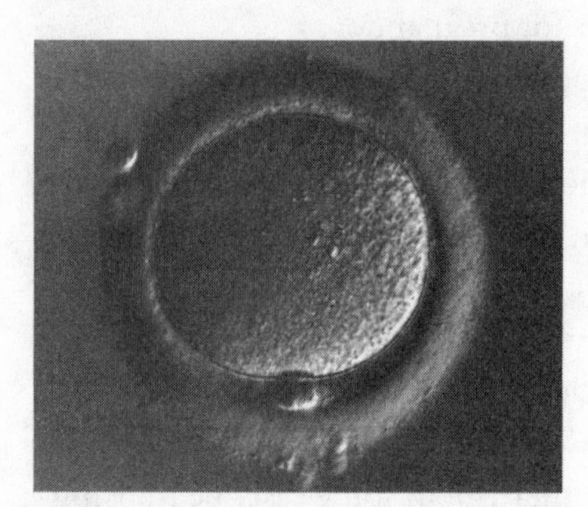

**FIGURE 11.5**
Mature M-II (metaphase-II) egg that has released its polar body (6 o'clock position) and is ready to be fertilized.

from the sperm can then unite with the twenty-three chromosomes of the egg, resulting in a normal embryo with forty-six chromosomes (see fig. 11.3).

This genetic process of meiosis has two steps. In the first step, the germinal vesicle (GV) breaks down, and we no longer see a nucleus. This is called the M-I (metaphase I) egg (see fig. 11.4). In the second stage the nucleus divides, but in an odd sort of way. Rather than the duplicated chromosomes dividing into two separate cells, one pair is extruded from the substance of the egg in what is called the first polar body, a little bleb sitting on the outside of the egg itself (see fig. 11.5). This is the metaphase two (M-II) stage, and the egg is now genetically ready to be fertilized.

In these pictures you can recognize the germinal vesicle (GV) as one big nucleus sitting in the center of the egg. The metaphase-one (M-I) egg, which is a further step toward maturing and preparing for fertilization, has no nucleus apparent, and no polar body. The M-II egg does not have an observable nucleus, but it does have an observable polar body sitting as a bleb outside of the egg substance itself but underneath the zona pellucida. It is at this stage that the egg is ready for fertilization.

GV and M-I oocytes cannot be fertilized. Only the M-II oocytes can be fertilized. In order for the HCG to allow extrusion of the polar body and formation of the fertilizable M-II egg, a proper period of FSH stimulation preceding the HCG had to have been carried out in order to create in the egg what is called meiotic competence. Without this, the HCG cannot prepare the egg genetically for fertilization. Therefore, when the eggs are cleaned in preparation for the ICSI procedure, careful attention is paid to how many are GVs, how many are M-Is, and how many are M-IIs. If one were to inject or attempt to fertilize a GV or an M-I egg, there would be absolutely no fertilization. Therefore, properly performed ovarian hyperstimulation of the wife with gonadotropins (to get the best eggs) is necessary for a high pregnancy rate.

## Pitfalls of Sperm Injection

### *Avoiding Damage to the Egg Nucleus and Spindle*

The nucleus of the egg contains its DNA. If the injection pipette were to damage the egg's nucleus, the egg would degenerate, no differently than if a sword were placed through an animal's heart. Positioning the egg in such a way that the nucleus is at a twelve o'clock or six o'clock position ensures that the penetrating needle can't do any damage as it goes through. However, it is almost impossible to see the nucleus in a mature egg that is ready for fertilization. That is why the polar body is placed at the twelve o'clock or six o'clock position, so that the egg's invisible nucleus (which is right next to the polar body but just inside the egg membrane) will be free from harm. If, however, you made the mistake of putting the polar body at the three o'clock or the nine o'clock position, the nucleus would most likely be destroyed by the needle as it enters the egg.

### *The Membrane Is Invaginated by the Injection Pipette but Not Broken*

The egg membrane is so incredibly pliable that once the tough zona pellucida is entered, the continuing insertion of the pipette does not break this membrane easily. Because the egg membrane is so elastic, one might think that the sperm is being injected into the egg substance, when in truth it is still outside the egg's membrane. Several minutes later, after the injection pipette is removed and the invaginated egg membrane comes back to its normal position, you can then easily see the sperm sitting outside the egg in the subzonal space without having actually penetrated into the cytoplasm. Thus, in order to achieve fertilization by direct injection into the egg, some of the egg's substance (cytoplasm) actually has to be sucked into the injection pipette until one can see the membrane pop, indicating it is broken. This is all performed under four hundred times magnification. Only then can the sperm be injected into the egg. Without this delicate maneuver, the egg will not be fertilized.

### *Catching the Sperm*

Probably the most difficult aspect of the ICSI procedure is catching the sperm in the pipette. If you ever went fishing in a trout stream and saw some trout or salmon hovering around a pool, and if you were tempted to try to reach out and just grab these fish instead of using proper fishing techniques, you would then realize how incredibly difficult it must be to pick up a sperm. One time, while fishing in Alaska, one of my sons was extremely impressed when he saw a brown bear come down to the stream and casually pick up a salmon in its claws, eat it in one quick bite, and then go on to pick up another salmon, seemingly effortlessly. My son decided to try to dispense with all the complicated and expensive fishing gear necessary to trick a fish into biting the hook, and simply reached down to grab the fish that were right in front of him. After hours of frustration, he looked up at me, looked over at the bears, and said, "Boy, they're really good."

In order to make it easier to catch the sperm, we first slow them down by putting them in a very viscous solution of polyvinylpyrrolidone (PVP). This is a thick liquid plastic that was used for years as a plasma expander for patients who had lost blood. Dr. Van Steirteghem knew it would be much easier to perform the ICSI procedure if the sperm were placed in such a solution first in order to slow them down. Even the most infertile, miserable sperm move at a speed that makes picking them up with a micropipette and micromanipulator extremely difficult. Sometimes, however, the sperm are so weak that they don't require PVP. Even so, you still need PVP because otherwise the fluid moves so quickly in the tiny pipette that delicate control of the rate of injection (so as to avoid damage to the egg) is very difficult. Thus, there are two reasons to put the sperm in PVP: to slow them down so they are easier to catch, and to have a thick fluid that gives better control of the rate of injection into the egg.

### *Problem of the Sperm Swimming Around Inside the Egg Substance*

With standard fertilization, the moment that the sperm fuses with the egg membrane, the tail is immediately immobilized so that the sperm can no longer move. However, when a sperm is injected via ICSI into the substance of the egg, it is not immobilized. Left alone, it would swim around quite happily in the egg and thus destroy it. Therefore, the sperm must be paralyzed before they are inserted into the egg by ICSI. This is accomplished by picking up the sperm in the PVP droplet, lining it up perpendicular to the micromanipulation pipette, and then actually crushing the tail of the sperm between the pipette and the bottom of the petri dish, all under four hundred times magnification (see fig. 11.6).

This is really a remarkable sight. Imagine picking up a tadpolelike creature by the tail, which is as thin as 1/15,000 of an inch, and then crushing that tiny tail between the pipette and the bottom of the dish, all with finely tuned micromanipulator dials. Once the tail has been crushed, the sperm cannot move. When it is injected into the egg's sub-

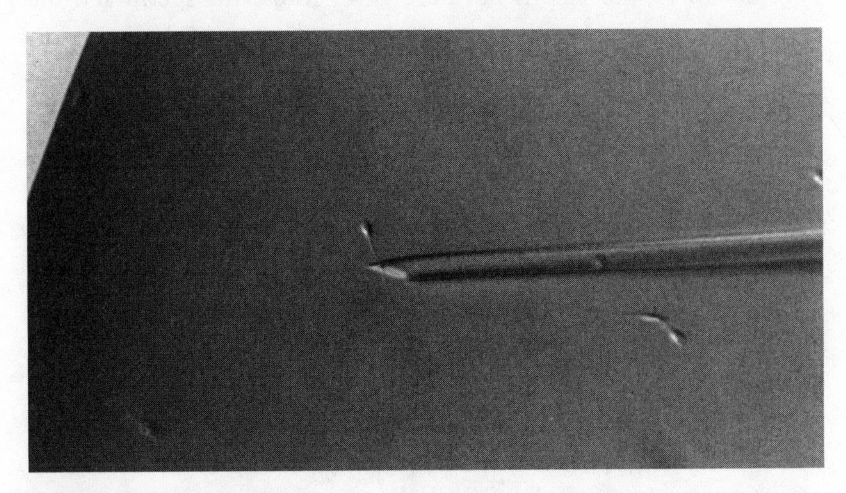

**FIGURE 11.6**

Under higher magnification, the sperm is immobilized by breaking the tail before it is picked up in the injection pipette.

stance, the sperm can then properly fertilize the egg because it cannot wiggle around within the egg and damage it.

There is another reason that the sperm's tail must be broken before it is injected into the egg. In normal fertilization the egg will not begin to develop into a dividing embryo unless it is first activated by the sperm's release of enzymes. After ICSI this activation will not occur unless the membrane is broken mechanically. This allows the sperm's enzymes to make the egg's membrane permeable to calcium, and that is what starts the fertilization process.

## Step-by-Step Details of the ICSI Procedure

### *Step 1: Preparation of the Eggs*

Egg retrieval is carried out by ultrasound-guided needle puncture thirty-six hours after the injection of HCG (as with standard IVF), and the eggs are placed in a petri dish to be prepared for the ICSI procedure. Normally, eggs are surrounded by a gooey, cumulus mass of gelatinous material, as well as a tighter layer of granulosa cells closely attached to the zona pellucida. This gelatinous mass makes it impossible to handle the egg or even to see the interior of the cytoplasm very well. These outer vestments of the egg must be cleaned off first. With standard IVF (or GIFT), this step is not necessary because the sperm and the eggs are simply put together in a droplet in the petri dish, the sperm manages to work its way through this gooey mass on its own, and the next day it is easily cleaned off. But with ICSI, the cleaning has to be performed before the injection procedure on the same day the eggs are retrieved.

We clean the eggs using an enzyme called hyaluronidase and aspirate the eggs in and out of glass pipettes that are about the same size as the diameter of the egg. The eggs must be put in the hyaluronidase mixture for only half a minute, to avoid damaging them. After that initial chemical action of the hyaluronidase, the outer gooey mass and granulosa cells can then be dissected off micromechanically by sucking the eggs in and out of these pipettes many times over a course of several minutes. After the eggs are properly washed, they are placed into a tiny microdroplet of media in a petri dish. Only eggs that are M-II, i.e., that have extruded the first polar body, can be injected with sperm.

### *Step 2: Preparation of the Sperm*

There are many methods of washing the sperm and obtaining the purest fraction of the best-quality sperm. We have discussed this in detail earlier in the book. We tried all of these different methods in our early work with ICSI. However, it is now apparent that the method of sperm preparation, which is so critical for regular IVF, has no importance whatsoever for the ICSI procedure. Individual laboratories' convenience and preference is all that matters in how they prepare the sperm for putting it in the petri dish, because there is absolutely no need to depend upon sperm physiology in order to achieve a proper fertilization with ICSI.

However, there is one warning: The only requirement is that for the sperm's DNA to result in fertilization, the sperm must be alive. The slightest motility, even a rare, occasional, barely observable twitch, is all that is necessary to verify that the sperm is still alive. If the sperm have truly died (most commonly from "old age"), then the DNA rapidly deteriorates so that normal fertilization is then impossible, even with ICSI.

### *Step 3: Setting Up the Injection Dish*

There are different ways of organizing the eggs and the sperm in the petri dish. The classical method is to place a droplet with 10 percent PVP and a droplet with regular culture media in the center of the dish, surrounded by eight microdroplets of culture media with one M-II egg placed in each one of those culture droplets. All the droplets are then covered with mineral oil (to prevent the evaporation of $CO_2$ and any drop in temperature) to maintain a stable condition for the eggs while they are outside the incubator. The media is buffered with a chemical called Hepes, which keeps the acidity (the pH) constant despite the media being exposed to air rather than the safe 5 percent $CO_2$ environment of the incubator. A microdroplet of sperm suspension is placed in the center of the PVP droplet, and sperm swim out into the PVP. Sometimes the sperm are of such poor quality that they cannot swim into the PVP. In that case, we place sperm in the droplet with regular culture media. After the sperm are picked up from that droplet, they can then be individually placed in the PVP.

### *Step 4: The Pipettes Used for Injection*

The glass pipettes used for ICSI are ultrafine microscopic "needles" made by placing very tiny, thin-walled glass capillary tubes into a computer-controlled microelectrode "puller." The glass of this tiny pipette is heated, and the two ends of the pipette are pulled apart in a carefully computerized fashion in order to give a precisely determined outer and inner diameter of microscopic dimensions. There are two main types of pipettes. One is the holding pipette, with which the egg is held by suction during the procedure. This pipette is much larger than the injection pipette. The injection pipettes are obviously much finer and very sharp. They have a diameter of about 1/5,000 of an inch. After the injection pipette is "pulled," it is placed in a microgrinder whetstone, and its tip is carefully ground to a 50-degree angle. The pipette is then bent with a heated forge under a microscope at an angle of about 35 degrees, to make it easier for it to reach over and into the petri dish. These glass injection and holding pipettes are extremely delicate. Any accidental touch of the tip will break them instantly and will require going to all the trouble of making another one.

### *Step 5. Picking Up the Sperm, Breaking the Tail, and Injecting It into the Egg*

Moving sperm will always eventually find their way to the periphery of the microdroplet, and swim along the outer edge. One can then micromechanically bring the glass injection pipette down to the edge of the microdroplet and pick up individual sperm, one at a time, as they swim along this edge. When the sperm are extremely weak and few, we use the principle of microfluidics to separate out the few good sperm for injection. We just create an M-shaped line of culture media in the bottom of the petri dish and place the droplet of semen at one end. Only the best sperm can eventually negotiate their way around all these angles to reach the other end of the M. It is then easy to pick them up and crush the tail.

The egg is then picked up with the holding micropipette and held in place while the injection pipette is used to rotate the egg so that the polar body is at the twelve o'clock position. The injection micropipette is then manipulated to enter the egg at the three o'clock position.

The pliable inner membrane does not break easily. Some of the egg material actually has to be sucked into the injection pipette in order to break the membrane. If this maneuver is performed without great delicacy and skill, the egg can be immediately destroyed. The instant that the membrane is broken, the sperm and the tiny amount of egg material that has been sucked up in the needle are then injected back into the egg, and the injection needle is removed from the egg.

### *Step 6: Checking for Fertilization and Cleavage*

After all of the eggs in the injection dishes have had a single sperm inserted into them, they are placed into a separate microdroplet of a culture dish, which is put back into the incubator. This culture dish will be the home for the egg over the next two or three days as it grows and develops, before it is put back into the patient.

Within four to six hours of the sperm injection, if the egg was successfully fertilized, the second polar body will extrude, indicating that the second meiotic division has been initiated by the penetration of the sperm. Within fourteen to twenty hours, we will be able to see the nucleus of the egg and the nucleus of the sperm clearly juxtaposed. This is called the two-pronuclear (2PN) egg, and it is the absolute indication that successful fertilization has taken place (see fig. 11.7).

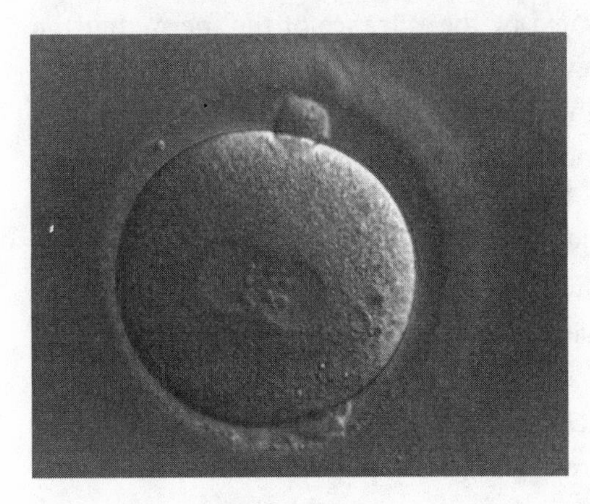

**FIGURE 11.7**

A 2PN fertilized egg twenty hours after ICSI. The second polar body was extruded at four hours, and the two pronuclei within the egg, one male and the other female, appeared at sixteen hours after ICSI.

The normal laboratory routine is to check each of the injected eggs early in the morning on day one after injection, and to look for 2PN fertilization. On average, whether with regular IVF or with ICSI, 60 to 70 percent of the eggs will exhibit 2PN fertilization. This 2PN fertilization is normal, which means that there is a single set of chromosomes from the mother and a single set of chromosomes from the father.

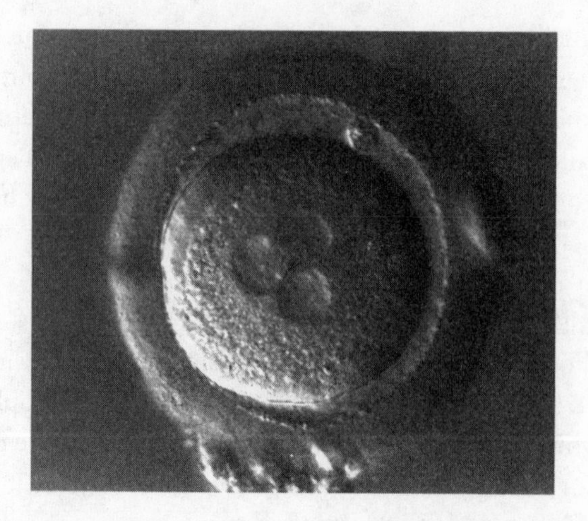

**FIGURE 11.8**

A 3PN fertilized egg twenty hours after ICSI. Since the second polar body was never extruded, this egg has two female nuclei and only one male nucleus. Three sets of chromosomes instead of two are not compatible with life.

Abnormal fertilization is seen in about 5 percent of eggs, no differently than with conventional IVF, and takes several forms. There may be only one pronucleus. This rather common form of abnormal fertilization means that the egg was activated by the entrance of the sperm, but the sperm nucleus itself never developed. This is a so-called parthenogenic fertilization (i.e., fertilization without sperm). In humans and in higher animals, these relatively common parthenogenic activations never develop very far, and never turn into offspring.

What appears to be a 1PN fertilization is sometimes really normal, because one of the pronuclei was simply obscured by the other one lying directly over it. In that occasional case, a 1PN–appearing embryo may cleave normally and result in a baby.

Another form of abnormal fertilization is the so-called 3PN egg (see fig. 11.8). In this case, there are actually three pronuclei seen on day one. This type of egg can develop much further than the 1PN, and can even lead to a chemical pregnancy, but these eggs will ultimately be miscarried because they are not programmed to develop normally. With 3PN fertilization, the egg never completes its second meiotic division. Therefore, the embryo has three sets of twenty-three chromosomes instead of the normal two sets. Such a fertilization is incompatible with life.

Careful notations have to be made about the normalcy of fertilization of each of the eggs in each of the microdroplets. It is very important that none of these microdroplets or eggs be confused or mixed up, and meticulous records and pictures of all eggs and embryos are essential. Many laboratories will skip these steps or be very casual about them in the rush to handle large volumes of eggs, but such a casual approach is not advisable.

The embryos must be inspected very carefully on day three to determine which ones are really viable, which ones are only divided cells that are not viable, and which ones will not result in a true embryo or fetus. To have the greatest chance of developing into a successful pregnancy, the embryos on day three should ideally have six to eight equal-size cells, they should have very few fragments surrounding these cells, and they should have a single nucleus observable in each of those cells (see fig. 11.9).

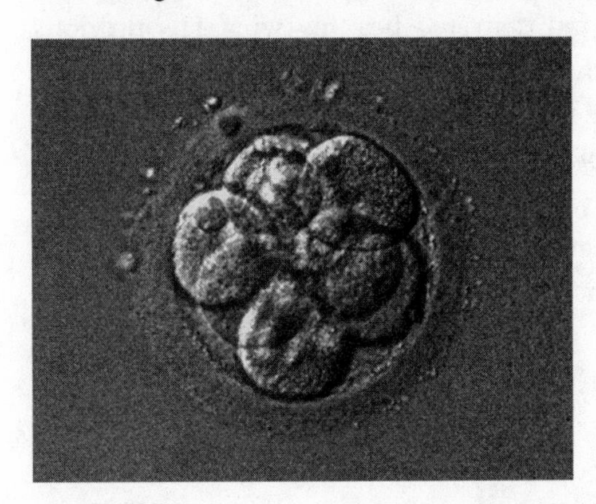

**FIGURE 11.9.** A normal day-three embryo with eight equal-size cells (blastomeres).

The majority of human embryos are abnormal and cannot develop into a baby. This is as true with spontaneous conception as it is with IVF or ICSI. It is just the human condition. Embryos that have all normal features have a good chance of being normal and developing into a baby. Thus, only the few embryos that are potentially capable of resulting in pregnancy are placed back into the woman on day three.

## ICSI for Male Infertility Versus Trying to Increase the Sperm Count

Previous therapies for male infertility caused by deficient sperm production have revolved around efforts to try to increase the sperm count, either through drugs like Clomid or Pergonal, or with testosterone, vitamin prescriptions, testicular cooling with cold, wet jockstraps, or varicocelectomy. A whole variety of ineffective treatments were designed to try to raise the sperm count, but these treatments were all destined to fail because the sperm count is genetically determined in each man and cannot be affected by any of these foolish therapies.

I remember a twenty-seven-year-old man with sperm count reports that consistently read "only an occasional weakly motile sperm." The patient had been declared absolutely sterile by a urologist, who had performed varicocelectomy, treated him with Clomid, then Pergonal, then testosterone rebound, and then even made him put ice around his scrotum to cool off the testicles every evening before he went to sleep — or tried to go to sleep. Obviously, none of these foolish treatments improved the sperm count. In the first ICSI cycle we performed for him, his wife became pregnant and delivered healthy twins. His previous doctors had hoped that with all kinds of conventional and ineffective treatments they could make him produce normal, mature sperm. But that was, of course, impossible.

There was a farm couple who had gone through the usual expensive, worthless male infertility treatments for five years, all of which was paid for readily by health insurance companies. The man had two surgeries, including a varicocelectomy on both sides and an unnecessary testicle biopsy. Their doctors then recommended a crossover vasoepididymostomy, even though the patient had no obstruction and was simply making a deficient number of sperm. He went through every kind of medication, and his wife went through fourteen cycles of IUI. Their insurance paid for all of this. On the other hand, when the time came to actually do ICSI, which is what they needed all along, insurance didn't pay. The wife produced only four eggs, three of which were injected with the ICSI procedure, and only one of which resulted in an embryo. This single embryo was transferred, and she became pregnant and had a happy, healthy baby girl.

A potentially disastrous case resulting from inappropriate treatment of the male involved a patient who was a prominent doctor from another city. His sperm count was twenty million per cc with 40 percent motility (not really all that bad), but he was told by the chief of urology at a university hospital that his sperm count was not high enough and that he needed a bilateral varicocelectomy. Following his bilateral varicocelectomy, the sperm count went down to zero, and one of his testicles completely disappeared. Obviously, the spermatic artery had been damaged in both cases. The remaining testicle had severe damage, but luckily recovered enough eventually to give him two to five sperm in the ejaculate. This extraordinarily low count, which many would consider the equivalent of zero, was fortunately more than enough for him to be able to get his wife pregnant with an ICSI procedure. But attempts to try to raise his sperm count, which wasn't so low in the first place, almost cost him any chance of ever fathering a child.

## Obstructive Azoospermia

It is amazing that ICSI even works for men with absolutely no sperm in the ejaculate. Azoospermia (the complete absence of sperm in the ejaculate) is caused either by obstruction or by failure of sperm production. Let's first talk about obstruction.

Between 1985 and 1992 we developed techniques of sperm retrieval (TESE and MESA) combined with IVF for men with obstruction. However, sperm retrieved from the epididymis or testes have very low fertilization potential with conventional IVF. Testicular sperm has virtually no motility except for very weak twitching, and was thought to have no fertilizing potential at all. But in November of 1992, we organized the first St. Louis–Brussels shuttle, which heralded a new era in which even men with zero sperm could now father their own genetic child. Dr. Paul Devroey and I (in Brussels and in St. Louis) came up with an idea that has completely transformed the treatment of male sterility caused by azoospermia. We were operating on a Dutch man to try to retrieve epididymal sperm, but once we got through the dense scar tissue caused by multiple previous surgeries, we found there was no epididymis whatsoever, so no sperm could be retrieved. However, we knew this meant an opportunity to try a crazy idea that had never been dreamed of before. We could take a small biopsy from the testicle, squeeze out the few nonmotile sperm that were present, and inject these premature testicular sperm into the eggs. To our shock, this resulted in fertilization rates no different than with normal ejaculated sperm and created beautiful-appearing embryos. The Dutch man's wife delivered healthy twins, a boy and a girl. This was the first couple to have babies using testicular sperm.

A St. Louis couple perked up when they heard about this. In the mid-1980s when I had first operated on the husband, I found that his epididymis had already been completely destroyed on both sides by an antiquated attempt to attach an "artificial spermatocele" to his epididymis in order to retrieve sperm. What we had found was a completely destroyed epididymis on both sides and a testicle encased in scar tissue that was incapable of releasing sperm. So we tried using testicular sperm, again not expecting great results. Yet this man and woman are now happy parents of beautiful twins. I had told them ten years before, in no uncertain terms, that their case was hopeless.

## Nonobstructive Azoospermia

In December of 1993, six months after Dr. Devroey and I performed the first successful ICSI with testicular sperm for irreparable obstruction, a lightbulb went off inside both our heads. I suddenly realized that a study I had done on quantitation of testicular biopsy in 1981 held the clue that would now allow us to help men who apparently produce no sperm at all. In 1981, we were simply trying to determine, for academic reasons only, whether counting all of the spermatids (immature sperm) in a testicle biopsy specimen could predict what the sperm count should be. It was a purely academic attempt to see whether we had enough understanding of spermatogenesis to predict the sperm count in any man by looking quantitatively at his testicle biopsy. This study from 1981 gathered a lot of dust in scientific libraries, and had very little clinical usefulness until the lightbulb went off in December of 1993.

In 60 percent of men who were completely azoospermic there were occasional sperm actually seen on their biopsy. In the 1980s, we considered this to be so rare a sperm that we weren't surprised that it correlated with seeing zero sperm in the ejaculate. Dr. Devroey and I then suddenly realized in 1993 that in the majority of azoospermic men, who appeared to have no sperm production at all, there must nonetheless be a tiny amount of sperm in a small focus somewhere in the testicle. In 1981, we had no comprehension of the enormous significance of the fact that most men who are thought to be making no sperm at all are really making an occasional sperm. In 1993, Dr. Devroey and I embarked upon the study of a large series of such patients, which were seemingly hopeless cases because of the absence of spermatogenesis. We decided to explore their testicles to see if a few sperm could be retrieved from these sterile men and used for successful ICSI.

The results were absolutely astonishing. We tried this technique on patients with azoospermia caused by maturation arrest, Sertoli cell–only syndrome, cryptorchidism (undescended testicles), previous cancer chemotherapy, and scarred fibrosis as a result of surgical trauma. Basically every kind of hopeless case you could imagine underwent testicular biopsy on the same day that the wife's eggs were retrieved for ICSI. In 60 percent of cases (just as would have been predicted from our testicle biopsy study in 1981), only a few sperm were found. But these were sufficient to yield normal fertilization and pregnancy rates not much different than if the man had a normal sperm count.

One of the first patients was a man from South America who had cryptorchidism (undescended testicles) as a child and was completely azoospermic with tiny testicles, no bigger than the tip of your little finger. We were able to retrieve from those tiny testicles enough sperm to get his wife pregnant with twins. The added twist to this case was that a cancer was found in those testicles at such an early stage that it could be removed while it was still 100 percent curable. Another case was a man whom I had told fifteen years earlier (he was a part of that original 1981 study) that there was no hope because he had maturation arrest, which we knew was genetic and not curable with hormones or any other treatment. Fourteen years later, we found fifteen sperm and were able to obtain five good embryos; he and his wife now have a happy little girl.

## Should ICSI Be Used for All IVF Cycles?

There has been a great deal of clinical debate about which couples should have conventional IVF and which couples should have ICSI. If a couple has gone through an IVF cycle in which none of the eggs were fertilized because of poor sperm quality, using ICSI in subsequent cycles makes the fertilization rate completely normal. The pregnancy rate and delivery rate is no different than in couples undergoing conventional IVF in whom there is no fertilization problem. However, what about couples who appear to have an adequate amount of sperm? Many of them will not have successful fertilization with conventional IVF, and it will not be apparent until they actually undergo the IVF procedure. In the United States so much emotional and financial energy is invested into just a single IVF cycle that no couple wants to learn via their IVF procedure that the husband's sperm is unable to fertilize the wife's eggs.

Of course, they can plan on ICSI in a subsequent cycle, but certainly it would have been better to have performed ICSI in the first place. The question is, can we tell by any testing or observations on the sperm beforehand whether or not the couple should have conventional IVF or ICSI?

Studies from Norfolk, Virginia; Scotland; Egypt; England; and Brussels have all failed to show any significant difference in overall ART results in couples undergoing regular IVF with normal semen parameters versus those undergoing ICSI. Embryos derived from ICSI versus those derived from conventional IVF are quite similar in the percentage of chromosomal errors. In other words, ICSI itself does not confer any increased risk or benefit to the embryo for either genetic or chromosomal errors. However, a very carefully controlled study from Brussels, demonstrated that there was complete fertilization failure in four times as many couples undergoing conventional IVF as in couples undergoing ICSI. Although the incidence of fertilization failure in the absence of an apparent male infertility problem is approximately 4 percent using conventional IVF, it is rare using ICSI.

This puzzling failure of fertilization despite what appear to be completely normal semen parameters was partly explained in the year 2000 by an amazing study performed by Dr. Liu and Dr. Baker in Melbourne, Australia. They found that fertilization failure with completely normal-appearing sperm usually resulted from a specific failure of the sperm to penetrate the zona pellucida of the egg. Everything else they tested in the sperm of these couples with fertilization failure was normal. Thus, it should not be surprising that 2 to 4 percent of couples undergoing conventional IVF have fertilization failure despite what appears to be completely normal-appearing sperm. In fact, the best test for determining this defect is a trial of IVF to see whether the sperm can fertilize. But this academic knowledge is not of much interest to the couple who is spending more than ten thousand dollars on their IVF procedure.

There is always a hot debate between andrologists, who wish to subject the sperm to increasingly more expensive tests to try to determine if fertilization failure will occur, and those who take a more pragmatic view. No matter how assiduously the sperm is tested, with very careful selection of couples who undergo conventional IVF versus those who undergo ICSI, there is still a complete failure of fertilization in anywhere from 2 to 4 percent of IVF cycles. In skilled hands there is no negative impact caused by fertilization using ICSI versus conventional IVF fertilization. Furthermore, in view of the huge expense and emotional investment for couples preparing for just a single IVF cycle, fertilization failure is an emotional tragedy that simply must be avoided. In my opinion, once a couple decides to go through the rigors of an ART cycle, they should be undergoing ICSI.

The only possible disadvantage to using ICSI for every single IVF case would be the extra cost that some clinics charge for performing ICSI. For that reason, we consider ICSI to be a routine accompaniment of any IVF procedure, and we do not charge one penny extra for it. If the couple would rather not have ICSI, for whatever emotional reason, then of course we will perform conventional IVF. Otherwise, we routinely perform ICSI in all our IVF cycles. We have become proficient enough at ICSI that doing ICSI for all our IVF cycles does not increase our cost, and therefore should not increase the patient's cost.

CHAPTER 12

# Will My Baby Be Normal?

IVF is big. The one millionth IVF baby was born in 2003. By 2005, there were more than two million IVF babies. In the United States alone, at least one hundred thousand IVF cycles are performed and more than forty thousand IVF babies are born every year, accounting for more than one percent of U.S. newborns. In Europe, almost 4 percent of babies are the result of IVF. Although one hundred thousand IVF cycles per year in the United States may sound like a lot, all evidence shows that if the government or insurance companies were to pay for IVF treatment as they do for other medical treatments, there would be a tenfold increase in the number of IVF cycles performed in the United States. Although the average IVF program in the United States might perform several hundred cycles a year, if there were insurance coverage for IVF, these same programs would be doing up to two thousand cycles a year. That means that if it were not for financial limitations, there would be approximately one million cycles of IVF (resulting in four hundred thousand babies) performed every year in the United States alone.

Infertility is an epidemic not only in the United States. Already there are many millions of IVF cycles performed yearly throughout the world. The Australian government pays for IVF cycles and considers ART an important part of health care. In Melbourne alone, there are more than six thousand IVF cycles performed every year. In just one IVF center in Tel Aviv, Israel, more than four thousand IVF cycles are performed per year, and in Amman, Jordan (where perhaps the second-largest IVF program in the world is located), there are well over six thousand cycles performed every year in just one institution. In Tokyo, one program run by a single doctor does thirteen thousand IVF cycles per year. In any very large city with a population of more than ten million, one would have to estimate that the number of IVF cycles done each year would exceed twenty thousand. Thus in the coming decade there will be many millions of IVF babies. Will those babies be normal?

The infertility epidemic is rampant in every modern society where women put off childbearing into their late twenties or midthirties. Approximately 25 percent of couples in any modern population in the world are infertile. Not only are infertility and IVF on the rise but about 30 percent of IVF children are twins, and 2 percent to 5 percent are triplets. Thus, for every million pregnancies, there are likely to be almost a million and a half babies. So if you think a million IVF babies born to date is a lot, there are plenty more on the way.

Huge numbers of our IVF patients clearly attest that their children are beautiful, normal, and intelligent. There are literally a million such happy anecdotes. Even women forty-six to fifty-two years old who had completely run out of eggs, after many years of facing their childlessness, finally chose donor eggs with IVF as their only alternative. These couples will attest to how normal their babies are, and what a joy and inspiration their children brought into what they referred to before as an "incomplete life."

Nonetheless, there have been worrisome reports spread throughout newspapers, magazines, and TV about possible risks and an increase in abnormality or genetic problems with children born from this reproductive technology. You need to understand these scary stories in context. All pregnancies carry a risk (usually small) of an abnormal child. Every mother who has ever conceived naturally, without having to resort to any treatment, will tell you that her biggest fear for nine months was whether the baby would be normal. No expectant mother can breathe easily until she has counted her baby's toes. Even then, throughout the child's life, the next biggest fear for mom and dad is whether their child is developing normally. This is a risk that every couple has to undertake if they wish to be parents, whether they are fertile or not, or whether they need infertility treatment or not. But are the risks of having an abnormal child via infertility treatment any greater than in a normal, fertile population, and if so, how much greater?

Numerous population studies involving hundreds of thousands of children from a variety of countries, born from normally fertile couples without treatment, have consistently revealed that 3 percent of all children are born with some kind of congenital abnormality. Many more are born without abnormality but develop some sort of childhood disease. Many of these problems can be corrected with pediatric surgery. Other defects don't even require correction, such as being born with an extra toe or an extra little finger. Defects that are readily correctable with surgery include cleft lip (which is cosmetically of concern, but can be repaired well), club foot, undescended testes, or hypospadias (when a male child has a normal penis, but with the opening positioned at the base rather than the tip). These "defects" can all be repaired quite routinely with modern pediatric surgery.

However, there are more frightening abnormalities, such as heart defects, which require major surgery; brain or spinal cord defects; and a whole host of other serious malformations. These malformations often have no specific genetic diagnosis and just represent relatively common errors in fetal development. They are simply the risk you take in deciding to have children, irrespective of whether or not you undergo any infertility treatment. All would-be parents are concerned about these risks, and they need to understand them. The question that scientists have been studying meticulously and methodically ever since the beginning of IVF is whether or not the reproductive technologies will result in an *increased* risk of any of these problems, and if so, which ones. In this chapter, I will discuss in detail how you can figure out your chances for getting pregnant with IVF treatment, as well as the odds (with or without IVF) of having a healthy child.

## IVF Statistics and Your Biological Clock

Universally, pregnancy rates begin to drop modestly in women over the age of thirty-two, and by age thirty-seven, they begin to drop quite precipitously. Figure 12.1 of this chapter demonstrates that the pregnancy rate per cycle for IVF, remarkably, can be superimposed exactly on the graph from chapter 3, comparing the decline in total number of eggs in the ovary with age (fig. 3.6). Similarly, the graph showing decline in IVF pregnancy rate with age can be superimposed on the graph in chapter 3 showing the decline with age in the number of antral follicles (fig. 3.9).

Figure 12.2 is a graph that is exactly the reverse of the pregnancy rate curve, showing the increased incidence of miscarriage with IVF pregnancies according to age. For women less than thirty-five years of age, there is a 15 percent chance of miscarriage. This is found in every population of fertile women. However, as a woman begins to progress beyond

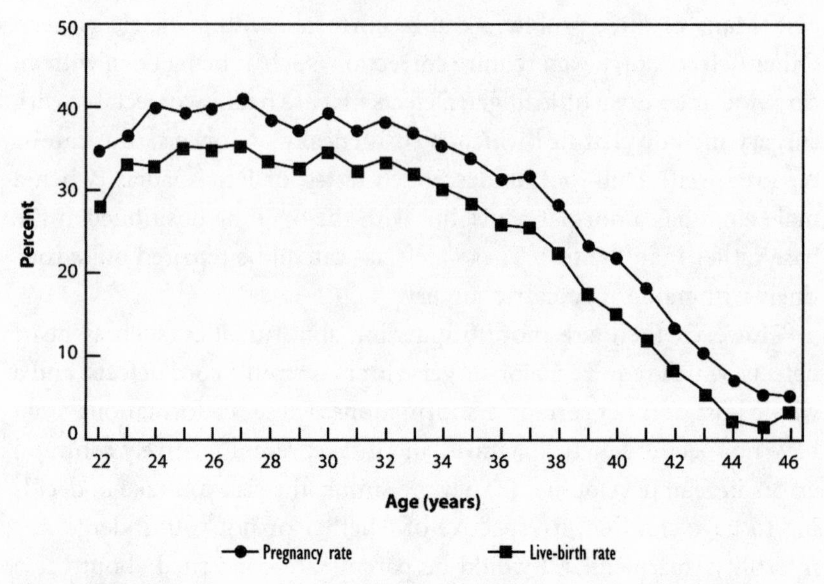


**FIGURE 12.1**

Pregnancy and live-birth rates for ART cycles by age of woman, 2000. Combined overall CDC Atlanta data of all IVF programs in the United States.

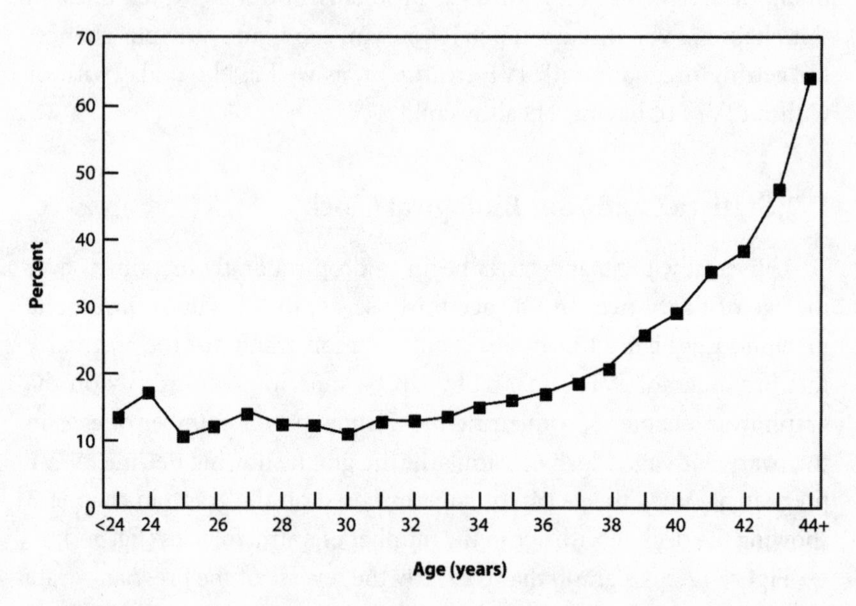


**FIGURE 12.2**

Miscarriage rates among women who had ART cycles by age of woman, 2000. Combined overall CDC Atlanta data of all IVF programs in the United States.

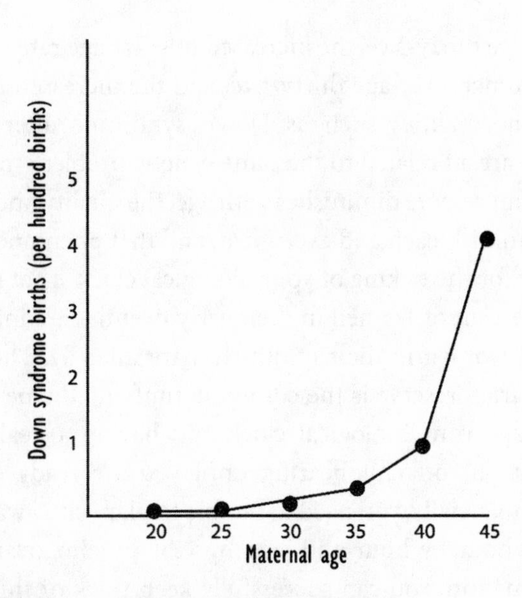


**FIGURE 12.3.** Maternal age and frequency of Down syndrome.

age thirty-five, her risk of miscarriage begins to rise, at first gradually and then quite drastically. By age forty-four, if she is lucky enough to get pregnant naturally or with IVF (it doesn't matter which), she has a 68 percent chance of miscarrying.

There is a big discrepancy between pregnancy and delivery in women over thirty years of age who have fewer than ten eggs. The older such a woman gets, with smaller numbers of available eggs, the greater the chance that she will miscarry even if she does get pregnant. This means that when only a few eggs are remaining in your ovary, those that are left are often of poorer quality. A look at figure 12.3 compares the risk of having a child with Down syndrome to a woman's age. Down syndrome (formerly called mongolism) represents a specific chromosomal error where the embryo has three copies of chromosome 21 instead of the normal two copies. This extra genetic material on chromosome 21 is what causes all the features of Down syndrome, which include reduced height, a simian crease in the eyes, reduced life span, and markedly retarded intelligence. This most feared of all congenital abnormalities occurs in over 1 percent of women aged forty, and in over 4 percent of women who have a child at age forty-five (as you can see from the graph).

These three phenomena — a reduced pregnancy rate with IVF in women over age thirty-five, the increased miscarriage rate with or without IVF in women over age thirty-five, and the increased risk of chromosomal abnormalities such as Down syndrome after the age of thirty-five — are all related to the same genetic problem in your ovary. As your ovarian reserve diminishes with age, the quality and quantity of those eggs diminish each and every year, and that phenomenon is what is responsible for the ticking of your biological clock. That is the reason why only 2 percent of women in their early twenties are infertile, while 25 percent of women in their midthirties are infertile. The inexorable decline in ovarian reserve is the common, unifying theme for learning how to manage your biological clock and having a healthy, normal child. As you put off childbearing until you are ready emotionally, socially, and financially, you need to be able to plan with awareness what is happening hour by hour and year by year in your ovary. With the proper information, you can successfully keep track of this, plan your life, and avoid the terrible surprise you may receive by finally deciding to start your family after your clock has already run out.

Figure 12.4 demonstrates an attempt on the part of the CDC to try to figure out whether or not the live-birth pregnancy rate across a wide variety of IVF programs, good and bad, throughout the United States can be related to any specific diagnosis of the cause of the infertility. What those bars show (allowing for the usual variation and noise in any study) is that in trying to prognosticate success of treatment, the so-called diagnosis, the only thing that matters is diminished ovarian reserve. In other words, all that matters in determining pregnancy rate with treatment is whether or not you have a lot of eggs left. Whether your doctor tells you that he or she thinks your tubes are a problem, or that you don't ovulate properly, or that you have endometriosis, or that your husband has a sperm problem, or if nobody can figure out what your problem is, or if you have multiple factors (whether multiple female factors, or multiple male and female factors), none of this useless diagnostic categorization predicts your chance for having a healthy, live baby. It is only your age and your ovarian reserve that matter.

As your number of eggs diminishes with time, the ability of those remaining eggs to perform the complex process of meiosis (where the forty-six chromosomes become twenty-three) is hampered. Your egg must have exactly half the number of chromosomes that it began with (twenty-three) so that its chromosomes can combine with the sperm,

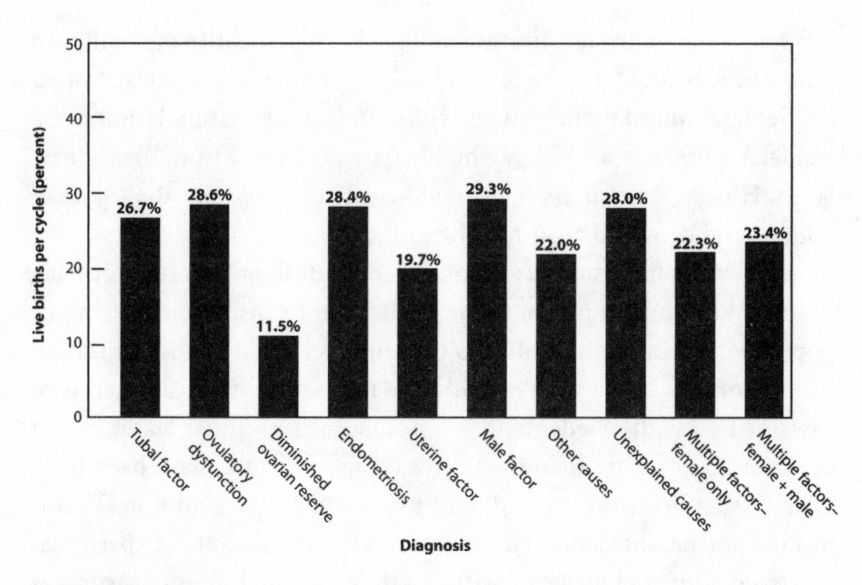


**FIGURE 12.4**

Live-birth rates among women who had ART cycles by diagnosis, 2000. No difference for any diagnosis except "diminished ovarian reserve." Combined overall CDC Atlanta data of all IVF programs in the United States.

which also has to have half the number it began with (twenty-three), in order to result in an embryo with the normal number of forty-six chromosomes. Indeed, all the cells in your body must have forty-six chromosomes, twenty-three from the egg and twenty-three from the sperm. In the aging ovary, as the number of remaining eggs diminishes the likelihood of chromosomal errors increases. On average, this problem increases precipitously at age thirty-seven. However, it occurs at different ages in different women. You need to know how much reserve *your* ovary has, and at what age *you*, in particular, need to worry.

## Fears About IVF Offspring Not Related to Age

A frightening story came out in the *L.A. Times* on January 24, 2003. You need to know how to deal with and analyze reports like this about the alleged negative consequences of IVF. This newspaper reported an alleged link between several rare medical abnormalities, including retinoblastoma and Beckwith-Wiedemann syndrome, and IVF. Just to cover themselves, the authors of the article did say toward the end: "The link between in vitro fertilization and birth abnormalities may still turn out to be spurious," and "several fertility experts pointed out that other studies have found no heightened risks." In fact, the retinoblastoma risk was later quietly debunked by a highly respected study from the Netherlands. However, the press had nonetheless accomplished their goal of selling good copy and creating unwarranted fears.

Beckwith-Wiedemann syndrome is extraordinarily rare, occurring in only about one in fifteen thousand natural births. Therefore, in any population of one million births (the number of in vitro fertilization babies born by 2003) there would have to have been at least sixty-two cases of Beckwith-Wiedemann syndrome. In the United States in just one year alone, more than thirty-five thousand babies have been born via IVF, so at least four would have to have had this condition. That is just the normal incidence. However, as soon as one mother experiences the tragedy of a child born with a rare congenital anomaly, such as Beckwith-Wiedemann's, she will naturally go to the Internet and look for others who have had the same problem. The Brussels group has reported detailed, meticulous IVF follow-up on almost six thousand cases, and in that report, there was not one instance of Beckwith-Wiedemann syndrome. Of course, by the time fifteen thousand babies have been studied, there is most likely going to have to be a case of Beckwith-Wiedemann. But to evaluate whether you should be fearful of trying to have a baby with IVF technology, you need to compare your risks to that of a normal, fertile population.

An equally alarming article in the March 2003 issue of *Popular Science* attempted to terrify the public about the dangers of IVF, claiming that IVF is an unregulated procedure. In reality, IVF is the most carefully monitored and regulated field of medicine. Press hysteria was aggravated by the publicity-seeking claim of an off-the-wall, cultist religious group, the Raelians, that they were going to start to clone human beings. Cloning is not even remotely akin to what is performed in an IVF lab.

Because such hysteria can be generated by unknowledgeable sources, you will have to engage in some serious study on this issue in order to have peace of mind and be comfortable with whatever steps you decide to take, whether going through IVF, conventional fertility treatment, or simply remaining childless. In this chapter, I will give you the tools, the information, and the resources to decide for yourself.

## First Published Studies on Risk to Offspring from IVF or ICSI

First, let's discuss scientific reports which caused concern that ICSI or IVF might have dangerous consequences for the offspring. In a 1998 study from Sydney, Australia, children at one year of age conceived via ICSI were compared to a group conceived by routine in vitro fertilization, and to a similar-sized group conceived naturally. There were eighty-nine children in the first group, eighty-four children in the second group, and eighty children in the naturally conceived group. The Sydney paper found no significant difference in the incidence of major congenital malformations, abnormalities, or health problems among ICSI children, IVF children, and children conceived naturally. However, this report stated that 17 percent of children conceived by ICSI had either mildly or significantly delayed development at the one-year mark compared to only 2 percent of a control group of children conceived by IVF, and only 1 percent of children conceived naturally. This report stirred up considerable alarm and seemed to contradict the general, worldwide experience of infertility doctors and their patients. In fact, if anything, our observation of ICSI and IVF offspring is that, on average, they are much more intelligent and advanced in development than what we would see in the general population (I'll explain the reason for that later).

Five years later, in 2002, at a meeting of the European Society for Human Reproduction, the same group reevaluated and reexamined these children and found absolutely no developmental difference. There was no difference in intelligence or the incidence of health problems among any of the groups of children arising from ICSI, from conventional IVF, or from spontaneous conception. At the same time that the Sydney paper came out in 1998, the Brussels group had carried out a similar study for developmental milestones for children aged two years. Their results indicated that neither the ICSI nor the IVF children had any lower score than the general population, and there was no indication of ICSI children having slower mental development than their counterparts from fertile parents. In 2001, the medical journal *The Lancet* published a study of children recruited from twenty-two different fertility centers throughout the United Kingdom. The study looked at neuromuscular development, intelligence, postnatal health, and congenital abnormalities in children conceived by ICSI, conventional IVF, and natural conception. They found no increased incidence of major congenital abnormalities in the ICSI group or the IVF group compared to the spontaneously conceived group of children. More important, there was no difference whatsoever between the ICSI or IVF offspring and the controls in neurodevelopmental scores or intelligence. So, at this point, there was no basis for fearing that there would be any difference between the children derived from ICSI versus those derived from spontaneous conception.

Then, in 2002, a series of alarming studies was published in the *New England Journal of Medicine.* One report came out of Western Australia. It involved 301 infants conceived with ICSI, as well as 837 infants conceived with conventional IVF. Those two groups were compared to 4,000 naturally conceived infants. It was simply a chart study, and no one had actually examined the children. This study claimed that 8.6 percent of the 301 children conceived by ICSI and 9 percent of the 837 infants conceived with conventional IVF had major birth defects diagnosed at one year of age. They compared this to the 4.2 percent diagnosed with congenital abnormalities from the naturally conceived group. I will discuss later in this chapter how that paper was completely in error.

In the same issue of the *New England Journal of Medicine,* an article was published by the CDC from Atlanta, stating that "among singleton infants conceived with IVF or ICSI, there was twice the incidence of low birth weight as in naturally conceived singleton infants." Oddly, among twins, who would be expected to have a lower birth weight anyway, IVF and ICSI children had no greater incidence of low birth weight than the general population. That seemed to make no sense. It was strange that among singletons there would be a greater risk of low birth weight with IVF and ICSI patients than with the general population even though among twins there was no greater risk of low birth weight. (Of course, lower birth weight in itself is not a terrible consequence, unless it is associated with an increased risk of developmental and other health problems.)

Reading between the fine print of this otherwise concerning paper, one can see that this lower birth weight in singleton ICSI-IVF offspring was found only when there was a greater number of fetal heartbeats in the early ultrasound monitoring. In other words, these were twins that reduced to singleton, and so they would be expected to have lower birth weight. Thus, even singleton children with lower birth weight are only a result of the multiple-birth problem, and there was no developmental problem associated with this slightly lower birth weight. Let me explain.

In order to increase the chance of pregnancy in IVF and ICSI, usually several embryos are placed into the uterus just to increase the chance of a pregnancy occurring, since the majority of human embryos are not going to develop. This means that there is, of course, a higher risk of multiple pregnancies, as with any infertility treatment (even the simplest fertility pills). This means it is possible for more than one embryo to implant. It is well known and established that high-order multiple pregnancies (greater than two) create a greater risk of premature birth and low infant birth weight. Thus, the lower birth weight of these ART offspring *cannot, in any respect, be attributed to any problem with ICSI or IVF* itself, nor to the propensity of these parents to have low-birth-weight children. Low birth weight is simply a risk associated with carrying more than one baby. In IVF programs that do not carelessly transfer large numbers of embryos, there will be no difference in birth weight among either singletons or twins compared to a naturally conceived population of singletons or twins.

## Risks Associated with Multiple Pregnancy

Clearly, the biggest issue for infertile couples to confront is the risk associated with a multiple pregnancy. However, this risk of multiple pregnancy can be completely controlled in IVF and ICSI, whereas with the general administration of fertility-promoting drugs, there is very little control. This means that IVF and ICSI are *safer* than the routine administration of fertility drugs. The popularly discussed septuplets from Iowa, whom I discussed in chapter 8, were, in truth, a medical tragedy, but not a tragedy related to IVF. The mother of the septuplets never underwent IVF. Indeed, if she had gone through IVF, the doctors could have carefully chosen the one or two best embryos to replace and could have frozen the extras so that she would have had a normal singleton, or at most twin, delivery. The big danger associated with IVF as compared to natural conception in a fertile population is the issue of transferring too many embryos, with the danger of more than two or three such embryos implanting. This results in low-birth-weight infants and premature delivery. But it is important to remember that this has nothing to do with any intrinsic problem in the mother or father, or with IVF or ART.

Nonetheless, modern obstetrics is quite a remarkable science. Normal infant birth weight is somewhere between 5 1/2 and 9 1/2 pounds. In the past, premature infants with birth weights under 4 1/2 pounds were at severe risk, but now even infants of only three pounds have an excellent prognosis for survival without any obvious abnormality and free of any serious handicaps. Neonatal intensive care units that began to spring up in the 1960s, and that represent the standard of care throughout the United States, have even allowed the survival of infants weighing less than one pound, delivered as early as twenty-six weeks of pregnancy. It is truly one of the miracles of modern medicine that these extremely low-birth-weight infants can survive, and many appear to develop normally without serious handicaps. However, their condition is tenuous, the health risks are enormous, and infants born at less than thirty-two weeks or under three pounds are often at a clear disadvantage. That is why it is advisable to do whatever is possible to avoid carrying anything more than twins.

The best follow-up study of extremely low-birth-weight (premature) infants appeared in the *New England Journal of Medicine* in 2002 from Children's Hospital of Cleveland. It reported the outcomes of extremely low-birth-weight infants born twenty years earlier. They compared 242 survivors among *extremely* low-birth-weight infants, averaging only 2.3 pounds at birth, with 233 controls from the same population base in Cleveland who had normal birth weights. It was quite remarkable that these very-low-birth-weight infants on average had IQ scores only five points lower than their normal-birth-weight controls. An editorial (in that same issue of the *New England Journal of Medicine*) coming out of the Harvard School of Public Health entitled "Premature Infants Grow Up" remarked about the relative success of these children. In fact, the extremely premature children were "almost as successful as the members of the normal birth weight comparison group in completing school." The editorial noted that "despite academic and other developmental challenges, most of these adolescents who had very low birth weight have academic achievement at least equal to that of their normal birth weight peers." *Moderately* low-birth-weight children (those between three pounds and five pounds at birth) have *not been shown to have any more problems* than normal-birth-weight controls.

I was sitting at a baseball game with the son of a friend of mine one summer, and he introduced me to his roommate from college, a Phi Beta Kappa and a star on the tennis team. He is an extremely big fellow, and I teased him a bit about his size. It was then that I found out that twenty years earlier, he had been born prematurely, at a weight of only two pounds, and his parents and pediatricians had never expected him to survive. Yet here he was, intelligent enough to be Phi Beta Kappa in his third year of college, and a star tennis player. So large population studies do not necessarily reflect individual cases.

Although I would warn very strongly against any practice that would encourage the proliferation of low-birth-weight infants, such as a triplet or greater pregnancy, I must confess that of the ten triplet pregnancies that we have had in the previous decade (which worried me greatly), all have gone past thirty-two weeks of pregnancy and resulted in healthy children without any measurable handicaps. But such a good result requires enormous expense and continuous care during pregnancy from a skilled team of super-high-risk specialists.

## Incidence of Birth Defects in ICSI and IVF Offspring Compared to Spontaneously Conceived Children: The Brussels Study

Our greatest resource in studying this issue comes from the Dutch-speaking Free University in Brussels, an institution I have personally worked with for well over a decade. From the very inception of their IVF program in the early 1980s, the Brussels group has had a transparent methodological approach to following up every single pregnancy and every single child born from their IVF procedures. Every pregnant mother was offered amniocentesis with chromosome testing of the fetus. Every single newborn baby was examined in detail by pediatric specialists, neurologists, and geneticists. This examination and follow-up was carried out on a precise yearly basis, and any treatments necessary were carefully documented and recorded in a massive computer database. The details of their follow-up on each pregnancy and each child (almost ten thousand babies) over the course of these decades gives us the information we need in order to be comfortable with IVF. Such a prospective study (rather than anecdotal news stories) is the only way to discern what increased risk, if any, you take by embarking on IVF.

First, I will discuss the incidence of congenital abnormalities (obvious defects visible at birth), and in later sections I will discuss the issue of chromosomal abnormalities (defects in the chromosomes that would only be detected with genetic study by CVS, amniocentesis, or the study of the infant's cord blood at the time of delivery).

There seems to be a running battle between the Western Australia Epidemiology group and the Dutch-speaking Free University in Brussels, Belgium. The Western Australia group stated that children born as a result of ICSI were twice as likely to have a major birth defect than naturally conceived children in the general population. The Brussels group responded that the cases classified by the Western Australians as major congenital abnormalities were so minor as to have never been diagnosed in a routine population register of babies that were not specially being studied. For example, there were several cases of minor cardiac abnormalities, which are very commonly present at birth but often go undiagnosed in the general population because they are so minor and usually correct themselves by three to six months of age. When the Belgians eliminated those cases from the Western Australian evaluation, once again the incidence of congenital abnormalities (about 3 to 4 percent) was no different from what is routinely reported in a standard population of newborns conceived from a fertile population.

The Belgians have studied IVF and ICSI offspring in such detail and in such a transparent manner that they have the greatest credibility. In 2002 they reported impeccably detailed evaluations of 2,899 infants resulting from ICSI and 2,999 infants resulting from conventional IVF between the years of 1983 and 1999. This is the most detailed and reliable follow-up study ever performed on the health and genetics of infants conceived through IVF technology.

First, we will look at birth weight in ICSI as compared to birth weight in IVF offspring in almost six thousand births (see table 12.1). Of singleton births, only 1.5 percent of ICSI infants were very low birth weight (less than three pounds), and only 1.8 percent of IVF children were very low birth weight (less than three pounds). This was similar to the 2002 U.S. study from the CDC referred to on page 280. In a normal population, 1.4 percent of infants would be expected to have very low birth weight. It was readily apparent that neither IVF nor ICSI increased the risk of premature delivery or of low-birth-weight or very-low-birth-weight infants, other than what could be observed as simply a consequence of multiple pregnancy. Note that the Brussels group had a very low incidence of multiple pregnancy, far lower than the United States, because of a more conservative approach to the number of embryos they transfer during an IVF cycle.

**TABLE 12.1**

**Comparison of 2,889 ICSI Offspring to 2,995 IVF Offspring (Prematurity and Birth Weight) — 2002**

| | ICSI CHILDREN | IVF CHILDREN | EXPECTED IN NORMAL POPULATION |
|---|---|---|---|
| Average birth weight | **2806** | **2920** | **16,730** |
| Singletons | 3224 | 3176 | |
| Twins | 2394 | 2382 | |
| Triplets | 1762 | 1769 | |
| Quadruplets | — | 1373 | |
| Prematurity (<37 weeks) | 902 (31.8%) | 867 (29.3%) | |
| Singletons | 126 (8.4%) | 140 (9.0%) | |
| Twins | 669 (54.6%) | 600 (47.6%) | |
| Low birth weight (<2,500 g) | 760 (26.7%) | 784 (26.5%) | |
| Singletons | 106 (7.1%) | 121 (7.8%) | 1,197 (7.5%) |
| Twins | 593 (48.1%) | 568 (45.1%) | |
| Very low birth weight (<1,500 g) | 125 (4.4%) | 167 (5.6%) | |
| Singletons | 22 (1.5%) | 28 (1.8%) | 239 (1.4%) |
| Twins | 64 (5.2%) | 96 (7.6%) | |

BONDUELLE ET AL., 2002

Only 3.4 percent of ICSI offspring and 3.8 percent of IVF offspring had any major congenital abnormality. There is also no difference in the incidence of these abnormalities related to the origin of the sperm, whether ejaculated or surgically retrieved from the testis or epididymis. In both ICSI and IVF offspring, as well as in the general population, there are slightly more boys than girls.

Looking at the minor malformations, which don't require surgery and result in no functional loss, again there was no difference from a normal population. Minor malformations include hairy ears, bilobe earlobes, large ears, moles, various septal defects in the heart that close and correct spontaneously over the first few months of life, phimosis of the foreskin, a fifth finger, irregularity of toe length, etc. An enumeration of everything that could possibly be slightly off of perfect could scare any couple into not wanting to try to have children at all, but this is part of life. In any event, there clearly was no difference noted in this huge series of almost six thousand infants between the health of offspring of fertile couples and the offspring of ICSI and IVF procedures. For couples who wish more detail, I recommend they look up the scientific paper, which is located in the journal *Human Reproduction,* 2002, volume 17, issue no. 3, pages 671 to 694. However, I can summarize by saying that there is no greater risk of congenital abnormalities or other illnesses in children born via IVF or ICSI compared to those born via natural conception other than those related to high-order multiple pregnancy.

However, what still concerned people was that there might be some subtle intellectual or chromosomal genetic deficit of their babies not readily apparent at birth without careful genetic study. There is no difference in developmental rates or intelligence of any of these children from a normal, naturally conceived population. However, the risk of chromosomal errors that might not be immediately recognized on physical exam remained to be studied.

## Understanding Genes and Chromosomes

It is critically important for all women having children at a later age to understand potential genetic or chromosomal errors that may not be readily apparent as congenital birth defects. Remember, we have said that when a woman is scraping the bottom of her ovarian pool of eggs, there will be a larger percentage of eggs that have chromosomal errors. This not only prevents pregnancy, but also increases the risk of Down syndrome or recurrent miscarriage. A similar phenomenon might occur with sperm from men who have extremely low sperm production, and thus might ICSI offspring have a similarly increased risk of chromosomal abnormality? To fully explore this, you first need to have a simple lesson in genes and chromosomes.

Genes are composed of long chains of DNA. The function of DNA is to direct by code the production of proteins. The amount and type of proteins that are produced under the direction of DNA determine your entire body structure and chemistry. That is how genes work. Your body, and the body of every animal on this planet, is made up of a variety of proteins, and these proteins are constructed from just twenty amino acids. There is an almost unlimited variety of amino acids that can be synthesized by chemists. However, in nature, on planet Earth, everything that is alive is composed of just twenty of those many hundreds of possible amino acids. This set of twenty amino acids is absolutely the same for all living beings on Earth, whether a fruit fly, an elephant, or a human. The reason that all of us are so different simply lies in the different ways that these amino acids are sequenced, which determines the characteristic protein structures of that particular being. The chemical structure of DNA is also the same for all animals on the earth. There is no difference between the chemistry of DNA in you or in a worm. In that sense, we are all the same.

In fact, DNA is nothing more than a long polymer, a molecule that just goes on and on in one long chain. Plastic is such a chain molecule. DNA (like plastic) is also a chain molecule consisting of four main ingredients: adenosine (A), thymidine (T), guanine (G), and cytosine (C). In scientific journals these ingredients are routinely referred to simply as the four letters A, T, G, and C.

The sequence in which these four basic "letters" occur in a vast sequential array on the DNA molecule represents a code that instructs the cell exactly which way to sequence its amino acids so as to construct each particular protein. This DNA code was first deciphered in 1967. Each of the twenty amino acids that make up a protein is matched by a very specific, definite codon, a sequence of three of the four DNA letters arranged in a specific order. The specific code whereby DNA instructs the sequence of amino acids to construct proteins is universal in all animals on Earth, and is no different in you and me from the toad, the guinea pig, or even a lowly bacteria.

There are 64 possible different ways in which these four letters (A, T, G, C) can be arranged, grouped three at a time, but only twenty amino acids they need to encode. Therefore, several different three-letter combinations can each encode the same amino acid. However, not all of these sixty-four codons produce a specific amino acid. There are several "nonsense" codons that serve as stop signs or start signs, telling the gene at what point to begin laying down the amino acids to create a protein, and at what point to stop. Thus, most amino acids are matched by several possible codons, and there are a few codons that have no amino acid match.

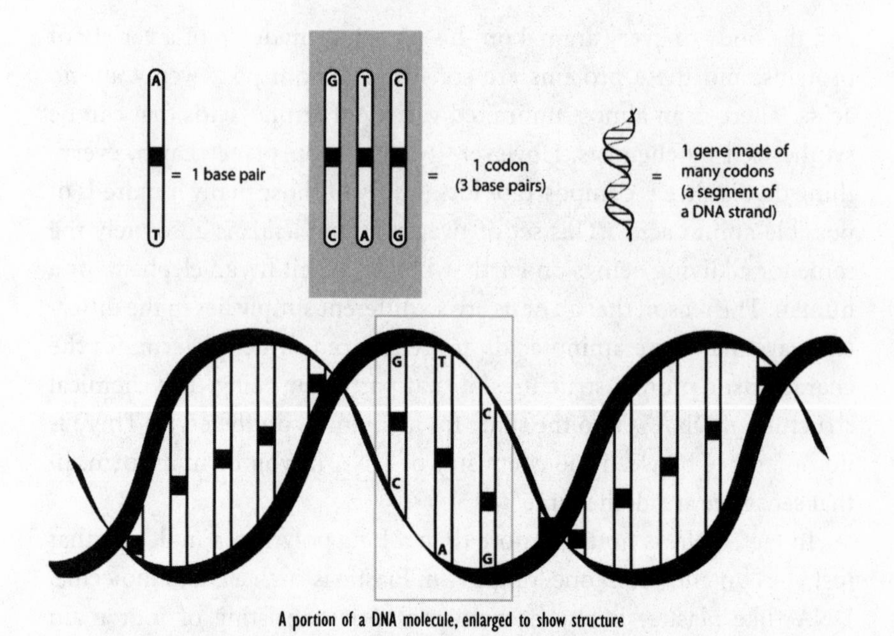


**FIGURE 12.5.** The relationship between genes and DNA.

These letters of DNA, which encode for amino acid sequence and, therefore, protein structures, are often referred to as nucleotides, or base pairs. Either way, in most scientific journals, they are simply referred to as the letters A, T, G, and C. It is the sequence of these three billion letters of A, T, G, and C from our father's sperm and our mother's egg that determine, at least structurally, who we are. Each molecule of DNA actually comprises two separate chains of letters wrapped around each other in a double helix, much like a spiral staircase (see fig. 12.5). The nucleotides, i.e., A, T, G, and C, comprise the coding side of this double helix. The other side is just a generic sugar molecule. A single length of DNA is composed of two sets of base pairs that are intimately attached and identical to each other. The A of one strand is always attached to the T of the other strand, and the G of one strand is always attached to the C of the other strand. A base pair is simply an A lined up with a T, or a G lined up with a C. Wherever there is a T, its opposite mate is an A, and wherever there is a G, its opposite mate is a C. This complementary system allows DNA strands to duplicate themselves exactly, the one strand serving as a template for the creation of another identical strand. It is this organization that allows a chromosome to divide into absolutely identical subunits during cell division so that every single cell of the ten trillion cells in our body is genetically, if not functionally, identical.

A chromosome is simply a huge, long chain of literally millions of base pairs of the A, T, G, and C components of DNA. Understanding your chromosomes will allow you to understand better how your fertility clock works and will help you decipher the otherwise confusing array of "scare" articles you may have read regarding whether to expect a healthy, normal baby.

Base pairs in a single strand of DNA merely represent one chromosome, and every cell in your body (except for sperm or mature eggs) has two sets of chromosomes. Each set of three base pairs represents a code and, therefore, is called a codon; thousands of these codons make up a gene. There are approximately a thousand or more genes in every one of your chromosomes, and each one of these genes consists of many thousands of DNA base pairs lined up in a specific sequence. Thus, all of life on Earth, no matter how complex and varying, is made up of these same four base pairs, which code in the same exact way for the same exact twenty amino acids to produce a variety of different proteins that account for the incredible variety of life.

Most of the cell's DNA is enclosed within the nucleus of the cell. The nucleus is about twenty microns in size, which is thinner than the diameter of a single hair. All of the genetic information that codes for what you are is crammed into this little package. A total of six billion base pairs, three billion for each set of chromosomes, are located in that tiny twenty-micron nucleus located within each cell. To gain an understanding of this remarkable feat of nature, just imagine this: If the chromosome were actually three millimeters thick (approximately 1/15 of an inch), then all of the chromosomes within a single cell would stretch all the way from the East Coast of the United States to the West Coast.

Each cell in your body has forty-six such chromosomes (two pairs of twenty-three) (see fig. 12.6). Forty-four of them are called autosomes because they have nothing to do with sex determination. The other two are the X and Y chromosomes. The chromosomes are arbitrarily numbered and designated in order of decreasing length. Thus, the largest human chromosome is chromosome 1, and the smallest human chromosome is chromosome 22. The human X and Y chromosomes are separately named because they are inextricably connected to each other throughout evolutionary time and must work together. The X chromo-

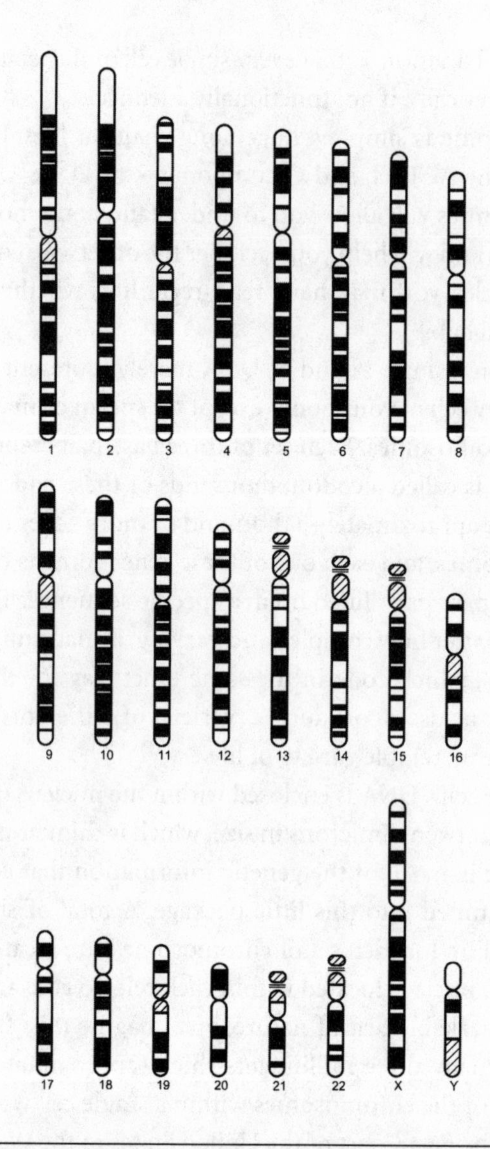


**FIGURE 12.6**

A diagram of all twenty-two human autosomal chromosomes, as well as X and Y. The dark-staining regions are densely repetitive DNA, and the light-staining regions are nonrepetitive sequences. These staining patterns are used to identify the chromosomes.

some's size falls between that of chromosome 7 and chromosome 8. The Y chromosome is very tiny, and it is the chromosome that determines whether the embryo will become a boy or a girl. It also harbors many genes specifically designed for proper sperm production.

## An Abnormal Number of Chromosomes Causes Down Syndrome and Miscarriage

Two copies of each chromosome are absolutely necessary for the embryo to develop into a normal fetus and a healthy baby. If there is an extra copy of one of these chromosomes, or a missing copy of one of these chromosomes, leading to perhaps forty-seven chromosomes or forty-five chromosomes in the fertilized egg, the embryo cannot possibly develop normally. That is why fetuses with three copies of chromosome 21, instead of two, either miscarry (80 percent of the time) or result in a Down syndrome baby. In fact, the reason that Down syndrome (trisomy 21) is so feared is that it is one of the few chromosomal abnormalities that is not programmed for complete death and miscarriage, but rather can result in an occasional, but abnormal, live offspring. A glance back at figure 12.6 will explain the reason that individuals with three copies of chromosome 21 can survive. Chromosome 21 is probably one of the smallest chromosomes, and has the fewest genes. Thus, an overdose of genes from an extra chromosome 21 would not be as likely to be lethal as an overdose of any of the other autosomes. Trisomy means three copies rather than two copies of a particular chromosome. A trisomy of chromosome 1 would not be compatible with embryo development because chromosome 1 is huge, and it harbors many genes critical for life function. You wouldn't even see errors in chromosome 1 in a fetal miscarriage because the fertilized egg simply would not develop far enough even to implant.

However, when chromosomes 13 and 18 are present in three copies instead of two, although ultimately lethal, this can occasionally result in advanced fetal development and even a stillbirth. In fact, any of the chromosomes larger than chromosome 12, if present in three copies instead of two, can result in pregnancy but will ultimately end in an early miscarriage. The reason for this miscarriage is not some defect in the mother's uterus or her inability to "hold the pregnancy." Rather, it is simply because the embryo was programmed for death from the very beginning. In contrast to trisomy (three copies of a chromosome) when there is only one copy of a particular chromosome (monosomy), this is almost always fatal, and with the exception of the sex chromosomes, it is unlikely to lead even to a hint of early pregnancy.

## How Your Aging Eggs Develop Chromosome Errors

How do these chromosomal errors occur? How does this problem of too many or too few copies of a chromosome occur in at least 15 percent of pregnancies even in young, fertile women, and in well over 60 percent of the pregnancies of older women? Actually, the majority of human embryos are chromosomally abnormal, and most of these abnormalities are present in the fertilized egg in the first few hours of life. These common chromosomal errors (where you have either one too many or one too few of a particular chromosome, or of several chromosomes) in 90 percent of cases are a result of how the egg prepares for fertilization by reducing its chromosome number from forty-six to twenty-three. In 10 percent of the cases, it is a consequence of how the sperm is produced in the testes (also when sperm precursor cells reduce their number from forty-six to twenty-three). This process of reduction from forty-six to twenty-three chromosomes occurs only in the egg or in the sperm (no other tissue in the body) as they are preparing for fertilization. This process is called meiosis. Most chromosomal errors that would result in a Down syndrome child, a miscarriage, or simply a failure to get pregnant arise from faulty meiosis.

I will now explain exactly how meiosis occurs and try to simplify this very complex process so that you can understand just how the chromosomes can get accidentally mis-shuffled, and what we can do about it. But it is a little tricky to understand, and those who aren't interested may wish to skip to the next subsection.

Take a look at figures 12.7 and 12.8, which show how most cells in your body divide and replenish themselves. During most of the cell's life, the chromosomes are very loosely entwined with one another in the nucleus and are working at directing the production of the various proteins, which take care of the cell's growth and metabolism. Your chromosomes, most of the time, look like a curly, jumbled mass of wires, similar to a Brillo pad, inside the cell's nucleus. However, when it comes time for the cell to divide, the chromosomes line up in an orderly way on a special structure called the spindle. When the cell divides, each chromosome duplicates, and one set of chromosomes goes on its way along the spindle to one cell, as the other set of chromosomes goes on its way to the other cell. Every cell in the body needs to do this in order to divide. This process of identical cell division, with exact duplication

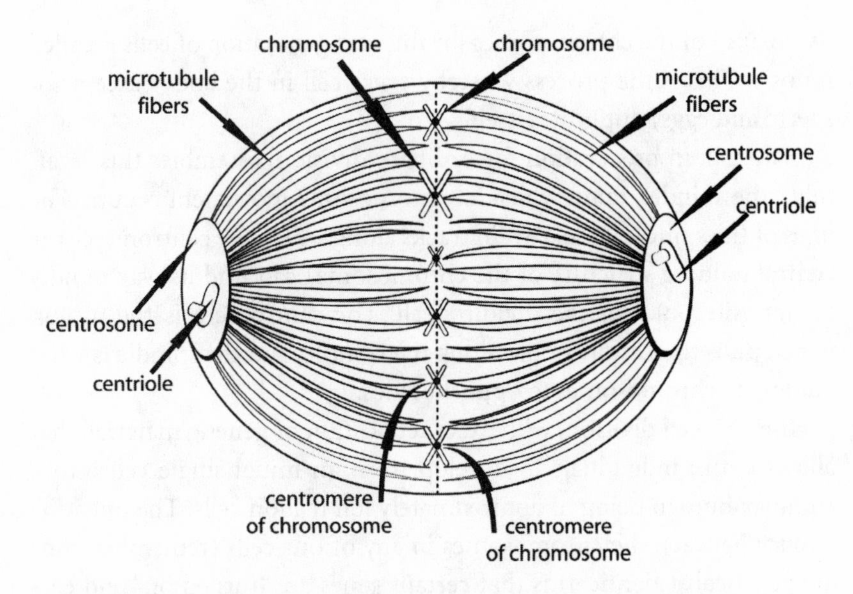


**FIGURE 12.7.** Mitotic cell division: chromosomes lining up on spindle prior to separation.

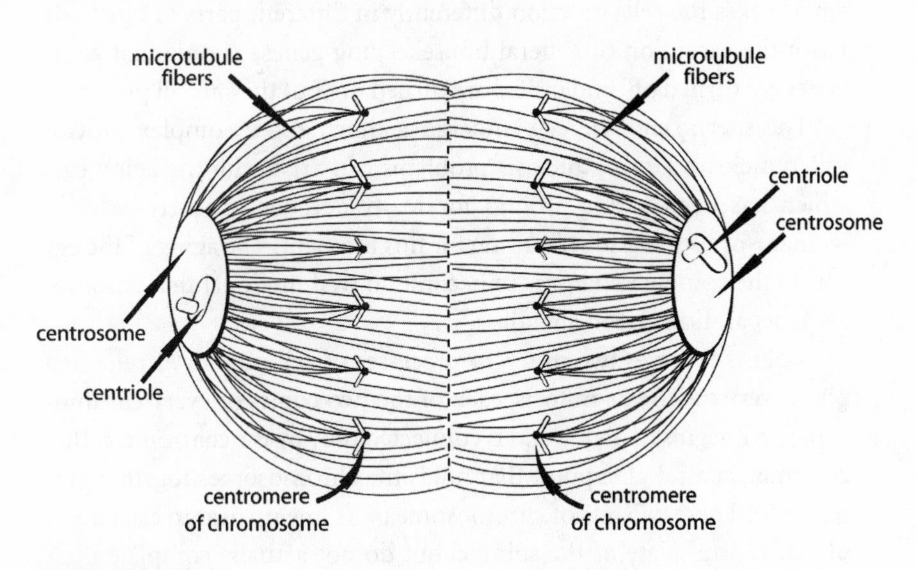


**FIGURE 12.8**

Mitotic cell division: spindle motor network for separating chromosomes at the time of cell division; chromosomes are now receding toward opposite poles along this spindle.

(Xeroxing) of the chromosomes for the next generation of cells is called mitosis. This is the process whereby every cell in the body (except for sperm and eggs) duplicates itself.

The cell, in preparation for ordinary division, assembles this "scaffold," the spindle, upon which all chromosome movement occurs. The lines of the spindle are like train tracks along which the centromere (the central holding structure of the chromosome) can find its way rapidly to opposite poles of the dividing cell. The centromere is the motor, which pulls the chromosome along the spindle, and the spindle is what guides the chromosomes to opposite sides.

It is this cell division, with exact replication of genetic material, that allows entire individuals to develop from an initial single cell into a complex human being of approximately ten trillion cells. The only difference between the chromosomes in any of our cells (remember, they are genetically identical) is that certain genes are "turned on" and certain genes are "turned off" depending on which tissue or body part they reside in. The genetic blueprint is the same in every cell in our body, and what makes the cells function differently in different parts of our body (with the exception of general housekeeping genes) is only that some genes are turned off, and others are turned on, but they are all present.

The sperm and the egg undergo a much more complex process called meiosis. During meiosis problems can arise with the aging egg, which has been sitting around for many decades (in forty-year-old women, for four decades) waiting for this moment. The aging of the egg causes the spindle apparatus to become so dysfunctional that chromosome separation gets mishandled.

Meiosis involves two different processes of cell division. In the first phase, very much like mitosis, each of the two copies of every chromosome pair begins to divide and is connected only by the centromere, that common, central glue point that holds the chromosomes together (see fig. 12.9). These two sets of chromosome pairs line up next to each other on the central plate of the spindle, but do not actually complete their division yet. Their duplication does not result in complete separation because the centromere holds fast and does not, itself, separate. These homologous chromosomes then exchange genetic material (in a process called recombination). Without dividing, they get pulled away from each other along the tracks of the spindle as their centromeres move to opposite poles. This is the so-called first meiotic division.

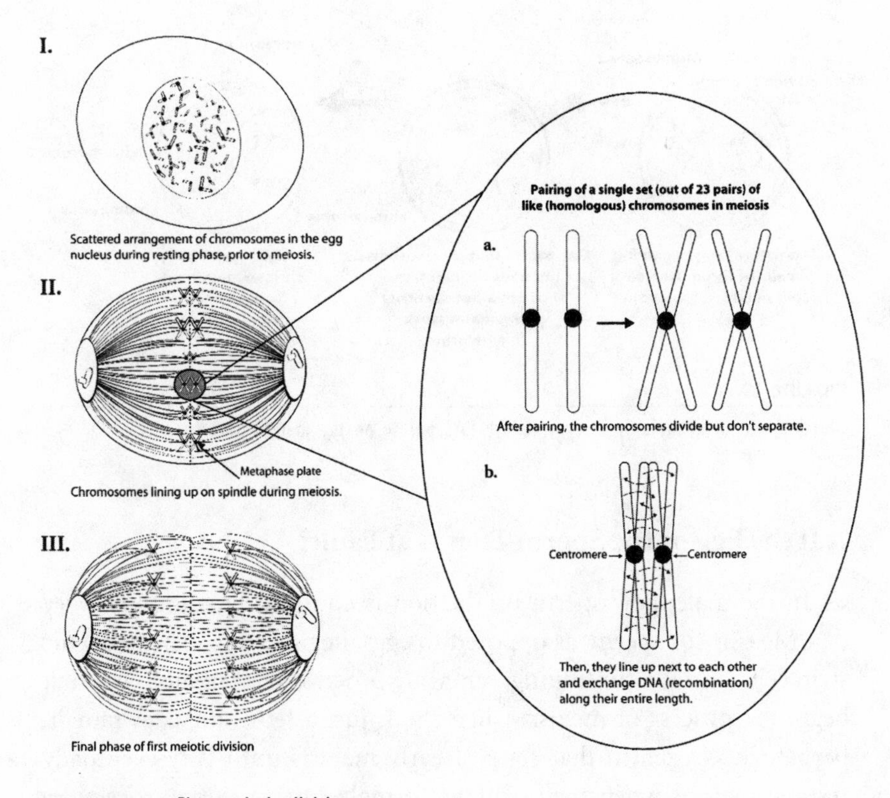


**FIGURE 12.9.** First meiotic division.

In the second meiotic division, the chromosomes that had originally divided but were still held together by their centromere finally finish their division as their centromeres divide. It is during the shuffle of these two phases of meiotic division, when chromosomes first become duplicated, then separate, and then divide later, that an error can occur in the number of chromosomes that wind up in the egg or the sperm. If the spindle is not working properly, because of an aging process inherent in the egg that becomes more and more exaggerated as the woman gets older, there may either be an extra copy of one or several of the chromosomes in the egg, or there may be a copy missing of one or several of the chromosomes (see fig. 12.10). That is the cause of increasing infertility with the woman's age, miscarriage, and chromosomal birth defects such as Down syndrome (see fig. 12.11).

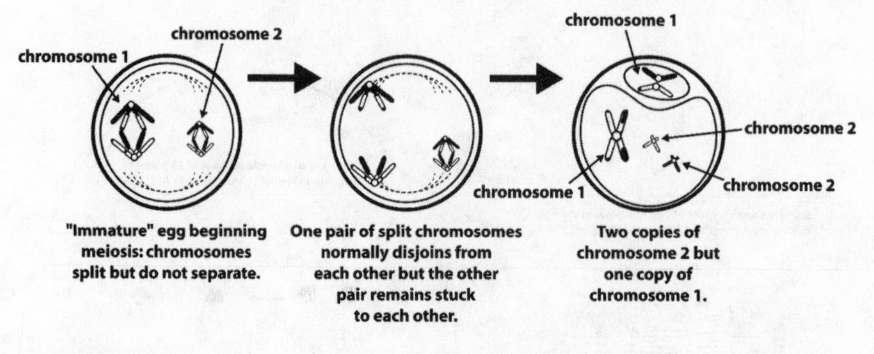


**FIGURE 12.10**

Development of aneuploidy in eggs: failure to separate on the meiotic spindle.

## Is It the Egg or the Sperm That Is at Fault?

In the male, new sperm production is continually going on every day. Meiosis for sperm, as opposed to eggs, begins with spermatogenic stem cells, and is a continuing, renewing process. The female's eggs first begin the process of meiosis when she is just a fetus; the eggs remain perpetually frozen in that state of early meiosis until they eventually resume meiosis when they ovulate. In males, the meiotic process, by contrast, is fresh and free-running, with cells progressing daily through meiosis in an uninterrupted fashion. In females, the long delay over many decades in completing the meiotic division is the reason for the dramatic increase in birth defects seen in older women. Ninety percent of chromosomal errors in human embryos come from the egg while only 10 percent come from the sperm.

There is, however, another important difference, specifically in humans, between male meiosis and female meiosis. The neck of the sperm has a round structure on it that joins the sperm head with the sperm tail. This is called the sperm centrosome. Every cell in your body must have a centrosome in order to pull the centromeres of the divided chromosomes to the opposite poles of what will become two new cells when it divides. Whether you're a male or a female, the centrosome of every cell in your body was inherited from your father's sperm. In the egg of the human female, however, there is no centrosome. In order to perform meiosis, the egg's chromosomes must bind themselves to the spindle, which has to be built from inside out without any assistance from a centrosome. After fertilization, the sperm centrosome (once it

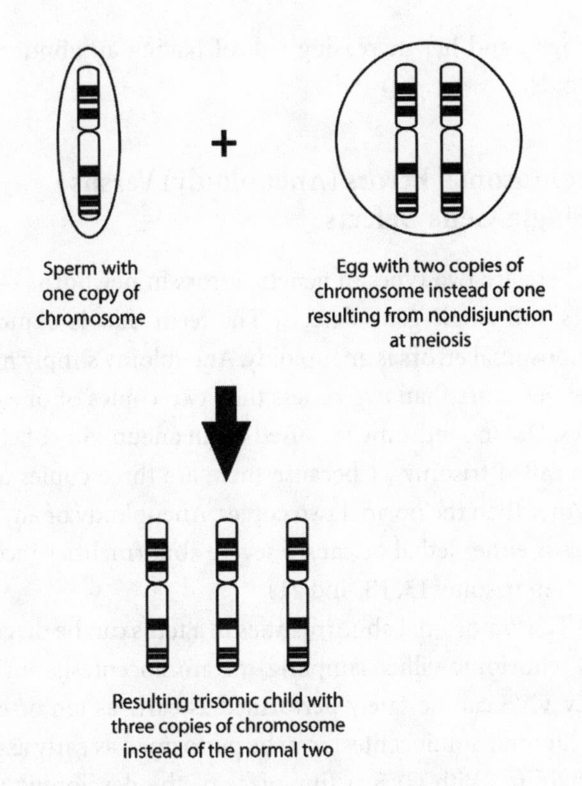


**FIGURE 12.11**

Diagram showing how three copies of a chromosome (instead of the normal two) can find their way to what becomes the trisomic Down's infant because of nondisjunction in the egg's meiosis, with two copies (instead of one) in the original egg.

enters the egg) divides and becomes the centrosome of the egg, which is necessary for all future development of that fertilized egg into a normal embryo, and subsequently into a baby.

The centrosome of the sperm is thus crucial for development of the fertilized egg through all of its embryologic and fetal stages. The centrosome remains necessary for the maintenance of all adult life. Cell division is the basis of all life, and it cannot occur without the proper, equal separation of chromosomes, which occurs because of this chromosomal motor, which comes from the sperm. Therefore, the entrance of an intact, normal sperm is essential for human embryo development.

Nonetheless, in more than 90 percent of cases, the cause of chromosomal errors in the embryo is the aging egg. The aging egg is the origin of the woman's biological clock. It is the cause of her infertility, her miscarriages, and her increasing risk of having an abnormal child as she gets older.

## Chromosomal Errors (Aneuploidy) Versus Single-Gene Defects

There are two types of genetic errors in newborns — chromosomal errors and single-gene defects. The term that is commonly used for chromosomal errors is aneuploidy. Aneuploidy simply means that there are either more than two or less than two copies of one of the chromosomes. Down syndrome is caused by an aneuploidy of chromosome 21, often called trisomy 21 because there are three copies of chromosome 21 rather than the normal two copies. Aneuploidy of any of the 22 autosomes is either lethal or causes severe abnormalities incompatible with life (as in trisomy 13, 18, and 21).

All chromosomal abnormalities in a fetus can be diagnosed by either CVS (chorionic villus sampling) or amniocentesis during early pregnancy. CVS can be safely performed as early as ten or eleven weeks of fetal life, and amniocentesis can be performed as early as fourteen weeks of fetal life. With CVS, a tiny piece of the developing placenta of the embryo is aspirated and classically the cells are cultured for several weeks so that the chromosomes can be stained and observed. However, a quick answer can be obtained by the next day using a direct staining process called FISH (which I will explain fully in the next chapter). Amniocentesis is very similar to CVS except that the needle is placed directly into the amniotic cavity of a somewhat more developed pregnancy. Amniocentesis is much more popular than CVS because it is easier and requires less-specialized training, though both are successful methods for diagnosing virtually any abnormality resulting from a chromosomal error. However, CVS will give you an answer much earlier in pregnancy.

Most aneuploidies result in an early miscarriage before CVS or amniocentesis can even be attempted. However, trisomies of chromosome 13, 18, and 21 will often survive far into pregnancy and can occasionally lead to birth. It is mostly for that reason that CVS or amniocentesis is advised for women over the age of thirty-five. Congenital anomalies not related to chromosome error are generally only diagnosable by ultrasound, and often at a later stage in the pregnancy (typically at eighteen weeks). The major reason most women undergo CVS or amniocentesis is to detect Down syndrome.

Chromosome analysis (karyotyping) will not pick up subtle gene defects that are often referred to as single-gene errors. Karyotyping only detects gross errors such as an abnormal number of chromosomes or a structural defect in a chromosome. Remember, there are about twenty-five thousand genes located in these twenty-three pairs of chromosomes. Each gene (except on the X) has two copies and consists of a sequence of many thousands of DNA base pairs. A mistake in just a single one of those base pair letters can result in a severe disease such as cystic fibrosis or muscular dystrophy. This will not show up on routine chromosome analysis because the DNA defect is tiny compared to a missing or extra chromosome. There are many, many single-gene defects, some of which you may have heard of, such as cystic fibrosis, Tay-Sachs disease, muscular dystrophy, sickle cell anemia, Gaucher's disease, Marfan syndrome, and hemophilia, just to mention a few. But unlike aneuploidy, they are very uncommon. These are diseases caused by specific defects in a tiny area of a gene that would go completely unnoticed with any karyotype analysis (i.e., chromosomal examination). They are caused by mutations rather than numerical chromosomal errors.

With aneuploidy, there is a numerical error in the number of chromosomes present, representing a huge chunk of DNA (possibly one hundred million base pairs) that is clearly visible upon microscopic examination. On the other hand, a mutation represents a tiny, submicroscopic defect in the organization of DNA letters within a specific gene. The most common single-gene defect is cystic fibrosis, which occurs in about 1 in 1,600 offspring. The remarkable aspect of these single-gene defects is that most of us are carriers for at least ten such fatal diseases. In fact, 4 percent of the Caucasian population are carriers of cystic fibrosis, even though only 1 in 1,600 children actually have the disease.

These single-gene diseases are nonetheless uncommon for two reasons. First, if the genes are recessive, the child must inherit the mutation from each parent, both of whom must be carriers. If just one healthy gene from one of the parents is present, then the child will be disease-free. Cystic fibrosis functions in this way. Thus, although 4 percent of the entire population are carriers for this disease, the chance that any two people who are both carriers will marry is 4 percent of 4 percent. That means that only sixteen out of ten thousand babies would be born to couples in which both mother and father are carriers. Furthermore, only one quarter of those babies would receive a defective recessive gene from both the father and the mother. Three quarters of those babies would either have no defective genes, or be carriers themselves. Thus, only about 1 in 1,600 children are actually born with this terrible disease, even though 4 percent of the population are carriers for it. There is a huge variety of these mutations, but only if we are very unfortunate, and happen to have married a similar carrier, is there a danger we could have an offspring affected by the disease.

On the other hand, there are also single-gene diseases caused by so-called dominant genes, which means that if just one, not necessarily two, of the genes you inherit from your father or mother is abnormal, you will have the disease. Classic examples of these are Huntington's, Marfan's, myotonic dystrophy, and polycystic kidney disease. These are terrible diseases that affect people who have just one abnormal gene out of the two. Even though the homologous gene is normal, they still have the disease. This means that if your father had Huntington's disease, there is a 50 percent chance that you will have it as well, depending randomly on whether you received your father's defective Huntington gene or his normal Huntington gene. Autosomal dominant disease, therefore, is usually only an adult-onset condition that occurs after the early childbearing years, and is genetically transmitted to half of the offspring.

## Chromosomal Translocations and Infertility

Aneuploidies, or numerical chromosome errors, as we have discussed, result from having either more or less than the normal two copies of any one of the chromosomes. Aneuploidy is caused by errors in meiosis in either the egg (90 percent of the time) or the sperm (10 percent of the time). However, aneuploidy can also occur from missegregation of chromosomes caused by a phenomenon referred to as translocation. This means that a portion of one chromosome is "translocated" onto another chromosome. Translocation is actually a normal part of evolutionary development in the creation of new species. About one in every four hundred adult men and women have such a translocation in their chromosomes, and they are completely normal individuals, suffering no genetic or health consequences. A translocation simply means that part of one chromosome has been broken off and moved to another. As long as there is no addition or subtraction of genes caused by this translocation, it doesn't really matter where the genes are located. As long as the nucleus of every one of your cells has the normal number of genes, even if the chromosomes have been split apart and rearranged like a randomly shuffled deck of cards, translocation has no negative consequence.

With reciprocal translocations, there is simply an exchange of chromosome material from one non-homologous chromosome to another. Thus, a chunk of your chromosome 13 might be located on chromosome 14, and a chunk of your chromosome 14 might be located reciprocally on chromosome 13. This has no negative effect on your health as long as there is no missing or extra chromosomal segment. In another type of translocation, called Robertsonian translocation, the centromeres of two chromosomes are fused, and so one entire chromosome is thereby completely attached to another entire chromosome. This type of translocation is only found with chromosomes 13, 14, 15, 21, and 22. Since there is no health consequence to you if you carry a Robertsonian or a reciprocal translocation, these chromosome errors are referred to as balanced, and these individuals are completely healthy.

Translocations occur throughout evolution, as large or small chunks of chromosomes can dislodge and become attached to other chromosomes. In fact, this is one of the major mechanisms whereby species differentiate, and the reason that you can't cross one species with another. The chromosomes simply would not match up. Occasionally, crossbreeding between closely related species is possible. For example, the crossing of a horse and a donkey yields a mule. However, because the chromosomal organization is essentially different in the donkey and the horse, the mule is sterile and cannot breed further mules.

So why are these translocations important to you and your desire to have a child? The problem is that at the time of either the production of sperm or the maturing of the egg via meiosis, an equal separation of chromosomes must occur, with one pair of chromosomes going to one pole of the dividing egg (or sperm), and the other equivalent set of chromosomes going to the other pole. If you have a balanced translocation, the chromosomes cannot separate off equally in meiosis (see fig. 12.12).

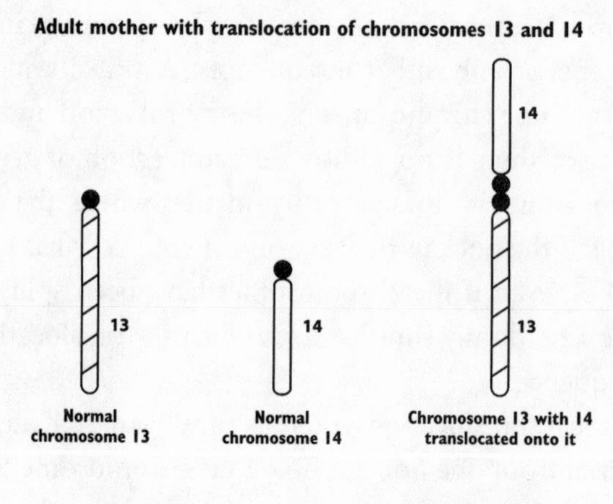


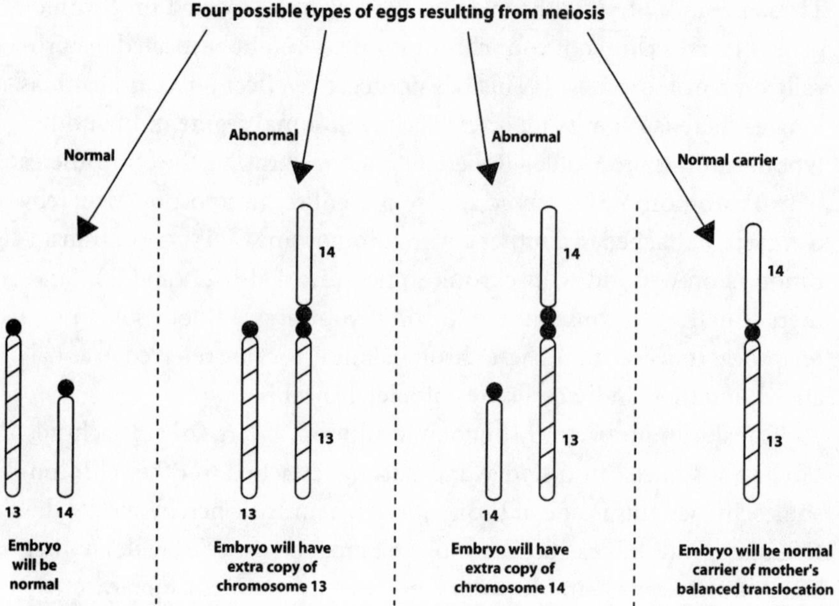


**FIGURE 12.12**

How balanced translocations in 1.3 percent of infertile parents lead to normal and abnormal embryos.

Thus, if chromosomes 13 and 14 are fused together (Robertsonian), there will be eggs that have the fused pair of both 13 and 14 as well as another extra copy of one of those chromosomes. In other words, the chromosomes have to be intact and paired so that an equal amount of chromosomal material goes to each sperm, or to each egg, during meiosis.

The simple math (although it doesn't always work out this way) would be that one quarter of the offspring would have inherited the balanced translocation from its parent and be no different from that parent. One quarter will inherit no translocation and will just inherit the normal chromosome of each one of the parents. However, half of the embryos resulting from a parent with a balanced translocation will have an unbalanced number of chromosomes (see fig. 12.12). The abnormal meiotic separation of chromosomes in the presence of translocations produces aneuploid gametes not because there is an extra or a missing chromosome in the fetus, but rather because there is an extra or a missing *portion* of a chromosome. This results in miscarriages as well as abnormal offspring. Fortunately, translocations are only found in a small percentage of the general population (about 1 in 400). But they are found in as many as 1.5 percent of infertile men and women. The offspring of these patients have a 50 percent chance of having the same problem as their parents and at least half of their conceptions will be nonviable.

## Sex-Chromosome Aneuploidies

Thus far, we have concentrated on explaining aneuploidy of the *autosomes.* Aneuploidy of the autosomes, i.e., chromosomes 1 through 22, leads to either a nonviable embryo that cannot implant at all, a viable embryo programmed to die sometime in the first three months (miscarriage), or, occasionally, a stillbirth or a child affected with Down syndrome (trisomy 21). However, aneuploidies of the sex chromosomes can be quite viable and may result in a real dilemma for every patient undergoing assisted reproductive technology with IVF or ICSI. ICSI offspring have a slightly increased incidence of sex-chromosome aneuploidy, so you need to understand it.

Sex-chromosome aneuploidy means that there is either an extra or a missing copy of the X or the Y chromosome. We know that two copies of the X chromosome makes a normal female, and that one copy of the X and one copy of the Y makes a normal male. The X and the Y chromosomes are very unusual compared to the autosomes. The X is rather large, between the size of chromosome 7 and chromosome 8, and contains more than one thousand genes. The Y chromosome is a very tiny, puny little mate by comparison, representing only 1 percent of the entire human genome. The Y chromosome is approximately the same size as chromosomes 21 and 22, which are also very small, and it is dwarfed by its corresponding mate, the X chromosome.

For many years, it was thought that the only purpose of the Y chromosome was to provide the male sex-determining gene (SRY), because women with two X chromosomes certainly don't need the Y, and even women with a single X chromosome (XO Turner's syndrome patients) can get along (with some handicaps) without a Y chromosome. Nonetheless, the Y chromosome has important genes on it, as exemplified by the fact that 99 percent of XO aneuploid embryos miscarry within the first three months and are completely nonviable. It is only a tiny minority of embryos with only one X chromosome (no second X, and no Y chromosome) that survive. Therefore, the X chromosome is absolutely essential for survival, but interestingly, only one copy of it is necessary so long as there is a corresponding little Y chromosome to accompany it.

This can best be understood in terms of the whole evolutionary history of the X and the Y chromosomes that has occurred in mammals for hundreds of millions of years. The X and the Y chromosomes actually started out as a pair of ordinary autosomes approximately the size of chromosomes 7 or 8. Before the development of the Y chromosome, the gender of the offspring in our ancient reptilian ancestors would be determined simply by the randomness of the temperature at which the egg was incubated. We see this today, of course, in alligators, crocodiles, and many turtles. However, once a sex-determining gene developed in our ancestral mammals, these two chromosomes could no longer pair at meiosis. This sex-determining gene ensured a balanced, fifty-fifty sex ratio in spite of all kinds of unpredictable vicissitudes of environmental temperature, but it also guaranteed the gradual atrophy and shrinkage of what would eventually become the Y chromosome. Chromosomes that do not pair during meiosis gradually deteriorate. But the evolving organism cannot survive with only one chromosome of a given pair. Thus, the evolving X chromosome developed a way to work overtime to make up for the loss of genes from its mate, the Y.

The female X chromosome works twice as hard as any other chromosome, making up for the absence of the vast majority of the genes from its deteriorating mate, the Y. However, this hyperproduction of the X chromosome, though saving the life of the male by making up for the deficiency of the Y, would be disastrous for the female (with two copies of X chromosome) were it not for another phenomenon called X inactivation. The female (XX) actually inactivates one of her X chromosomes so that she doesn't suffer from a gene overdosage. In this way, a normal XX female basically has only one of her X chromosomes functioning, and a normal XY male also has only one X chromosome functioning. This can help to explain why sex-chromosome aneuploid embryos can survive. You will have to decide whether they present enough of an abnormality for you to be concerned for your offspring.

The most common of these sex-chromosome aneuploidies is XXY, or Klinefelter's syndrome. The vast majority of men with sex chromosome trisomy, XXY, appear to be completely normal and healthy. In fact, they live completely normal lives and will go undiagnosed as having this sex-chromosome aneuploidy until they try to have children and discover that they have no sperm in their ejaculate. There are less common, more severe cases of XXY Klinefelter's whereby testicular function is so compromised that even hormone production is deficient, and such a patient would never go through normal puberty. He would need testosterone supplementation, usually via injection twice a month, in order to live a normal life. Furthermore, he would be sterile and unable to have his own genetic offspring. But the majority of XXY males are perfectly normal, except that they are infertile.

The earliest reported cases of Klinefelter's were not detected by routine genetic testing of an otherwise normal male coming in for an infertility evaluation. Therefore, only the more severe cases, in which there was obvious male hormone deficiency, were diagnosed in the early days. These men had all the signs of testosterone deficiency, including lack of drive, bone weakness, relative paucity of facial and pubic hair, deficient muscle mass, and a lack of proper pubertal development. That is why for many years, a controversy has raged about whether these XXY males have some sort of mild retardation. But we have seen more XXY men than perhaps any other center, and aside from their infertility, these men are 100 percent normal. Many are quite brilliant, no different than in any normal population of men.

Many years ago, I remember being shocked by a routine chromosome report showing Klinefelter's on a patient who was an extremely successful and highly regarded businessman and who never would have known he had an XXY aneuploidy were it not for the fact that he and his wife were trying to have a baby. Chromosome evaluations (karyotyping) in the past had not been routinely performed for infertile men. But as we began to routinely screen all of our infertile male patients, we discovered that 4 percent of our men with azoospermia (no sperm in the ejaculate) actually had Klinefelter's. There was nothing else wrong with them.

Sex-chromosome aneuploidies, regardless of age of the parents, are found in only 0.2 percent of infants (1 in every 500) in a normal newborn population. However, they are found in 0.8 percent (1 in 125) of offspring from severely infertile males requiring ICSI. This is approximately the same as the incidence of Down syndrome found in infants of thirty-eight-year-old women. Therefore, much like every woman over thirty-five who has to decide whether to have amniocentesis to determine whether or not the pregnancy is normal, every couple undergoing ICSI for severe male infertility has to make a similar decision, depending upon how much concern they have over the less than 1 percent possibility of a sex-chromosome aneuploidy. However, sex chromosomal abnormalities related to ICSI are very minor events compared to the risk of Down Syndrome in older women. All of these infants will appear to be completely normal at birth. The sex-chromosome aneuploidy may never even be discovered unless, during an infertility evaluation later in life, the man undergoes chromosome testing.

There are numerous other sex-chromosome aneuploidies that are less common than XXY. XYY males are fertile, and almost all of them lead normal lives. Most of them never even find out that they are XYY. In fact, XYY occurs in about 1 in 1,000 babies born in a normal population. Some poorly contrived studies suggested that the frequency of XYY is somewhat higher in prison populations than in a normal population. The suggestion has been made that XYY males may tend to be more aggressive than XY males because of the increased "maleness" of having an extra Y. In fact, this supposition is complete myth.

XXY males, as we have said, will grow up to be infertile, and the most severe (but least common) variety of the XXY males will need testosterone replacement to lead normal lives. The majority, however, will not need testosterone replacement, and will simply be infertile. Whether or not these XXY males are completely normal except for infertility is a crucial issue for couples undergoing ICSI, since up to 0.8 percent of ICSI offspring will have such a sex-chromosome anomaly. This is a potentially controversial issue, but we have interviewed so many of these

XXY men whose only problem was azoospermia that we feel that XXY children are just as likely to be rocket scientists as any other population of males.

Other sex-chromosome aneuploidies include XXX and XO females. Even with ICSI, the XO sex-chromosome aneuploidy is very uncommon at birth because it is usually lethal to the early embryo, and results in early miscarriage. But it poses a problem to prospective parents if such a pregnancy actually were to result in the birth of an XO baby girl. XO (also called Turner's syndrome) is extremely rare (0.01 percent) because these fetuses simply do not survive 99 percent of the time and miscarry very early. But when they do go to birth, these girls will grow up to be very short (less than five feet tall), some will have a webbed neck, and some will have one horseshoe-shaped kidney instead of two normally shaped kidneys. It is also alleged that they do not have high intelligence, but that is very disputable.

The head professor and chief of the Department of Genetics at the University of Amsterdam, who has studied this phenomenon extensively, relates a story that is now well known among geneticists. There was a female first-year medical student who was quite brilliant, already at the top of her class, listening to a medical genetics lecture. The professor went through a list of birth disorders and explained XO Turner's syndrome. The professor explained, "The Turner's syndrome female carries only one X chromosome due to a loss of one of the X chromosomes during meiosis, or early embryonic mitosis. She may be of shorter stature, possess rudimentary ovaries, thus making her sterile, have immature breasts and general development, and usually will be of below-average intelligence." This medical student knew that she had XO Turner's, and could not believe that this professor, who was well respected and learned, would be making such incorrect statements, at least as it applied to her. Afterward, she spoke to the professor and explained to him that she was at the top of her class and that she was a Turner's syndrome XO female. The next day, the professor apologized and said, "There is nothing written in stone about how these people will live their lives and what their mental capacity will be." This is a very famous anecdote, and it emphasizes that despite fears couples might have about discovering sex-chromosome errors in their offspring, either at amniocentesis or in early childhood, it is unlikely that many of these uncommon sex-chromosome aneuploidies will lead to any heartbreaking problems other than infertility.

## Severely Infertile Males and Sex-Chromosome Aneuploidy

Sex-chromosome abnormalities come from the sperm rather than the egg, and are not increased in older parents. They are *not* the result of the biological clock of the eggs, but rather of errors in meiosis of sperm.

It is the Y chromosome that determines, at approximately six weeks of fetal life, that the embryo will become a male. Even Y chromosomes that are missing large chunks (a type of chromosomal error called a deletion) that are easily visible with karyotyping, still are males. There is just one tiny region (the SRY gene) on what is called the "short arm" of the Y chromosome that is necessary to determine that the offspring will be male. Most of the rest of this tiny chromosome, the Y, harbors genes that are absolutely required for spermatogenesis in any species that has been shown to have a Y chromosome. Therefore, an individual with a defective Y chromosome, missing large chunks of its DNA, can still be a completely normal male, but cannot produce sperm. Uncovering how this Y chromosome and its corresponding X chromosome function has helped us understand the evolution of virtually all life on Earth. But the discussion of that incredible finding is complex and will require its own book. But I will give here a very simple summary.

During meiosis in the female ovary, when the woman's eggs are undergoing preparation for fertilization, all of her "like" (homologous) pairs of chromosomes, including her two X chromosomes, line up next to each other on the equatorial spindle plate in a uniform fashion. All of these like chromosomes, from 1 to 22, and also her two X chromosomes, adhere to each other and participate in this miraculous process called recombination. However, in the male testes, where sperm are being produced, the X and the Y chromosomes are so different that they cannot, and they do not, attach to each other or recombine along their entire length. Although homologous, they are really completely different chromosomes. The function of the SRY gene, located in the Y chromosome, is to determine, at six weeks of fetal development, that the indifferent gonad will turn into a testis (which begins the whole cascade of male rather than female development), and therefore it cannot get too intimate with the X.

But there is a tiny region at the tip of the Y chromosome that is identical to a similar region at the tip of the X chromosome, and at this tiny area near the tip, the X and the Y do line up, adhere to each other, and recombine. (See fig. 12.17.) In this tiny little area, the X and the Y chromosomes function exactly as though they were autosomes. Without this residual pseudo-autosomal region at their tip, the X and the Y could never line up with each other and would never undergo proper meiosis. In other words, without this tiny pseudo-autosomal region, nondisjunction of either the X or the Y chromosome in the male testes would be routine. Without this tiny little area reserved for the X and the Y to be just like each other and to stick together in the process of meiosis during sperm production in the testes, most of the sperm so produced would have numerical errors in the number of sex chromosomes allotted to them. There would be sperm that had two X chromosomes instead of one, and there would be sperm that had two Y chromosomes instead of one. There would be sperm that had no X or no Y chromosomes. It is this fragile, tiny area of homology between the X and the Y, pulling them together to undergo proper meiosis, that prevents the majority of all our offspring from having what we call sex-chromosome aneuploidy.

Remember, we said that in 90 percent of cases, or more, autosomal trisomies (like trisomy 13, 18, or 21) come from female meiosis, from the mother's side, when her egg is being matured. Two copies of chromosome 21 are left in the egg after meiosis rather than the proper one copy of chromosome 21, owing to a faulty lineup of chromosome 21 on the spindle. This is caused by aging of the female's meiotic spindle.

Sex-chromosome aneuploidies, i.e., extra copies or missing copies of the X or Y chromosomes, are not associated with increasing age in either the male or the female, and the vast majority originate in the testes, from errors in meiosis during sperm production. The reason for such errors in sperm production resulting in sex-chromosome aneuploidy is the intrinsically fragile nature of that bond between X and Y chromosomes in that tiny little region called the pseudo-autosomal junction. That is why there is a higher incidence of sex-chromosome abnormalities in the offspring of men with extremely low sperm count.

## Chromosomal Abnormalities in Infertile Men and Women, and in Their ICSI and IVF Children

Numerous studies of the chromosomes of infertile men with severely impaired sperm production and very low sperm counts have consistently demonstrated chromosomal errors in the blood samples of approximately 4 percent of these men. Out of almost eight thousand severely infertile men, either azoospermic or severely oligospermic, 3.8 percent had a sex-chromosome aneuploidy, most commonly Klinefelter's, and 1.3 percent had an autosomal translocation. Remember, a translocation means that one visible chunk of a chromosome has been chopped off and stuck to another chromosome, but there is no excess or deficiency of total genetic material. Thus, you might have a piece of chromosome 14 stuck on chromosome 13. A carefully documented worldwide study of almost ninety-five thousand newborns demonstrated only a 0.17 percent incidence of sex chromosomal abnormalities, and a 0.25 percent incidence of almost autosomal chromosomal abnormalities. Thus, there is a fifteenfold increase in the incidence of sex-chromosome aneuploidy and a fivefold increase in autosomal translocations found in infertile men as compared to a normal population. This poses a chromosome problem for a small fraction of the offspring of infertile men.

Therefore, we should look at the tiny risk that does exist for various chromosomal aneuploidies found in the offspring of ART patients and compare it to a normal newborn population. Table 12.2 summarizes the incidences of chromosomal abnormalities in more than fifteen hundred babies born from ICSI in Brussels, and compares it to control populations of more than ninety thousand spontaneous pregnancies among normal, fertile couples. There is a very low incidence of sex-chromosome aneuploidy in ICSI babies, but it is consistently three to four times what would be expected in a population of newborns conceived naturally. The incidence of autosomal chromosomal abnormalities was only slightly higher in ICSI babies than what is found in a population of babies of older women who conceived naturally. There was no significant increase in the risk of a simple, numerical abnormality like trisomy in these offspring over what would be expected based on the older age of the women who undergo ICSI. In other words, even in a population of fertile women who are over thirty-five and conceive naturally, the incidence of a trisomic or aneuploid pregnancy is about the same as that of women over thirty-five who conceive using ICSI (about 1 out of every 200 to 1 out of every 300 pregnancies).

TABLE 12.2

**Chromosome Abnormalities of ICSI Offspring in Comparison to Control Populations — 2002**

| TYPE OF CHROMOSOME ABNORMALITY | ICSI OFFSPRING (1,586) | SPONTANEOUS PREGNANCY (56,952) | SPONTANEOUS PREGNANCY (34,910) | AMNIOCENTESIS FEMALES >35 YEARS OF AGE (52,965) |
|---|---|---|---|---|
| De novo | (25) 1.58% | 0.45% | | 0.87% |
| Sex chromosome | (10) .63% | 0.19% | 0.23% | 0.27% |
| Autosomal | (15) .95% | 0.26% | 0.61% | 0.60% |
| Numerical | (8) .50% | 0.14% | | 0.33% |
| Translocations (de novo) | (7) .44% | 0.11% | | 0.19% |
| Transmitted | (22) 1.39% | 0.47% | | 0.33% |
| Balanced translocations | (21) 1.32% | 0.45% | | 0.27% |
| Unbalanced translocations | (1) 0.06% | 0.023% | | 0.07% |
| Total | (47) 2.96% | 0.92% | 0.84% | |

However, the incidence of de novo chromosomal translocation (brand-new translocations that were not simply inherited from either parent) is 0.44 percent, which is clearly four times higher than what would be seen in the normal population. The occurrence of these newly arising balanced translocations in ICSI offspring is still extremely low (approximately 1 in every 200 or 300 babies), but newly arising translocations are always worrisome because they can be associated with some microscopic chromosomal loss that is undetectable with karyotying, and could result in abnormalities. However, thus far, these children with de novo (i.e., new) autosomal translocations have been normal.

Remember, we said that men with low sperm counts have a higher incidence of having a balanced translocation (1.3 percent) than the general population (0.2 percent). Thus, it is not surprising that nearly 1.4 percent of ICSI offspring have a transmitted balanced translocation, which is inherited from the father. This in itself is nothing to worry about except that it is very likely that this child will have the same infertility problem as his father.

Of the ICSI offspring born with transmitted translocations (nearly

1.4 percent), 5 percent of them (1/1500 of all the ICSI offspring) will have an unbalanced translocation. Fortunately, most unbalanced translocations do not survive because they represent such a severe aneuploid defect, and they miscarry early. However, couples must bear in mind that a tiny number of ICSI offspring (1/1500) may have a dangerous unbalanced translocation. Again, put in perspective, most women who are approaching forty recognize they have approximately a 1 percent chance of having an aneuploid baby, and many choose to undergo amniocentesis or CVS for that reason. They still don't hesitate to try to get pregnant. The same counseling needs to be given to couples undergoing ICSI because of severe male infertility. The risks are very low, and are not related to the ICSI procedure itself, or even to the age of the woman, but rather to her husband's inherently poor sperm production.

The same Brussels study shows that this risk only applies to couples where the sperm count is severely depressed, i.e., less than twenty million sperm per cc. In cases of moderate male infertility (greater than twenty million sperm per cc), the total risk of chromosomal abnormality in the ICSI offspring is no different from a healthy, normal population spontaneously conceiving (0.23 percent).

These data demonstrate that there is no increased risk associated with the ICSI procedure itself. The only increased risk associated with having ICSI (or IVF) is related to the intrinsic potential, however low, for abnormalities in the sperm or the egg among infertile couples. Thus, the counseling and decision-making for infertile patients undergoing IVF or ICSI should be no different from the admonition given to any older woman or any man with a low sperm count who is planning to have children. These increased risks in older women for having children with chromosomal abnormalities, as well as the increased risk for men with extremely depressed sperm production, are nonetheless extraordinarily low.

## Transmission of Infertility to IVF and ICSI Offspring

It is clear that IVF and ICSI are extraordinarily well studied and quite safe. But will children conceived via IVF or ICSI inherit their parents' infertility? It would at first seem illogical for infertility to be inherited. You would think that infertile men and women would be less likely to have children and that infertility over generations would therefore be weeded out of any population. So I will explain that apparent contradiction in the rest of this chapter since transmission of infertility to your offspring is essentially the only major risk associated with infertility treatment.

With the male, this genetic determination has to do with the number of normal sperm he is genetically endowed to produce on a daily basis throughout his life. With the female, the genetic determination is related to how many eggs she will have at birth and, therefore, how quickly her biological clock will eventually time out. The number of eggs a woman is born with, which determines how much time it will take for her biological clock to run down, is most likely inherited.

### *Inheritance of Male Infertility*

The issue of male infertility is very poorly understood by the majority of urologists who might be counseling you. Before 1992, very few doctors suspected that male infertility, i.e., low sperm count or azoospermia, could be genetic in origin. However, all the treatments that had been advocated for male infertility, such as Clomid, testosterone, human menopausal gonadotropin, human chorionic gonadotropin, corticosteroids for sperm antibodies, cold/wet athletic supporters, vitamins, nutritional supplements such as Proxceed, and even the varicocelectomy operation, have failed to withstand the scrutiny of carefully controlled studies. In fact, by the early 1990s it became clear to more knowledgeable scientists that almost all cases of male infertility (with an occasional exception) were impervious to improvement with any known therapy.

Sperm counts are so extremely variable (because of the variation of sperm transport at the time of ejaculation depending upon mood and the period of prior abstinence) that a peculiar mathematical phenomenon called regression toward the mean has often confused urologists into believing in various treatments for male infertility. Figure 12.13 lays out a two-and-a-half-year history of consecutive weekly sperm counts performed in an otherwise fertile medical student. This classic example is found in the World Health Organization (WHO) manual on sperm count and is used to emphasize how easy it is to be fooled into thinking that therapy is having an impact. This medical student's sperm counts ranged from a low of one million per cc to as high as 172 million sperm per cc. The dotted line represents twenty million sperm per cc (which is

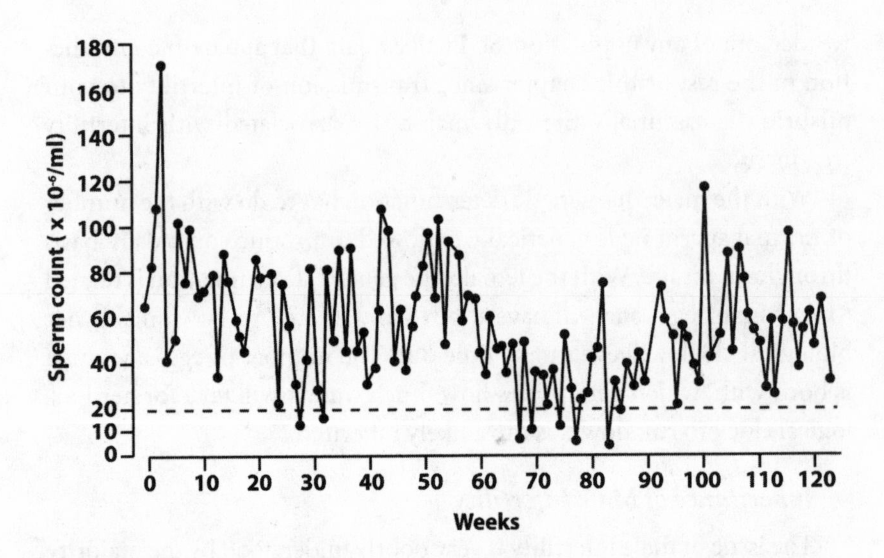


**FIGURE 12.13**

Variation of weekly sperm count over a two-year period in a single, normal male volunteer (WHO Manual, 1998).

arbitrarily defined by WHO as the threshold for normal sperm count). His sperm count at twenty-nine weeks was only twelve million sperm per cc, and at eighty-two weeks it was only one million per cc. In between those times, it ranged from two million per cc to 120 million per cc. Regression toward the mean, as described in chapter 7, simply means that with a highly variable measurement such as sperm count, if your initial evaluation is low, subsequent evaluations are likely to be higher. If your initial evaluation is high, subsequent evaluations are likely to be low. If you had put this medical student on any treatment (even sugar pills) during any of those periods, you might think either that you had improved his count with treatment, or that you had damaged it.

Whether you treat the male or do not treat the male, there is a certain percentage of couples every month who will get pregnant despite the husband's low sperm count. This is especially true with younger wives and shorter prior durations of infertility. Figures 12.14 and 12.15 summarize the control studies performed by Dr. Gordon Baker, in Melbourne (fig. 12.14), and Dr. Eberhard Nieschlag, in Germany (fig. 12.15). With or without treatment of the male, the two curves can be superimposed on each other. The pregnancy rate of the couple is not at

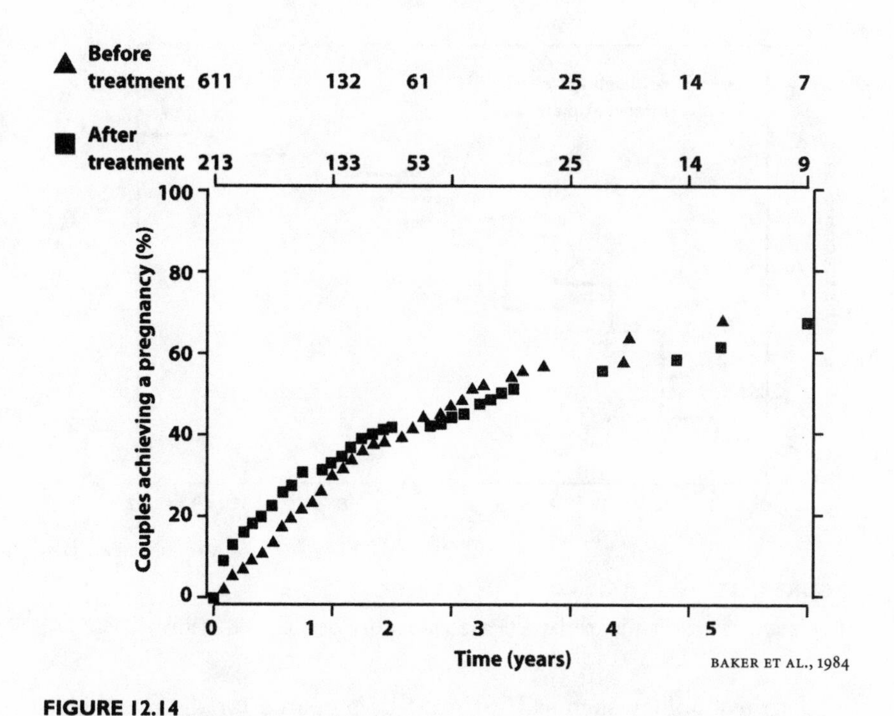


**FIGURE 12.14**

Pregnancy rate over time in couples with and without treatment of male infertility.

all affected by the treatment of the male. If the woman gets pregnant after the male is treated, you might mistakenly think that this worthless treatment worked. But these graphs show that results are not any better than no treatment at all. In other words, male infertility is impervious to all conventional treatment. These powerful studies forced us to accept that there had to be a genetic origin to male infertility and to diminished sperm production.

The initial hot spot to study was, of course, the Y chromosome. We are now certain that there are a great number of genes (at least sixty) on the Y chromosome, all interacting in a dosage-related way to control sperm production. If certain of these genes are missing, then the male will have defects in sperm production, and possibly no sperm production at all. If other genes are missing, the defect will be mild. It is the combination of this wide variety of genes, both on the Y chromosome (most likely also on the X chromosome, and even on the autosomes), that ultimately determines each man's sperm count. Thus, if male infertility is of genetic origin, couples who are now able to have children via

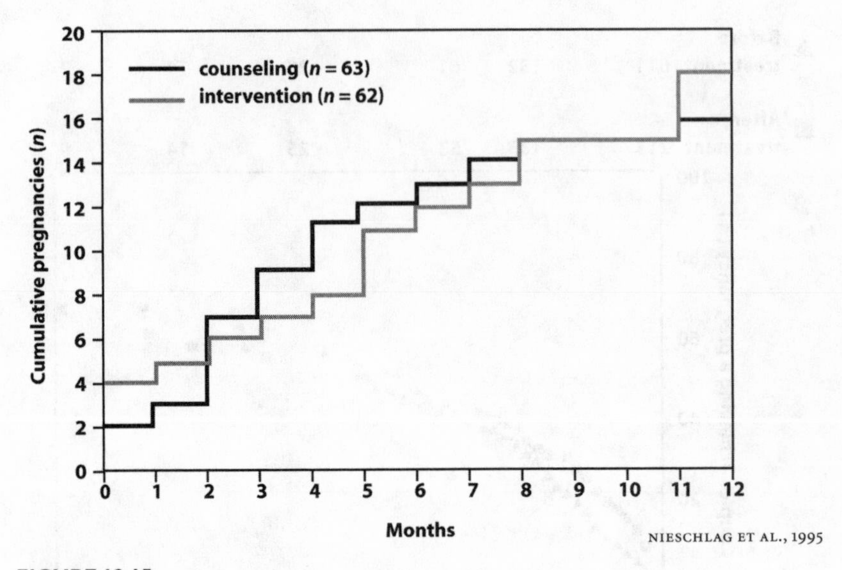


**FIGURE 12.15**

Pregnancy rate over time in couples with and without treatment of male infertility.

modern technology such as ICSI must be prepared for the possibility that their male offspring will also be infertile.

The Y chromosome is an extremely precarious place for all of these male infertility genes to be located (see fig. 12.16). There are vast arrays of identical DNA on the Y chromosome, making it easy for them to accidentally recombine with each other as though they were a pair of homologous chromosomes. When that happens, all the unfortunate genes that are caught in between just drop out and disappear. That is called a deletion. Figure 12.17 illustrates how the X and the Y only recombine at the very tip, while the rest of the Y virtually hangs in the

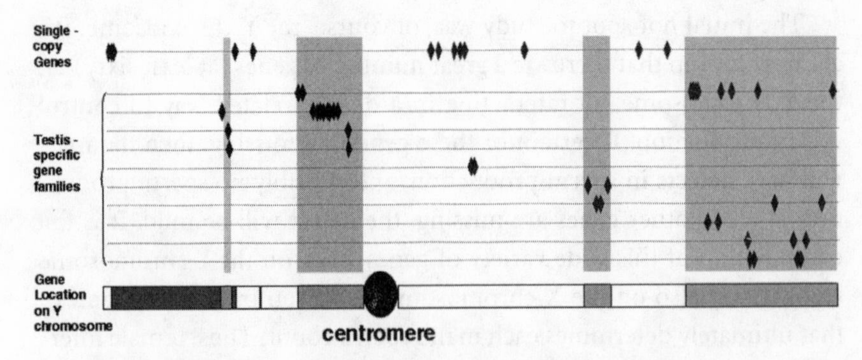


**FIGURE 12.16.** Multiple genes on Y chromosome affecting sperm production.

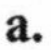
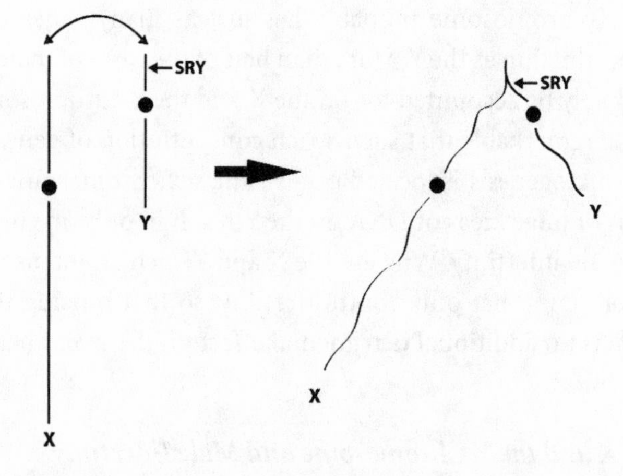


Normal "homologous" recombination occurs only at tips of X and Y chromosomes, not along their entire length (as occurs with all the other chromosomes)

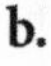
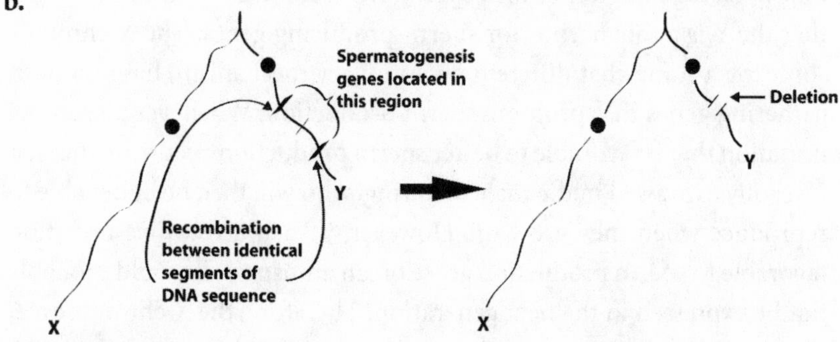


**FIGURE 12.17**

Illegitimate "homologous" recombination between like sequences on the Y chromosome during spermatogenesis causes dropping out of intervening spermatogenesis genes, and subsequent male infertility.

breeze. So these vast arrays of identical DNA sequences on the Y recombine with each other, and huge chunks in between, loaded with spermatogenesis genes, just disappear. That is how fertile males conceive male offspring who are infertile. While the normal fertile man is making sperm normally in his testis, an occasional sperm will suffer a Y deletion, and if that is the sperm that fertilizes the mother's egg, their son will be infertile. So the father of the infertile man is fertile, but the son derived from ICSI is sure to inherit the same spermatogenic defect as his infertile father.

The X chromosome probably has just as many genes controlling sperm production as the Y. More than half of the cases of male infertility can probably be accounted for on the X and the Y chromosomes alone. It is quite remarkable that such a rich concentration of genes that control spermatogenesis is located on just the sex chromosomes, and that deletions of huge areas of DNA on the Y result in only one health problem — male infertility. Why are the X and Y such an intense collection depot for genes that only control fertility, so that missing these genes usually has no additional detrimental effect on the man's health except for infertility?

### *The X and the Y Chromosome and Male Infertility*

Over 300 million years of evolution, the Y chromosome has gathered together copies of large numbers of genes from throughout the genome that work together to perform sperm production. The reason for this is that the Y is a safe harbor for sperm-producing genes. The X chromosome, by a somewhat different evolutionary mechanism, has also been gathering genes that promote sperm production. Whenever a recessive mutation that is favorable to better sperm production occurs on the X, it is readily expressed in the male offspring, who will then be better able to reproduce when they grow up. However, if such a recessive mutation favorable to sperm production arose on an autosome, it would probably not be expressed in the next generation. Therefore, the X chromosome, like the Y, but for different reasons, has a remarkable accumulation of genes necessary for sperm production.

For example, a patient of ours had an X-linked mutation causing failure of spermatogenesis. Both the patient and his brother inherited their severe infertility (azoospermia) from a mutation on one of their mother's X chromosomes. Both of their mother's brothers (maternal uncles) were also sterile, and they inherited this condition from their mother. Their sister also inherited one of grandma's mutated X chromosome genes and was a carrier on her X of the same gene for male infertility that her mother gave to all of them. In turn, her two sons both inherited their infertility from mom. Thus, half of the mother's sons would be likely to be fertile, and half would be infertile, depending on which X chromosome they inherited from mom. Therefore, his son derived by ICSI will be completely fertile, but all of his daughters will be carriers for male infertility, and half of his grandsons will inherit his problem.

On the other hand, a Y-chromosome deletion is transmitted identically to the man's male offspring in every case. Therefore, those parents, although quite happy with their otherwise completely normal male child, must understand that he will have exactly the same infertility problem as his infertile father. But the man's daughters will not even be carriers of infertility. Thus, the male's infertility will be transmitted to subsequent generations in different ways, depending on whether the defective gene that is causing the spermatogenic deficiency is located on the X chromosome, the Y chromosome, or on one of the autosomes.

Kallmann's syndrome is a rare, well-studied X-linked recessive-gene defect that causes male infertility. It is a specific form of male infertility in which the pituitary gland cannot secrete FSH or LH because the hypothalamus does not secrete GnRH. The testicles are normal, but they aren't receiving any gonadotropin stimulation. This deficiency will be transmitted from a fertile carrier mother to her son. If the gene defect were on the Y chromosome, then all of the male offspring would be infertile, and all the females would be normal and would not be carriers. However, if the gene defect causing male infertility is on the X chromosome (like Kallman's), then all of the female offspring will be carriers, all the male offspring will be fertile, and 50 percent of the male grandchildren will be infertile.

In 2001, Malcolm Faddy, Roger Gosden, and I published a mathematical model in *Nature Genetics* predicting the incidence of male infertility in successive generations based on a few simple mathematical assumptions (see fig. 12.18). Our mathematical construction predicted that if just 1 percent of the male population is currently infertile (a conservative figure) and if all such married males had access to successful ICSI treatment, then in about three hundred generations (or ten thousand years) the entire male population would be infertile.

If male infertility is genetic, why would it be so prevalent? In fact, it turns out that the origin of these Y deletions arises during the otherwise normal fertile father's sperm production. In about 1 in 100 sperm produced in every normal male's testes, a chunk of Y chromosomal DNA drops out during the recombination process. If that is the unlucky sperm (from any normally fertile father) that fertilizes mom's egg, then the baby boy will be infertile. In any normal man's ejaculate, with 200 million sperm, there are bound to be at least one hundred thousand such sperm every day that have a severe, large Y deletion that will result

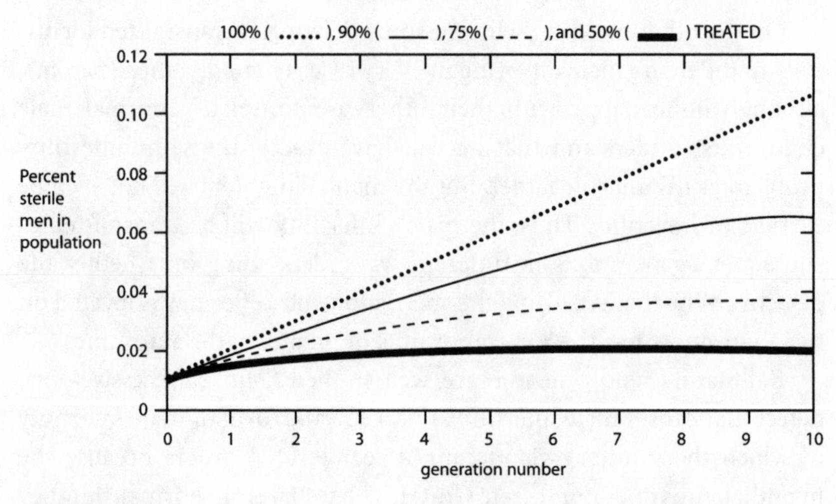


**FIGURE 12.18**

**Predicted incidence of male infertility in successive generations. Results are based on the percentage of men undergoing ICSI treatment for severe oligospermia or azoospermia. Faddy, Silber, and Gosden, 2001**

in sterility in his male offspring if it just so happens to be the sperm that fertilizes mom's egg.

Because the Y chromosome does not have a partner (except at its tiny tip) with which to "mate" and recombine during meiosis (as do all the other chromosomes), these areas of DNA identity on the Y wind up "mating" with each other. Since the Y does not have a homologous chromosome with which to join during the production of sperm, like the X does during the maturation of an egg, the different sequences of the Y that are identical to each other wind up recombining with each other instead. That is how genetic deletions which cause infertility occur.

There are a huge number of gene copies concentrated on the Y that together act in a dosage-related way to determine what your sperm count will be. If there is only a *small deletion,* taking out only a few of those genes or just some of the *genes that have duplicate, backup copies,* then the sperm count will only be moderately depressed. Such deletions have only a moderate effect on sperm count and are transmitted to the next generation without notice if the wife is young and fertile. However, deletions that are much larger and take out large numbers of these spermatogenesis genes result in severe defects in spermatogenesis, extremely low sperm counts (less than two million sperm per cc), or even no sperm at all in the ejaculate. These deletions are only transmitted to the next generation if a man with such a deletion is married to a very fertile woman, and they have children at a young age.

Therefore, severe male infertility usually arises anew within each generation of males as a new genetic defect transmitted to male offspring from completely fertile fathers. More moderate infertility is transmitted from a father with moderately low sperm count to his offspring, who will then have the same low sperm count as his father.

## Inheritance of Female Infertility

I discussed male infertility first because the genetics of male infertility at this point has been delineated so much better than that of the female. However, we are now right at the edge of recognizing the genetics of female infertility as well. The reason we understand the genetics of male infertility better is that it is so easy to get an objective measure, i.e., sperm count, to compare with chromosomal mapping. It seemed harder to get an objective measure of female fertility, and therefore, the female was harder to study genetically. But as the theme of this book continually reemphasizes, most (of course, not all) female infertility is simply related to age and the biological clock, and is strictly dependent upon the number and quality of eggs with which you were originally born. As I have said, less than 2 percent of couples in their early twenties suffer from infertility. It is only as the woman enters her late twenties that the infertility rate of the couple increases dramatically. Which women are lucky enough to still be fertile in their late twenties, thirties, and early forties depends to good extent on ovarian reserve. This is reflected in a woman's antral follicle count and is most likely predetermined by her genes.

Sperm count is regulated by a large number of sperm-production genes, which are present in multiple copies and work together in a polygenic fashion; sperm count does not deteriorate with age. Females, on the other hand, are endowed with a certain number and quality of eggs, and these factors determine their biological clock. The antral follicle count in any particular age group of females is equivalent to the sperm count in males. At last we have an objective clinical measurement in females that can be correlated to chromosome mapping and sequencing.

What is the evidence that the number of eggs with which you were born is genetically determined? As of yet it is early and preliminary only. The first clue came in the early nineties with a condition called fragile X. Fragile X syndrome is the most commonly inherited cause of developmental and mental retardation. It is an X-linked dominant condition transmitted from mother to son and sometimes from mother to daughter. The gene that causes fragile X is located in a region of the X chromosome that normally contains as many as thirty repeat segments of three DNA base pairs, CGG. However, in women who are carriers of fragile X, this region contains between fifty and two hundred repeats of this DNA sequence. This is called a premutation rather than a mutation because it causes no problem but is an unpredictable prelude to a true mutation. The carrier is normal and has only a premutation, but her offspring can have the fully expanded mutation, which consists of huge numbers of these triplet DNA repeats. If it is a daughter, she may be very mildly affected, but if it is a son, he will be born with the full-blown disease.

Ten percent of women who have the premutation on the X (who otherwise appear to be completely normal) develop premature ovarian failure (POF), meaning that they have a very small number of eggs and go into menopause well before the age of thirty-five. This indicates that the fragile X gene is a gene that plays an important, contributory role in determining the number of eggs with which a woman will be born. Subsequently, since 1998, studies in London and in Austria have demonstrated deletions on the X chromosome in otherwise normal women with premature ovarian failure.

Perhaps an even more telling clinical clue comes from females with XO, or Turner's syndrome, who have no eggs at all. The number of eggs with which a woman is born depends upon genes that will support her embryonic oogonial stem cells. Those genes direct the early egg precursors' migration to, as well as growth and development within, the primitive follicles of the ovary. In the same way, the number of sperm precursors in the man's testes depends upon genes that control the migration and sustenance of the male's primitive germ cells, which will become the sperm within the seminiferous tubules of the testes. With only a single X chromosome, it is impossible for a woman to be born with any eggs. Therefore, the genes essential for having a high ovarian reserve must be located on the X chromosome. We are just beginning to systematically study the genes that affect ovarian reserve. But just as we were correct to start with the Y in male infertility, we are probably equally correct to start with the X for studying the woman's biological clock. To whatever extent your ovarian reserve is directed by genes on the X chromosome, there would be a 50 percent chance of passing this trait on to your female offspring.

CHAPTER 13

# How to Make Sure Your Baby Is Normal: Preimplantation Genetic Diagnosis (PGD)

One of the benefits of infertility technology is that we are now able to help *all* couples, whether infertile or not, avoid having a child with genetic defects. By 2003, most of the twenty-five thousand or so genes in the human genome had been identified, if not characterized, and their DNA sequenced. Methods for molecular analysis of genes are becoming simpler, more efficient, and highly computerized. Because there are so many thousands of genetic diseases, almost all of which are heartbreaking, not to mention the "milder" genetic defects that can give one a propensity toward developing illnesses like cancer or heart disease later in life, genetics is clearly today's most important medical tool.

We can now prevent couples from having to face the horror of giving birth to children with otherwise devastating genetic defects such as Down syndrome, cystic fibrosis, muscular dystrophy, mental retardation, etc., that terrify every woman who ever gets pregnant. We can also solve the problem of recurrent miscarriage and better understand the genetic errors that can arise in older mothers. For example, pregnant women over thirty-five years of age often fear that they might have a child with Down syndrome. So they routinely have CVS or amniocentesis to detect such genetic errors. If the fetus is found to be genetically abnormal, they then face the heart-wrenching dilemma of deciding whether to undergo an abortion or to carry this abnormal child to term. We can avoid that dilemma by testing the embryo for Down syndrome before it is ever even implanted.

A patient of ours in her late thirties had undergone four IVF cycles in Europe without pregnancy. In her fifth IVF cycle (also in Europe), she finally became pregnant and was advised to have an amniocentesis because of the 1 percent risk of Down syndrome, or other possible trisomic chromosomal abnormalities that could lead to miscarriage or stillbirth. Amniocentesis carries a 1 percent risk of losing the pregnancy. Tragically, her amniocentesis became infected, and she had what is called a septic abortion, a massive infection of the pregnancy that would have resulted in her death if it were not aborted. The karyotype of the fetus showed that it would have been a completely normal forty-six XY baby boy. That is why she insisted on using preimplantation genetic diagnosis (PGD) in any future attempt to get pregnant with IVF. PGD eliminates the risk of endangering an established pregnancy by screening for abnormalities *before* the embryo is allowed to implant. This does not mean that PGD is foolproof and doesn't have its potential errors. But a patient who has already lost a pregnancy because of an amniocentesis would never consider doing amniocentesis again.

Couples who are afraid of amniocentesis can instead have the embryos' chromosomes and DNA tested before placing them back into the uterus. If an embryo is abnormal, it need not be replaced. It can even be frozen indefinitely (for ethical reasons) until a time when there might be a genetic cure for that embryo. Only the healthy embryos are then placed back into the wife, who is now reassured from the very beginning that she will most likely not have to face finding out (when she is perhaps three months' pregnant) that she is carrying a defective child. This technology of embryo testing will be one of the great areas of medical progress over the next twenty years, and could eventually allow us to prevent all genetic diseases.

This means that infertile couples using IVF and ICSI, whose offspring might be thought of as having greater risk for problems, could in fact be less likely to have an abnormal child than couples who conceive spontaneously. Even fertile couples who fear having an abnormal child can use this PGD technique. Using PGD should not be construed as creating "designer babies," an incorrect term used only by the press and not by physicians. We could not manipulate (even if we wanted to) the features or characteristics of an offspring. That is just pure fiction. All we can do is eliminate heartbreaking and devastating genetic disease.

## Preimplantation Embryo Biopsy with Genetic Diagnosis

With this bold new development, we can safely biopsy what would appear to be normal embryos before transferring them to the woman,

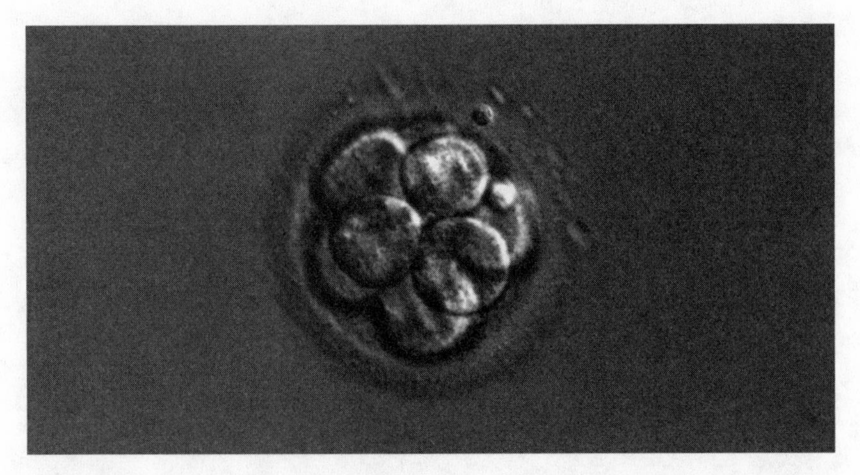

**FIGURE 13.1.** On the third day after fertilization, the embryo has divided into eight cells.

and we can test the DNA so that only truly normal, healthy embryos are transferred. This means that an embryo that would have developed Down syndrome would never be transferred. It means that parents who are carriers of severe genetic diseases like cystic fibrosis, muscular dystrophy, sickle cell anemia, Tay-Sachs, etc., no longer need to worry about having children with any of these heartbreaking genetic diseases.

### *What Is Embryo Biopsy?*

When an embryo reaches the third day of development, it normally has eight cells (see fig. 13.1). One or two of these cells, called blastomeres, can be removed from the embryo with the same sort of micromanipulation technique that is used for ICSI. The embryo will not be harmed, and it will go on to develop normally. Every cell of the embryo at the eight-cell stage is genetically identical to every other cell, and any group of those cells will develop normally on their own because they each have the same complete genetic machinery needed to become a normal embryo. A biopsy at this stage does not remove any genetic material that is necessary for the complete and normal expression of that embryo's genes. You can then subject those one or two cells to genetic analysis, which will reveal the genetic composition of the rest of the embryo. These genetic tests can be performed within a day or two, giving plenty of time to decide which embryos should or should not be transferred back to the patient.

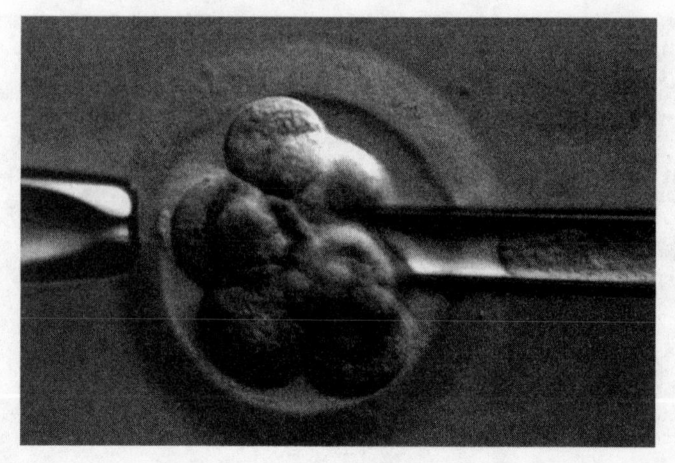

**FIGURE 13.2**

One or two cells (blastomeres) can be removed from a three-day-old embryo for DNA analysis, without harming it, to determine whether or not it is genetically healthy.

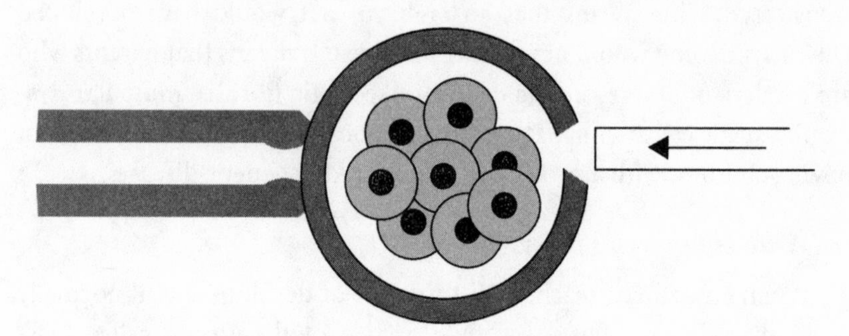

The 8-cell embryo is held by a holding pipette, and a hole is made in the zona pellucida.

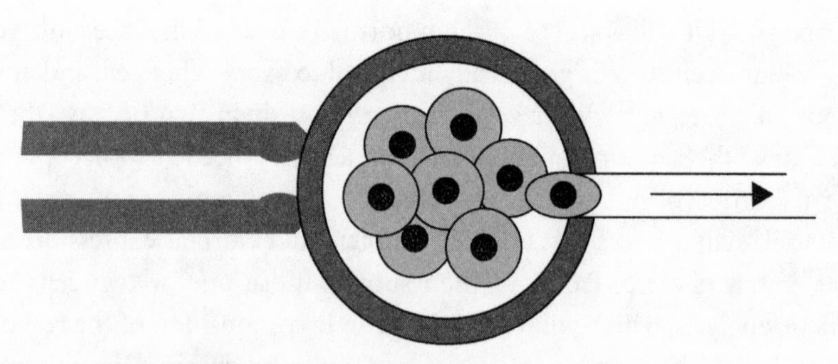

A blastomere is aspirated into a biopsy pipette.

**FIGURE 13.3.** Embryo biopsy.

The technique we use is illustrated in figures 13.2 and 13.3. A very narrow micropipette is used to drill a hole through the zona pellucida, using an acid-type solution. This has been demonstrated to do no damage to the embryo. Then one or two of the blastomeres from the embryo are gently sucked and teased out through that hole in the zona pellucida using a wider micropipette. These blastomeres that have now been removed from the embryo can then be tested genetically (see figs. 13.4 and 13.5). Their genetic complement is indicative of the genetic composition of the six to seven cells still remaining in the embryo.

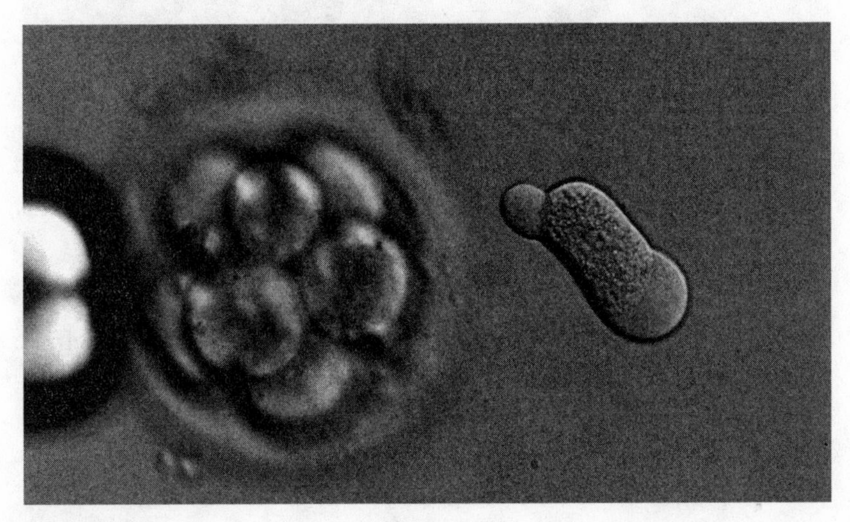

**FIGURE 13.4**

A single cell removed from what was an eight-cell embryo (which is now a seven-cell embryo).

## *Is There a Risk from Embryo Biopsy?*

We cannot be too casual about taking cells out of an embryo for analysis. The meticulous PhD thesis of Dr. Jiaen Liu in 1995 studied in great detail the effect of removing one, two, three, or more cells from an eight-cell, day-three mouse embryo. When more than half of the cells were removed from an eight-cell embryo, absolutely no live birth resulted. When just one cell was removed from the eight-cell mouse embryo, there was no significant effect on live-birth rate. When two cells were removed, there was about a 20 percent reduction in live-birth rate, and when three cells were removed, there was over a 50 percent reduction in live-birth rate. It is important to note that removal of up to

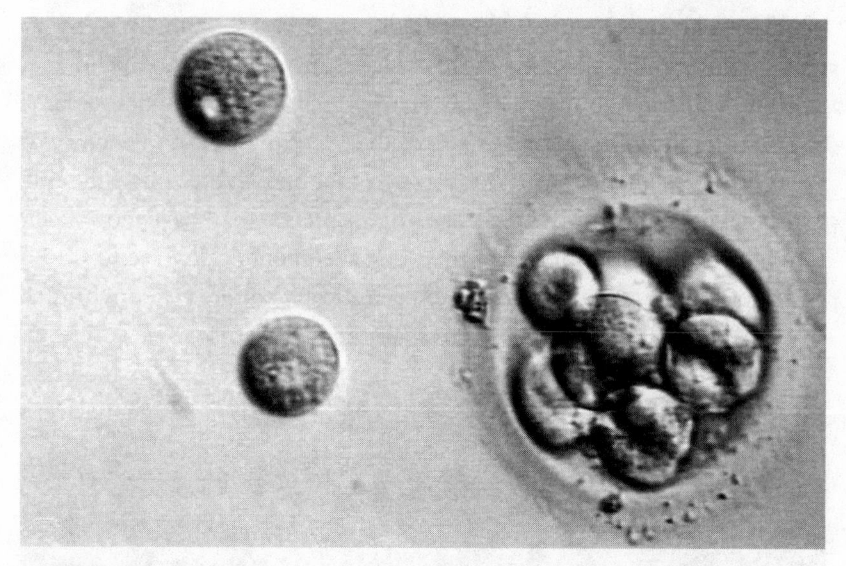

**FIGURE 13.5**

Two cells removed from what was a nine-cell embryo (which is now a seven-cell embryo).

three cells from the eight-cell embryo (in mice) had no negative effect on the initial pregnancy rate, but did have a dramatic effect on the incidence of live birth. This means that embryos with insufficient total volume might implant and result in a pregnancy but would not be capable of developing into a live offspring, thus leading to miscarriage. Because the most dramatic reduction in pregnancy rate occurred only when more than two cells were removed, many centers in Europe recommend taking two cells for diagnosis in order to be absolutely certain the diagnosis is correct. However, most centers in the United States will remove only one cell for diagnosis, because the effect of removing just one cell is likely to be negligible, but removing more than one cell can lower the pregnancy rate.

The question of how many cells can be safely removed from a day-three, eight-cell embryo before impairing its ability to develop normally has also been studied in the mouse in terms of how much cytoplasm can be safely removed from the egg (not just a cell from the embryo, but actual cytoplasm from the egg) before it becomes unable to develop. Dr. Ryuzo Yanagimachi, from Honolulu, performed a famous study on mice in which he removed from various mouse eggs one half of the cytoplasmic volume, one quarter of the cytoplasmic volume, and one eighth of the cytoplasmic volume. He and his group then performed conventional IVF on those volume-reduced eggs. They compared the IVF results using volume-reduced eggs to IVF results using control eggs in which no cytoplasm had been removed. For control eggs, 50 percent of the embryos resulted in live offspring, but when up to half of the cytoplasm had been removed, only 30 percent of embryos resulted in live offspring. They found that when more than half of the volume of the egg had been removed prior to IVF, although normal fertilization occurred, the resulting embryos could not develop past the two-cell stage.

They concluded that early embryos could tolerate reductions of small amounts of cytoplasm, and that some could even tolerate removal of as much as one half their total cytoplasmic volume, without compromising the prospect for pregnancy. These findings correlate with observations in humans with frozen embryos. When more than half of the cells of an eight-cell embryo are lysed (disintegrated) by the freezing, even if the embryo developed to a blastocyst stage, the inner-cell mass is half the normal size and not capable of development. Likewise, if 50 percent of the embryo is fragmented, it will not develop. That means that as embryonic mass is reduced, implantation and development are compromised. For this reason, embryo biopsy would never be performed before day three at the six- to eight-cell stage, and the least chance of harming the pregnancy rate requires that only one cell be removed for diagnosis.

There have been some studies from Europe that suggest that the pregnancy rate is no different if two cells are removed for biopsy compared to if one cell is removed. However, in these studies, the better embryos that were developing more rapidly had two cells removed, and the poorer embryos had only one cell removed. Therefore, it is impossible to judge from those European studies whether in any given embryo removing two cells is as safe as removing one cell. In fact, one has to be very cautious in performing embryo biopsy to make sure that excessive cellular material is not lost, thereby reducing pregnancy rate.

A radical approach to avoid all risk associated with embryo biopsy is to remove the polar bodies and to deduce that whatever genetic abnormalities are present in the polar bodies are not present in the egg (see fig. 13.6). The polar bodies are small blebs from the maturing egg, which contain the leftover set of chromosomes that is expelled from the egg after meiosis in order to reduce the chromosome number from forty-six to twenty-three. They would normally just degenerate soon after fertil-

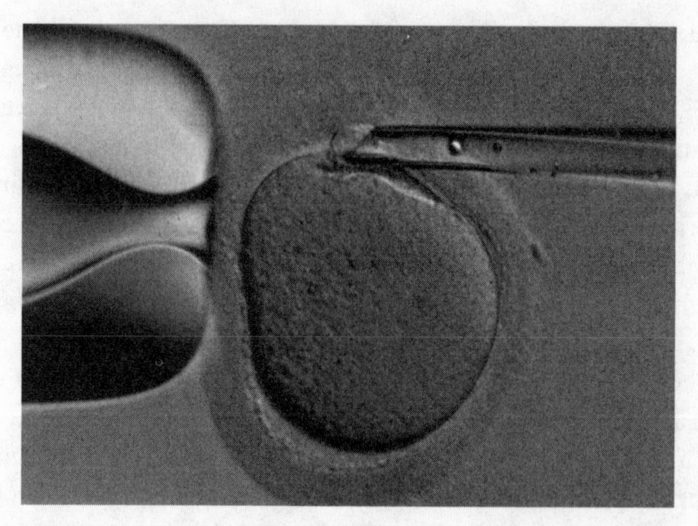

**FIGURE 13.6**

Removing a polar body from the egg prior to fertilization. This technique is the safest for the eventual embryo but is only useful when the mother is the carrier rather than the father, and results are sometimes difficult to evaluate.

ization. For evaluating aneuploidy, an abnormal number of chromosomes in the polar body means there will be an abnormal number left in the egg. For single-gene defects, by a reverse logic, an abnormal polar body containing the defective gene means that the egg itself does not have that defective gene. Both polar bodies must be removed and analyzed, before and after fertilization, and the results must agree with each other. Most authorities do not like to use polar body biopsy, because polar bodies are difficult to handle and the analysis of results can sometimes seem confusing at first glance. Further-more, it can reveal nothing about any abnormality coming from the sperm. However, in terms of not lowering pregnancy rate, polar biopsy may be the safest way to evaluate the embryo. If the polar body biopsy does not give an adequate answer, then on day three a single cell may still be biopsied from the eight-cell embryo to confirm the result, and this would be safer than removing two cells from the eight-cell, day-three embryo.

It is clear that some embryos with remarkable reduction in cytoplasmic volume can occasionally result in healthy pregnancies, and reductions in cytoplasmic volume do not increase the risk of having abnormal offspring. Despite our concern about removing more than one cell from the embryo, we have had remarkable pregnancies with healthy babies from frozen embryos in which half of the eight cells were completely lysed by freezing. We also have had healthy babies from embryos that developed to only four cells by day three, and from embryos that had as much as 50 percent fragmentation. It is just that in such cases, the pregnancy rate is much lower. A recent patient with recurrent miscarriage was scheduled for PGD, but her embryos developed so slowly that they had only four cells by day three. Therefore, we could not do the embryo biopsy. At her request, we transferred these embryos into her uterus without any genetic diagnosis. Nonetheless, she became pregnant and carried healthy twins.

In that same week, we did a frozen-embryo transfer on a patient who had only three out of six cells survive in one of the thawed embryos, and only four out of eight in the other embryo. After a day in culture, however, the surviving cells had divided; one was now a four-cell embryo and the other was an eight-cell embryo. Despite this relatively massive loss of cells (and what we thought was a dismal outlook for pregnancy), this patient delivered healthy twins. A third patient in that same week had gone through three previous IVF cycles with chemical pregnancy only (the equivalent of a very early miscarriage). She too had poor embryo development, with only five cells by day three, and we were very concerned about removing even one cell for PGD, but she insisted. One of those embryos turned out to have a normal complement of chromosomes (i.e., two copies of 13, 16, 18, 21, 22, a single X, and a single Y). We thought the prognosis was very poor, especially since the five-cell embryo, which was normal, had only developed to eight cells by the day of embryo transfer. Nonetheless, she also turned out to have a healthy pregnancy without miscarriage. Thus, we can never be too confident in our present state of ignorance of how to prognosticate for a patient. It seems that very challenged embryos, with very few cells, may occasionally turn into a normal, healthy pregnancy.

### *Fluorescent In Situ Hybridization (FISH) and Polymerase Chain Reaction (PCR) to Analyze the Embryo*

There are two major methods for analyzing the genetics of the embryo, fluorescent in situ hybridization (FISH), and polymerase chain reaction (PCR). FISH allows us to quickly and precisely determine which chromosomes are present and which are not present in the nuclei of the cells, as well as how many. The limitation of this FISH test is that

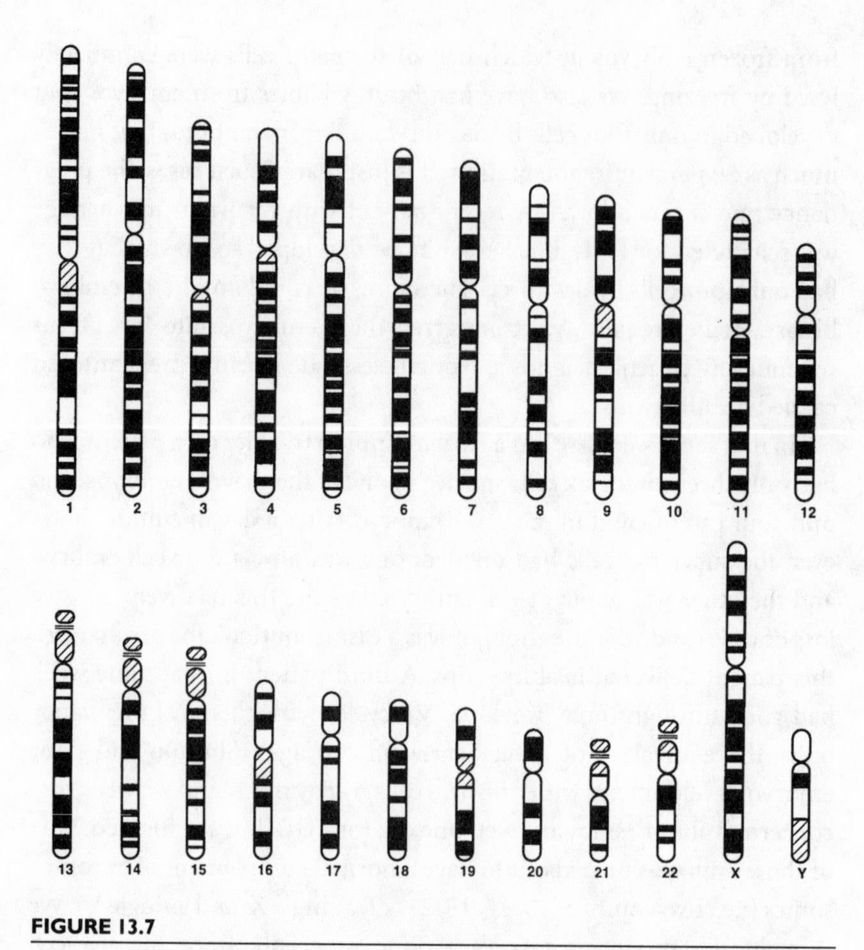


**FIGURE 13.7**

There are twenty-two pairs of autosomal chromosomes and one pair of sex chromosomes, which includes either an X and a Y in a male, or two Xs in a female.

we can't do a precise localization of a specific single gene defect, but its strength is that it can immediately give a broad picture of whether there is a normal or abnormal number of chromosomes. There are twenty-two autosomal chromosomes and two sex chromosomes. FISH can tell us which of those chromosomes are present and which are not (see fig. 13.7). For example, FISH could diagnose Down syndrome because you would see three instead of two copies of chromosome 21. However, you could not tell with FISH if there was a specific gene defect such as cystic fibrosis, Tay-Sachs, or muscular dystrophy.

To identify specific gene defects requires a test called PCR. PCR can detect specific genetic diseases such as cystic fibrosis, muscular dystrophy, Tay-Sachs, Marfan's, Huntington's, sickle-cell anemia, etc. A chromosomal analysis by FISH would never find such a small defect.

So there are two entirely different situations in which PGD can be used. One is for would-be parents who are carriers of a specific genetic disease and who don't want to transmit that disease to their offspring. They require PCR. The other is for infertile couples who must undergo IVF because of a failure to get pregnant naturally, previous recurrent spontaneous miscarriage, or the fear of age-related aneuploidy. They require FISH. FISH increases the efficiency of picking normal embryos so as to enhance the likelihood of a normal, live birth resulting from an IVF cycle and to minimize the risk of an older woman having a child with Down syndrome.

## PGD for Chromosome Defects

Genetic diseases caused by single-gene defects in carriers of specific genetic diseases can be prevented with PGD. However, PGD is much more commonly used for older women who are at increased risk for aneuploidy. A single gene is not large enough to be visualized under the microscope, but a whole chromosome may have one thousand genes, and the entire chromosome (or entire chunks of that chromosome) may be missing or overrepresented in aneuploidy. These errors occur during the process of meiosis in the egg or the sperm.

Chromosome errors are part of the whole issue of the decreasing fertility that occurs as the woman becomes older. These are not specific genetic diseases that carriers have to worry about transmitting to their offspring. Rather, these are defective pregnancies resulting from gross errors in separation of chromosomes as they are reduced from forty-six to twenty-three during the process of egg or sperm production. For conception to occur, twenty-three chromosomes from the husband's set of forty-six and twenty-three chromosomes from the wife's set of forty-six must meet at the moment of fertilization and become an embryo with a normal set of forty-six chromosomes. The process (meiosis) whereby primordial sperm cells and eggs lose half of their chromosome number as they become sperm and mature eggs ready for fertilization is very fragile. These defects are more likely to occur in the eggs of older women (and women with low antral follicle counts) and, to a much lesser degree, in men with severely reduced sperm production.

This process of meiosis becomes more and more difficult for the egg as it gets older. That is why eggs from older women are less likely to result in a viable embryo. That is also why older women are more infertile than younger women, and why older women have higher rates of miscarriage and of conceiving babies with abnormalities such as Down syndrome. Because men make fresh sperm on a daily basis, their sperm is unaffected by aging; therefore, men do not lose their fertility as they age.

### *How Defective Meiosis Causes Down Syndrome and Miscarriage*

Meiosis occurs nowhere else in the body except in the ovary and in the testis. Meiosis has two stages. In the first stage, like pairs of chromosomes line up next to each other, exchange genetic material, and then separate off into two different cells. The chromosomes duplicate but do not separate yet. In the second stage, the divided chromosomes finally separate. The egg does not perform this second meiotic division until the sperm fertilizes it. The second meiotic division (seen as the extrusion of the *second polar body*) occurs when the chromosomes that duplicated themselves in the first stage finally divide. This completes the reduction of the chromosome number from forty-six to twenty-three (see fig. 13.8). An error in the extrusion of the correct number of chromosomes in the first and second polar body is what causes Down syndrome and what causes older women to be infertile.

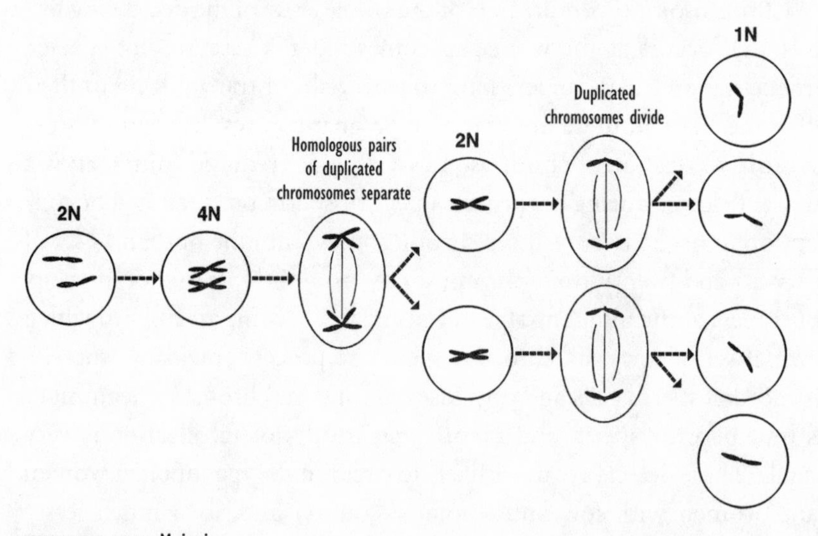


**FIGURE 13.8.** Meiosis.

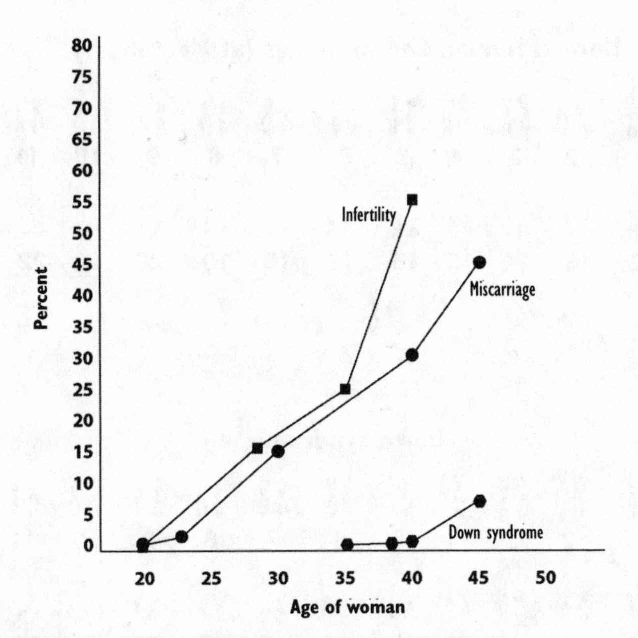


**FIGURE 13.8A.** Relationship of female age to aneuploid offspring.

Chromosomal errors are expressed in several different ways. Approximately 90 percent or more of early miscarriages are caused by a chromosomal error in the fetus. Miscarriage is a much more common expression of chromosomal error than Down syndrome (see fig. 13.8A). In Down syndrome, the baby has a total of forty-seven chromosomes, instead of forty-six, because it has three sets of chromosome 21 instead of the normal two sets (see fig. 13.9). This is because chromosome 21 failed to separate during the meiotic reduction division process in the egg (even though all of the other chromosomes did separate). This kind of chromosomal error, in which one of the twenty-three chromosomes has three copies instead of two, is called trisomy. When one of the twenty-three chromosomes has only one copy instead of two, it is called monosomy. Virtually all monosomies are lethal, except for those in the sex chromosomes, where one X can occasionally be compatible with a relatively normal life.

The public is most familiar with Down syndrome because about 10 to 20 percent of these fetuses do go to birth and result in an abnormal child. However, most fetuses with trisomy 21 miscarry, and all of the other autosomal trisomies miscarry or just do not implant. These chromosomal errors simply make it impossible for the embryo to remain

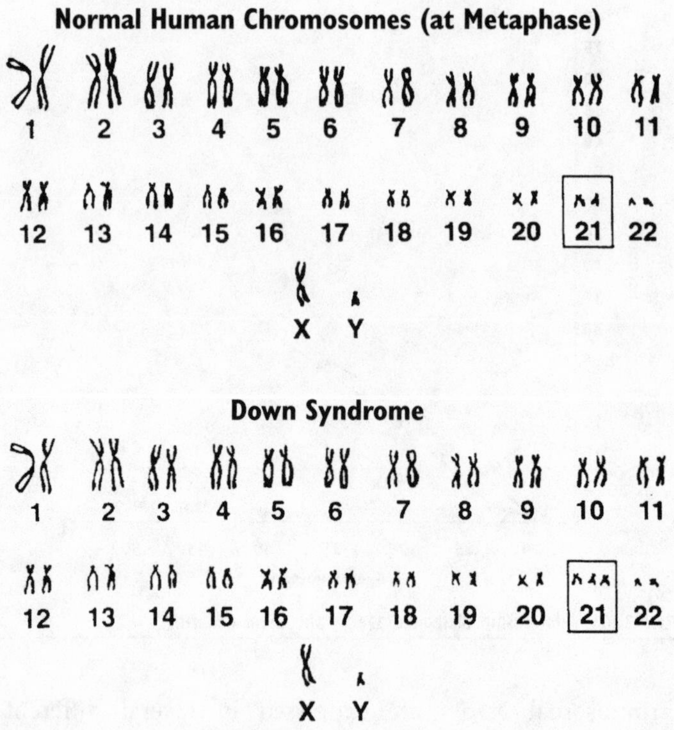

**FIGURE 13.9.** Normal human chromosome pattern compared to Down syndrome pattern.

viable. Thus, early miscarriage in the first three months of life seldom represents the loss of a baby but is an inevitable in utero death of an embryo that was never genetically viable to start with.

All of these conditions related to a woman's biological clock are caused by the same common problem: Older eggs have difficulty with proper chromosomal separation and organization. As a woman gets older, her fertility decreases as her rate of aneuploidy (chromosomal errors in her embryos) increases.

The type of aneuploidy that can occur in humans is random and variable from egg to egg. In some months, the woman will ovulate a normal egg, and in other months, she will ovulate an aneuploid egg. There will be a variety of different types of aneuploidy found in the different eggs over the course of time. In an ovulatory stimulation cycle for IVF, several different types of aneuploid embryos can be found in a single harvest of eggs, along with some normal ones. In general, when there is aneuploidy of the larger chromosomes, i.e., chromosomes 1 to

12, there is virtually never an implantation, and rarely even an early pregnancy. Aneuploidy of the smaller chromosomes, such as 13, 16, 18, 21, and 22, is more likely to result in a pregnancy but will still result in the eventual programmed death of the embryo and miscarriage. It is only the very small chromosomes, like 21, which have very few genes, that can sometimes result in viable but abnormal offspring.

### *Chromosome Errors and the Biological Clock*

If one were to test the early embryo for the *five* chromosomes most commonly in error in miscarriages (out of the twenty-four possible chromosomes), only 8 percent of embryos from women in their midtwenties would be found to have chromosomal errors. Three to four times as many embryos from older women would be found to have these chromosomal errors. If one extrapolates the risk of a chromosomal error among *all* of the chromosomes, half of embryos from women twenty-five to thirty-four years of age will be chromosomally abnormal, 84 percent of embryos from women thirty-five to thirty-nine years of age will be chromosomally abnormal, and almost all embryos in women forty to forty-five will be chromosomally abnormal. These simple age-related chromosomal errors (aneuploidies) explain the increased rate of miscarriage in older women, and also explain the lower pregnancy rates in older women. Although the majority of human eggs (especially in women over age thirty) are chromosomally abnormal, only about 5 to 10 percent of human sperm are chromosomally abnormal.

If you recall from an earlier chapter, we described the meiotic spindle as a set of railroad tracks along which the chromosomes separate. The chromosomes line up on an equatorial plate in the middle of the egg as it prepares to divide, and separate off so as to reduce the chromosome number from forty-six to twenty-three. This process is organized by a structure in the cell called the centriole. The centriole pulls the chromosomes along the spindle to opposite sides of the cell (in this case the egg) and then literally pulls the single cell apart as it divides into two. As the egg is matured, the spindle serves as a system of tracks upon which the chromosomes must travel to get to the opposite poles. Dr. David Battaglia, in Oregon, demonstrated that in women ages twenty to twenty-five, 17 percent of their eggs have an abnormal spindle. In women ages forty to forty-five, over 80 percent of the eggs have an abnormal spindle. The spindle apparatus of the egg is completely disorganized in the majority of older women, so that the chromosomes can't possibly find their way to opposite poles without getting mixed up.

Nothing about the IVF process or ICSI increases the risk of chromosomal abnormalities. It is simply the result of the aging of the woman's eggs. Ironically, if we want to be assured of having a healthy child, IVF (with PGD) is the solution to, rather than the cause of, genetic problems.

### *It Is Not Always the Egg*

Even in normal fertile men with high sperm counts, approximately 5 percent of the sperm will have an abnormal number of one of the chromosomes. In men with extremely low sperm counts, as many as 10 to 20 percent of the sperm will have an abnormal number of chromosomes, and usually this involves the X or the Y chromosome. That is why offspring resulting from ICSI have about a 0.7 percent incidence of sex-chromosome abnormalities as opposed to the normal 0.14 percent. This increased risk of sex-chromosome abnormalities does not result from the IVF or ICSI procedure, but rather from the fact that men with low sperm counts, just like women who have a low number of eggs, have an increased risk of sperm aneuploidy. However, this risk is still tiny compared to the percentage of abnormal eggs in older women.

A second problem related to the sperm of severely infertile men is that the centrosome, the little bead that connects the head of the sperm to the tail (right at the neck), is much more frequently defective in men with very poor sperm production. This centrosome becomes the centriole, which is the organizing motor for cell division in all cells of the resulting embryo. All of the cell divisions that take place in our body through life are organized to occur in an orderly fashion because of this centriole, which we inherited from our father's sperm. Therefore, a centriole defect does not result in a uniform error of just one chromosome too many or one chromosome too few. Rather, centriole defects cause a chaotic missegregation of chromosomes in the embryo so that any given cell might have one, two, three, or even more chromosomes that have an abnormal copy number. For example, a trisomy 21 resulting from an aging egg means that every cell in the embryo is normal except for an extra copy of chromosome 21. When there is a defective sperm centriole, every cell in the embryo has a different chromosomal error. There might be three copies of chromosome 21 in one cell and three copies of chromosome 16 in another, and perhaps one copy of chromosome 18 in another cell, etc. This is called chaotic mosaicism, meaning there is a mixture of different chromosome abnormalities in the various cells of the embryo.

Aneuploidy is an error in copy number of a particular chromosome, consistent throughout all the cells of the embryo. It is caused by an error in meiosis of the maturing egg, and therefore is increased dramatically in older women with a deficient number of eggs. However, chaotic mosaicism (different types of defects involving multiple chromosomes) is found consistently in a constant percentage of embryos no matter what the age of the woman.

### *Embryo Quality and Chromosome Abnormalities*

An aneuploid chromosomal error does not cause any abnormality in the appearance of the eight-cell embryo on day three. It simply programs it for failure to develop further, for early miscarriage, or for an abnormal birth. Thus, in an older woman it is common to see what appear to be normal embryos when in fact genetic analysis would show them to be chromosomally abnormal. However, chaotic mosaic chromosomal errors usually do result in abnormal-looking embryos as well as easily observable defects in early embryo development that are incompatible with life. It is only the simpler aneuploidy errors that increase with the woman's age, and these embryos "appear" normal during routine IVF. Older women, or women with recurrent miscarriages, may have perfectly normal-looking embryos that in a twenty-one-year-old would give an extremely high chance for pregnancy, but in a forty-one-year-old would give a very low chance for pregnancy.

Gross abnormalities in appearance indicate that an embryo is chromosomally chaotic and not viable. But a normal appearance does not eliminate the risk of Down syndrome or other chromosomal trisomies in an older woman. It does eliminate many of the embryos with multiple chromosomal errors that could never develop into a baby. But a sophisticated chromosomal analysis of the embryo is necessary to rule out the risk of Down syndrome and many other trisomies that result in miscarriage.

You can tell a great deal about the embryo's viability simply by evaluating the number of cells (blastomeres), the equality or inequality in the size of those cells, the percent of embryo that is composed of noncellular fragments, and whether or not there is a nucleus (or the presence of several nuclei) in the cells of the embryos. But you cannot diagnose the chromosomal errors that lead to miscarriage and abnormal births without PGD.

Table 13.1 summarizes the dilemma confronting all IVF centers when trying to determine which embryos to place back into the woman. Thirty-seven percent of embryos that look perfectly normal are actually chromosomally abnormal and cannot possibly result in a viable offspring. On the other hand, 80 percent of embryos that look abnormal are chromosomally abnormal. These figures are derived from studies in which only five chromosomes were examined. It would have been technically too difficult in a single cell of a human embryo with the technology currently available to reliably examine all twenty-four chromosomes. By extrapolating, one would have to guess that if we were able to examine all twenty-four chromosomes, at least half of the normal-appearing embryos would be chromosomally abnormal. So by simply analyzing the appearance of an embryo, we can estimate only to a limited degree its potential for further development.

**TABLE 13.1**

**Poor Embryo Quality and Chromosomal Abnormalities**

| TYPE OF CHROMOSOMAL ABNORMALITY | INCIDENCE OF CHROMOSOMAL ERRORS IN NORMAL-APPEARING EMBRYOS | INCIDENCE OF CHROMOSOMAL ERRORS IN POOR-APPEARING EMBRYOS |
|---|---|---|
| Aneuploidy | 17.3% | 8.8% |
| Polyploidy and haploidy | 2.1% | 26.6% |
| Mosaics | 17% | 43% |
| **Total chromosomal abnormalities** | **37%** | **80%** |

VERLINSKY ET AL., 2002

What is the frequency of chromosomal abnormalities in normal- and abnormal-appearing embryos as related to the woman's age? Again, these figures are lower than what would be expected if all twenty-four chromosomes could have been evaluated. This limitation would underestimate the rate of chromosomal abnormality. There are very few chromosomally normal embryos to be found in women over thirty-nine years of age, and the older the woman gets, the less reliable is the evaluation of the appearance of the embryo. In younger women, only a small percentage of normal-appearing embryos are chromosomally abnormal. However, in older women, the majority of normal-appearing embryos are chromosomally abnormal.

There is a specific type of chromosomal abnormality that is constant in the embryo regardless of the woman's age, and there is a different type of chromosomal abnormality that consistently increases with age. The incidence of aneuploidy, i.e., a simple error in a single chromosome that is uniformly distributed throughout all the cells of normal-appearing embryos, as we mentioned, increases dramatically with age. However, abnormalities involving several chromosomes are infrequent in normal-appearing embryos and do not increase at all with age.

There is not much of an increase in abnormal-appearing embryos with age, either those that stop growing over the first day or two in culture, or those that grow very slowly, or have multiple fragments. At any age the vast majority of abnormal-appearing embryos are chromosomally abnormal (chaotic mosaics), and there is no increase in the percentage of these poor-quality embryos as you get older. Whether in your early twenties, or early forties, you will have about the same percentage of abnormal-appearing embryos, and most of those will be chromosomally chaotic.

In some women of any age there is an intrinsic inability to form normal embryos. Certain women simply produce beautiful embryos whenever they undergo IVF. If they are older, these normal-appearing embryos are more likely to be aneuploid. These normal-appearing embryos are likely to be either normal or have one consistent chromosomal error (aneuploidy). However, some women repeatedly make poor-appearing embryos, whether the husband's sperm or donor sperm are used. If these are younger women, eventually there may be a normal embryo that will result in a pregnancy, and some of these women can still have a baby. But when women in this situation are older, they are very unlikely to ever get pregnant.

This consistency of embryo quality, or appearance, in any given couple, regardless of age, can be caused either by intrinsic defects in the woman's eggs or by defects in the sperm's organizing centrosome. Good-quality embryos result in higher pregnancy rates, but in older women, even good-quality embryos are likely to be chromosomally defective and still yield low pregnancy rates.

## Preventing Specific Genetic Diseases

### *PGD to Prevent Down Syndrome: FISH*

The biggest fear of most pregnant women is that their child will be abnormal, and the most common abnormality they worry about is Down syndrome. As we have explained already, Down syndrome is caused by an extra copy of chromosome 21 resulting from defective meiosis in the egg. It is not caused by a single or specific gene mutation, but rather by an incorrect number of whole chromosomes. These children are severely retarded mentally, and they usually die before their thirtieth birthday. The frequency of Down syndrome is related to the age of the mother. Women who are in their twenties have about a 1 in 2,000 risk of having a child with Down syndrome. Women who are thirty-five have a 1 in 500 risk, and women at age forty have a 1 in 100 risk. In women over forty-two years of age, the risk goes up to 5 percent.

Several years ago, I saw a thirty-one-year-old couple who had been infertile for more than eight years. They had undergone conventional infertility treatment involving stimulation of ovulation and intrauterine insemination (IUI). As a result of that conventional treatment, the wife became pregnant but delivered a baby with Down syndrome. One doesn't expect to find Down syndrome in young women, because it is so much more frequent in older women. However, because of this history, her risk of having another Down syndrome child in a future pregnancy, or of having an embryo with any other chromosome trisomy, would be very high despite the fact that she was young.

Prior to seeing us, the couple then went through IVF at another center without any preimplantation genetic diagnosis. She became pregnant again, but this time, as might be expected, she miscarried. Thus, both of her pregnancies resulting from infertility treatment were aneuploid. When this couple finally came to us, it was apparent that they needed IVF with PGD to determine which embryos were normal and which were not. We obtained a total of only eight eggs, seven of which were mature (M-II), and they were each injected with a single sperm. All seven of those eggs fertilized, and by day two all of those embryos appeared to be normal except for one. The other six embryos developed relatively normally to day three (with five to seven cells). All six of those embryos underwent biopsy on day three, with one cell removed and analyzed by FISH. Five of those six embryos developed normally to day five with very healthy-looking blastocyst formation.

However, only one of the five normally developing embryos was chromosomally normal, a male. We transferred only that one normal embryo. The wife became pregnant with a singleton and delivered a normal, healthy baby boy. This couple was a typical example of couples who are infertile at a relatively young age and who are highly prone to chromosomal errors resulting in either a failure to get pregnant, an abnormal pregnancy that usually will miscarry, or sometimes an abnormal birth. By using PGD with FISH, we were able to select the one normal embryo that would result in a healthy baby boy.

### *PGD for Preventing Autosomal-Recessive Gene Disease: Cystic Fibrosis*

Cystic fibrosis is the most common genetic disease caused by a specific gene defect. Unlike Down syndrome, it is caused by a tiny mutation in a single recessive gene. Autosomal recessive genetic diseases, such as cystic fibrosis, Tay-Sachs, sickle-cell anemia, etc., are among the most common single-gene defects. These are caused by small errors in the DNA sequence of crucial recessive genes not located on the sex chromosomes.

If an inherited disease is recessive, as the vast majority of them are, you would need to inherit a recessive gene from each parent in order to have the disease. This means that parents who are perfectly healthy can be carriers of a lethal trait. Their offspring will be healthy so long as the other parent isn't a carrier for the same trait. If both parents are carriers for the same disease, then the child has a 1 in 4 chance of having that disease. Cystic fibrosis (CF) is the most common of these recessive autosomal diseases. Four percent of all of us are carriers of this dreaded gene defect. In the past, most children with cystic fibrosis died before reaching adulthood, although with modern medical treatment, the average life expectancy is age thirty. Some people with milder versions of the disease are lucky enough to live with this condition much longer. This genetic disease is caused by failure of the cells of the lungs and the pancreas to produce a protein called CFTR, which allows for proper fluid transport across cell membranes. Children missing this protein have sticky, viscous fluid throughout their lungs, which makes it progressively harder for them to breathe, and so they slowly suffocate. They also have inadequate secretions of the pancreas, which is required for proper digestion of food.

The gene that is defective in cystic fibrosis patients is relatively enormous (about 230,000 base pairs), and it is located on chromosome 7 (a fairly large chromosome). There are many different varieties of error in the cystic fibrosis gene, but just one tiny amino-acid error in this 1,480-amino-acid protein is enough to wreak complete havoc with the pulmonary system and the pancreas. Routine genetic testing for CF carrier status is available throughout the civilized world now, and it can be performed relatively cheaply on anybody's blood, or even via a cheek swab. It will soon be tested routinely on the vast majority of married couples.

To prevent carriers of cystic fibrosis mutations from having diseased children, we again use embryo biopsy, but in this case, we cannot use FISH. For specific gene defects like cystic fibrosis, we need PCR. FISH will only give us the broad chromosomal picture, such as which chromosomes are present or missing, and is useful for detecting Down syndrome or determining sex. But for a single-gene defect, PCR is required.

The PCR test allows us to amplify from a single cell of the biopsied embryo that specific speck of DNA that has the tiny mutation. If the cell is normal, that speck will not amplify. PCR is a technique that has revolutionized genetics and the unraveling of DNA. At high temperatures the enzyme Taq polymerase causes DNA to copy itself. The specific DNA sequence (like a disease mutation) is added to the Taq polymerase, and then the temperature is raised and lowered twenty to thirty times. This will amplify the specific sequences of DNA that there is concern about. With embryo biopsy and PCR, there is no reason in the modern world for any child to be born with this frightening disease.

Cystic fibrosis is an absolutely amazing example of how random and unpredictable our genetic construction is. You only need a small degree of functioning CF gene to produce a tiny amount of CFTR protein, to protect you from having this fatal disease. However, you also need this CFTR protein to make a vas deferens in early embryo development. Male CF patients and even carriers may have no sperm in the ejaculate because of the absence of a vas deferens. In a way that no one really understands, you would need complete production of a large amount of this CFTR protein when you were a six-week-old male fetus in order to make a vas deferens, and you need only a small amount of CTFR protein to prevent cystic fibrosis. It does not appear that there is any understandable relationship between keeping the secretions in our lung and pancreas properly liquid and the development of a vas deferens in the early embryo. In this way, the human genome is thus far inexplicable. The same genes can have a variety of different functions at different times in our life, with no obviously coherent organization on our chromosomes.

Our first case of PGD for cystic fibrosis came in 1993, when a man with congenital absence of the vas deferens applied for the first St. Louis–Brussels series of ICSI for men with azoospermia. Although we knew he was a CF carrier for the delta F-508 mutation, we were horrified when we routinely tested his wife and discovered that she also was a carrier of the delta F-508 cystic fibrosis mutation. It was enough of a miracle that we were able to fertilize her eggs with sperm we retrieved microsurgically from her husband's testes. But now we also had to test two cells from each of the five 8-cell embryos that resulted from this early ICSI procedure. Two of the five embryos tested normal, and three would have produced a baby with cystic fibrosis. We transferred to the woman's uterus the two normal embryos only, and she delivered a healthy baby (without cystic fibrosis) nine months later.

### *PGD for Preventing Muscular Dystrophy: X-Linked Versus Autosomal-Dominant Disease*

There are basically two types of muscular dystrophy, the X-linked and the autosomal dominant. One type is inherited as a recessive defect on the X chromosome of the mother, and is transmitted from mother to son, much like hemophilia. These include Duchenne's, Becker's, and Kennedy's disease, named after the physicians who first described them. The other type of muscular dystrophy, called myotonic dystrophy, is not inherited recessively and is not on the X chromosome. It is inherited as a dominant trait on chromosome 19.

With Duchenne's muscular dystrophy, the child is born with a rapidly developing muscular deterioration, which results in death in his teen years. As the child gets older, from early years to age five or ten, the parents must bear the agony of seeing what appeared to be a normal baby boy become confined to a wheelchair by age twelve. The child then completely deteriorates and dies by the age of sixteen. Becker's muscular dystrophy results from a defect on the same dystrophin gene, but it is mild and limited enough that such a patient could have a relatively normal life.

The first case of successful embryo biopsy for Duchenne's muscular dystrophy took place in Brussels. The major advance made by this Brussels team was to demonstrate that you didn't have to solve this problem by allowing only girls to be born, and discarding boy embryos. Since Duchenne's is X-linked, daughters of a Duchenne's carrier will either be carriers like their mother, or not have the defective gene at all. In any event, they would be healthy. Half of the boys would be normal (having inherited the mother's normal X chromosome), but half would have the disease. Some doctors recommend PGD just to determine the sex of the embryos, and only transfer girls. I do not believe that such sex selection is the right way to handle this problem. With PCR, we are able to specifically choose all healthy embryos, whether boys or girls.

Another example of X-linked muscular dystrophy is spinal bulbar muscular atrophy (Kennedy's disease), which is caused by an excessive number of CAG triplet repeats in the androgen receptor gene on the X chromosome. This disease is also inherited from the mother, who is a carrier but doesn't have the disease herself. It is transmitted to 50 percent of her sons, depending on whether the son inherits her abnormal X chromosome or her normal X chromosome. Thus, 50 percent of her sons will have the disease, and 50 percent of her daughters will be carriers.

The other type of muscular dystrophy, which is perhaps more common, is myotonic dystrophy, which is autosomal dominant. With an autosomal-dominant gene defect, one parent is the carrier of the defective gene, and that one parent actually has the disease. If the child inherits that gene from the one parent, then the child will also have the disease. These are usually adult-onset diseases that don't preclude the genetically affected individual from having a child when younger and then manifesting the disease later in adulthood.

Fifty percent of these children will inherit the disease from their parent. Those who inherit this genetic defect from their diseased parent will appear healthy at first, but they will eventually manifest the disease when they grow up. Both males and females can transmit the disease equally, and both male and female children are just as likely to get the disease. There is no gender specificity because these defects are inherited on one of the twenty-two autosomes.

These autosomal-dominant diseases are really terrifying because they only manifest in adulthood, after the beginning of childbearing age. Thus, someone who thinks he or she is completely normal can begin to manifest these symptoms in his or her twenties, thirties, or forties, and die prematurely, often suffering an agonizing and debilitating death. These autosomal-dominant diseases are caused either because the gene defect results in the production of a toxic protein, or because two copies rather than one copy of that particular gene are needed for its particular function. The most famous of these dreaded diseases is Huntington's.

This is just one of a number of progressive neurodegenerative diseases that are all caused by the so-called triplet repeat. This means that a specific group of three base pairs (or letters) of DNA are repeated in a very specific region of the gene. These areas of triplet repeat are relatively unstable. Over the course of generations, subsequent children have a gradually increasing number of triplet repeats until, at some point, the region undergoes a huge expansion, and the offspring then has the disease.

Thus, the mother or father may have a premutation of fifty to one hundred repeats on the myotonic muscular dystrophy gene on chromosome 19, representing an omen to any future offspring but not sufficient to cause the disease. All of the cells in the body of these carriers have a safe number of triplet repeats, and so they are healthy. However, if their eggs or sperm suffer from an expansion of these triplet repeats, it would cause an abnormal child to be born. Since this is autosomal dominant, only one parent is a carrier, and if a defective chromosome 19 is transmitted to the child by this one parent, that is sufficient to cause the disease. So every child of such a parent has a 50 percent chance of having the disease.

A patient of ours had gone through the terror of conceiving a child with the severe congenital form of myotonic muscular dystrophy. This was a happily married couple in which the male actually had a mild form of myotonic muscular dystrophy caused by a triplet repeat of 133 sequences. A normal myotonic dystrophy gene would only have five to fifty CTG repeats. Both the husband and his father had this same premutation (133 CTG repeats) on chromosome 19, and so the couple had hoped that their offspring would only have the same mild version of the disease that the father and grandfather had. But to their utter horror, amniocentesis had demonstrated a massive expansion from 133 repeats (a premutation) to 444 triplet CTG repeats, meaning that the child would have a severe congenital form of the disease not compatible with life. For that reason, they decided not to risk any future pregnancy without using PGD.

When we performed their PGD, it was impossible to detect the mutated myotonic dystrophy gene because PCR in a single cell would not be able to find such a huge number of triplet repeats. Therefore, we had to check the embryo for the husband's normal genes, which had to have a different number of triplet repeats than the wife's. Thus, if we found that the embryo had the husband's normal gene, that meant that the embryo did not get his abnormal gene.

Both of the wife's normal genes had five CTG triplet repeats. The husband had one normal gene with eight CTG triplet repeats, and his abnormal gene had 133 (the premutation). This meant that we could use PCR to try to detect the gene with eight triplet repeats, and if this gene was not present, then we knew that the baby would have severe myotonic dystrophy. Thus, we only picked the embryos in which we could detect the normal eight triplet repeat gene of the father.

In the first IVF/PGD cycle attempt, nine eggs were obtained, seven eggs were fertilized, only two embryos developed to day three, and only one of those embryos was free of the disease. She did not get pregnant in that cycle. In her second IVF/PGD cycle, two embryos were normal, and she became pregnant and delivered a healthy baby girl who inherited one of her mother's two healthy genes and her father's healthy gene, meaning that this little girl was completely disease-free. This couple had been so emotionally devastated by conceiving a child with myotonic dystrophy in their first pregnancy that they had decided they would never have any more children if PGD were not available.

### *PGD for Preventing Marfan's Syndrome*

Marfan's syndrome is an autosomal-dominant genetic disease in which seemingly healthy children grow to be young adults who are at risk of sudden death because of a defect in the connective tissue in their body. It is a disease that undermines the formation of the connective tissue that holds our body together. They have a tiny point mutation on the fibrillin gene on chromosome 15 involving a GC substitute for CT. This results in the replacement of the amino acid arginine with the amino acid proline in this one specific tiny area of what is a huge protein consisting of thousands of amino acids. This one little typographical error in a gigantic array of DNA letters prevents the body from being able to construct its connective tissue properly. If the father has this disease, his offspring, whether male or female, have a 50 percent chance of having the same disease. If the mother has the disease, she is very likely to die from pregnancy. PGD with IVF and gestational surrogacy is the perfect answer to the otherwise frightening outlook for such couples.

A twenty-six-year-old woman who was engaged to be married in eight months came into my office with her fiancé to see if there was any way to safely have children. She had been diagnosed at six years of age with Marfan's syndrome after learning she had a leaky heart valve. Her father had Marfan's syndrome and almost died, but was saved by an emergency operation on his aorta (the main artery of the chest) and on his heart valves. Her mother was perfectly normal. Her brother was born with Marfan's and required emergency heart surgery and repair of the aorta at age twenty-three (just three years before she saw me). Her father's brother died suddenly from Marfan's because he failed to have the corrective surgery in time. She knew that it would be fatal for her to try to bear children. Furthermore, any of her offspring would have a 50 percent chance of having the same problem she had.

Her forty-eight-year-old mother, who did not have Marfan's, offered to carry her baby, thus precluding the risk of her dying because of pregnancy. They came to us proposing we do IVF using her eggs and her fiancé's sperm, and then place the embryos into her mother to carry the baby. However, they were still in a dilemma about the 50 percent possibility that their babies would have Marfan's.

We suggested preimplantation genetic diagnosis, i.e., only transferring embryos that did not have Marfan's syndrome. We retrieved sixteen eggs and injected the fifteen that were mature with her husband's sperm. Fourteen of them fertilized. Thirteen of those fourteen developed into eight-cell embryos on day three, and a single cell was taken from each one of those embryos and tested for Marfan's. But testing for Marfan's is even more complicated than that.

The actual Marfan's gene mutation is very hard to characterize in individual patients. So we tested blood samples from everyone in her family who was still living. We identified what we call linked markers, or DNA fingerprints, on the Marfan's gene by comparing chromosomes from the patient, her brother, and her father, all of whom have Marfan's syndrome (presumably from the same gene mutation), and from her husband and her mother who do not have Marfan's. By selecting the embryos that did not have the same linked markers as the wife, her brother, or her father, we could be sure that the embryos we were transferring did not have their gene mutation. In fact, using this technique of linked markers, virtually any genetic disease can be tested for (even if the specific gene defect is not capable of being characterized yet) so that only healthy embryos need be transferred back into the patient. We wound up transferring three healthy embryos without Marfan's defect to the patient's mother, who became pregnant and delivered healthy twins, one boy and one girl. Neither of these children has Marfan's syndrome, thanks to the PGD procedure.

*Genetic Prevention of Early Onset Alzheimer's*

PGD can go way beyond simply avoiding obvious genetic diseases in young children. It can also be used to prevent the tragedy of having a child who appears to be healthy when born, but who would run a high risk of developing terrifying diseases later in life. One disease we all dread is early onset Alzheimer's, in which a relatively rapid onset of senile dementia occurs. Some types of Alzheimer's can develop as early as the late thirties, and are therefore even more dreaded than the more common later onset Alzheimer's that begins in the sixties and seventies. Early onset Alzheimer's disease is another example of autosomal-dominant familial disease, and it is similar in its genetic transmission to Marfan's, Huntington's, and myotonic dystrophy. It is caused by a mutation in one of three different genes found on chromosome 14, chromosome 1, or chromosome 21.

A woman in her late twenties who had such a mutation in the amyloid precursor protein (APP) gene on chromosome 21 knew she faced Alzheimer's in her future and wanted to make sure her child would not be in a similar predicament. She was not a patient of ours, but her story is quite powerful. Her father had died relatively young and had a history of memory loss and psychological disorientation prior to death. Her older sister developed Alzheimer's in her forties, but she was still alive and functioning reasonably well. One of her brothers had the same mutation, and he had suffered from a much milder and less progressive form of Alzheimer's. One could seriously question whether it was wise to help this woman become pregnant because of her short-term expectancy of remaining competent. Using IVF and PGD, only embryos that did not have the defective Alzheimer gene were transferred. As a result, she conceived a child that did not have this mutation, and who will not have to face the same frightening future her mother or grandfather did.

### *Huntington's Disease*

Huntington's disease is a form of programmed brain death that affects about 1 in every 10,000 individuals, and is caused by inheritance of an autosomal-dominant gene defect on chromosome 4. The famous folk singer Woody Guthrie died of this disease. It usually begins in the late thirties, and starts with progressive development of uncontrolled and jerky movements as well as deterioration of thinking and sudden changes in emotional temperament. It is a horrible, agonizing death. The type of gene defect causing Huntington's is similar to other neurodegenerative diseases; it does not result from an error in a specific letter in the DNA sequence, but rather from an expansion of a triplet repeat sequence of DNA over and over again above the number that the gene should normally have.

Normally, the Huntington's gene on chromosome 4 has anywhere from eleven to thirty-four copies of a specific DNA sequence of the letters CAG. CAG codes for a specific amino acid, glutamine. Whenever there are more than forty repeat copies of CAG, producing more than forty copies in a row of glutamine on the Huntington's protein, this mutated protein causes the terrible neurological disease of Huntington's.

If one of your parents died of this disease, you have a 50 percent chance of having it as well. The genetic defect does not need to be present in both parents in order to be passed on because the disease is autosomal dominant.

Young adults whose parent had Huntington's disease usually do not want to know if they will suffer the same end, and are very resistant to testing. They refer to it as toxic knowledge. However, these same would-be young parents who have a 50 percent chance of getting the disease later in life (and who don't want to know about it ahead of time) definitely do *not* want their children to have it. This is where IVF with preimplantation embryo genetic diagnosis will eliminate their fears of having a child with Huntington's, while maintaining (if they so wish) their ignorance of whether or not they themselves will have it.

### *Predisposition Toward Cancer and Rh Disease*

With the discovery of the BRCA gene mutations that cause early onset breast and ovarian cancer, women who have a high probability of developing these cancers at an early age (inherited from their parents) can now undergo PGD with genetic testing to make sure their offspring do not have that same high risk of developing cancer when they grow up. Women who have a parental history of breast or ovarian cancer and who have the BRCA gene mutations are wise to undergo early removal of their breasts even before the cancer develops. But they don't want their daughters to have to go through this. With PGD, only the embryos without the BRCA mutations are transferred.

Women with Rh disease, who are sensitized to their own child's Rh factor, can now also have healthy children. A small number of Rh-negative women who are given Rhogam at the time of delivery of their first child to prevent Rh disease become sensitized to Rh anyway, and future offspring who are Rh-positive will be at enormous risk of dying in utero. With PGD, such women can undergo IVF, and only the Rh-negative embryos that will survive pregnancy without such problems are transferred back to her. Fifty-five percent of men who are Rh-positive have only one out of two genes for Rh. If the Rh-negative woman becomes pregnant from such a male partner, 50 percent of her embryos will be positive like the father and will undergo serious Rh-factor disease in utero. Fifty percent will be negative like the mother. In this instance, PGD is not being used to select healthy, viable embryos that will result in healthy offspring, but rather is being used to select embryos that will survive the pregnancy by not eliciting a deadly Rh reaction in the mother.

## X-Linked Disease

There are about six thousand known hereditary diseases in the human. More than 350 of these are X-linked, which means that they are carried as a recessive trait on the X chromosome and are not expressed as a disease in women, only in men. The classic example of X-linked genetic disease is hemophilia, a blood-clotting disorder that the czars in Russia suffered because of inbreeding. Hemophilia is caused by deficiency of clotting factor 8 in the blood. Any couple in which the wife is a healthy carrier of an X-linked disease like hemophilia, Becker's or Duchenne's muscular dystrophy, retinitis pigmentosa, or fragile X has a 50 percent chance of having male offspring with the disease.

There are many other relatively common hereditary diseases carried on the X chromosome that are perhaps not as well known as hemophilia. Retinitis pigmentosa is a condition that, in its mild form, simply means color blindness, but in the serious form of the disease can lead to complete loss of vision. Men with this condition become more and more blind as they get older. The male offspring of these men will be completely normal. However, the daughters of such men will all be carriers of the disease, and their grandsons have a 50 percent chance of having the disease.

The most common genetic cause of mental retardation is fragile X syndrome. Fragile X is also an X-linked recessive disorder. Mothers who are carriers will transmit this disease to 50 percent of their sons, and 50 percent of their daughters will be carriers. Fragile X simply means that the FMR-1 gene on the X chromosome has a CGG triplet repeat defect similar to what we described in Huntington's and myotonic dystrophy. This gene on the X chromosome must be functioning properly to allow normal mental development. About one third of these female carriers have a mild form of the condition, and about two thirds of female carriers are completely normal. All males with this gene defect have a severe form of the disease. This disease is caused by a triplet repeat expansion of a gene on the X chromosome. In this case, it is a CGG nucleotide repeat, which codes for the amino acid arginine. On the fragile X gene there are *normally* six to forty-nine repeats of the CGG code for arginine. When there are fifty to two hundred copies of this DNA repeat, whether in a male or female, the individual is completely normal, but trouble is on the way for future generations. As soon as a generation appears in which there are more than two hundred copies of this DNA triplet repeat, the male baby will exhibit fragile X.

This is one of the commonest forms of mental retardation in male offspring, second only to Down syndrome. About 30 percent of women who are carriers of this fragile X mutation have some mild degree of learning problems themselves because half of all their X chromosomes are inactivated randomly (see chapter 12). The reason is that for most X-linked diseases, it does not matter if half of the person's cells have a good X chromosome and half have a bad X chromosome inactivated. As long as there is some normal X chromosome function, that is enough for the female not to have the disease. For fragile X syndrome it is safer for the female to have two normal X chromosomes.

For some odd reason, when the father passes this premutation on to his children, it does not expand and remains a premutation. However, when a woman who is a carrier of this premutation (which she might have inherited from her father) has children, they often suffer an expansion beyond two hundred CGG repeats, and if so, her male offspring have the condition.

A twenty-five-year-old woman came to see us with her mother prior to getting married, because her brother had fragile X syndrome and suffered severe retardation. She had greater than two hundred CGG repeats in one copy of her FMR-1 gene, as did both her mother and her brother. She and her mother were completely normal, but it was clear that any male offspring she had would be mentally retarded, and that there was an unpredictable possibility that even a female offspring might be somewhat affected. She had been on birth control pills since seventeen years of age to avoid any risk of getting pregnant. Now, married, she can utilize PGD and have completely normal children without the fear of this dreaded genetic defect.

## PGD for Human Leukocyte Antigen (HLA) Tissue Typing: Having a Baby Who Can Save the Life of Her Dying Sister

Perhaps the most controversial use of PGD, which was documented in the *Journal of the American Medical Association* in 2001, involved a family whose six-year-old daughter was dying of an autosomal recessive condition called Fanconi's anemia. The parents of this dying six-year-old were carriers of the FANCC mutation on chromosome 9, which causes a shortage of blood cells and a predisposition to leukemia. With Fanconi's anemia the bone marrow does not function properly, and the sufferer will eventually die. Each parent had a copy of this recessive gene; they were normal, but their little girl had received the mutated genes of each parent. They were not going to allow themselves to have a spontaneous pregnancy ever again because there was a 25 percent risk of having another child with this condition. So they underwent IVF with PGD, *not only* to avoid having another child with this terrible genetic disease, but also to select an embryo that would be a genetic tissue match for their dying daughter. In this way, as soon as the child was born, a small amount of umbilical cord and placental blood (which is normally discarded at the time of birth) could be given to the dying sister in order to save her life. This transfusion, much like a bone marrow transplant, provides rich stem cells, and it created a whole new blood supply and immune system for the dying six-year-old girl. Her life was saved because PGD allowed the parents to be sure that their next healthy child would be a perfect HLA-compatible tissue match for their otherwise dying daughter.

Of thirty embryos that were tested in four different IVF attempts, six were homozygous (meaning they had both of the Fanconi gene mutations and would have the disease), and twenty-four were normal. Only five of these twenty-four normal embryos were found to be HLA compatible. Two of these embryos were transferred in the first IVF cycle, but no pregnancy occurred. One was transferred in each of the next three cycles, and a pregnancy occurred in the last cycle, with a normal embryo that was a perfect HLA match for the sister. The remaining healthy embryos that were not HLA compatible were frozen and saved for future pregnancies. This whole concept might sound extremely scary, but careful thought by many ethics committees decided that it was the correct thing to do, not only to bring a new life that was healthy into the world, but also to save the life of a child who otherwise would have died.

## DNA Fingerprinting, Single Nucleotide Polymorphisms (SNPs), Linked Markers, and PGD

Not all mutations, which are misspellings in the genetic code, are bad. In fact, there are at least three million variations (mutations) in the human genome code that don't appear to have any obvious impact on health. A variation in genetic code that doesn't have a major effect on health is called a polymorphism. Obviously we are all different, and these differences, which are not considered defects but are simply variations from one individual to another, may very well be tied in to this prevalence of polymorphisms. Polymorphism is simply a DNA variation from the routine that we don't call a mutation because it doesn't appear to have any disastrous consequences. The final sequencing of the human genome uncovered about three million polymorphisms that involved just a single letter of DNA. These are called single nucleotide polymorphisms, or SNPs. These and other vast arrays of polymorphisms have been used in forensic science and discussed greatly in the popular press as so-called DNA fingerprints. Many of the three billion base pairs that represent the human genome do not have clearly definable genes. The majority of the genome contains letters, or base pair sequences, that have no obvious immediate meaning to us. There are tremendous variations of the sequences of DNA in the "meaningless" area of the genome that are absolutely specific for every single individual, much like fingerprints.

These differences are not significant to the person's health or to any clearly definable characteristics, any more than the fact that each zebra has completely different stripe patterns from all other zebras on the face of the planet. In the same way, each human has different fingerprints from all other humans. DNA fingerprinting is simply a technique for quantifying the polymorphic regions of our DNA. This process has become a very reliable technology, and it is certainly acknowledged by most scientists in the field as easier than classical fingerprinting for forensic or legal purposes.

We also use these nonpathologic, individual variations in DNA sequence as linked markers for PGD. It is critical to avoid errors in the genetic diagnosis of an embryo, yet you have only one cell to examine. Therefore, it is wise not only to look for the mutation (which might not amplify) but also to establish with certainty which parental genes are in the embryo. DNA fingerprinting allows us to do this, and to be remarkably accurate in the diagnosis.

## Conclusion

The biggest fear of all women striving to have a child is the possibility of birth defects or genetic disease in the offspring. With IVF and PGD, carriers of genetic disease no longer have to be fearful of the prospect of giving birth to a diseased infant. There is not now, nor is there ever likely to be, any prospect of this turning into a "designer baby" phenomenon, because humanity is so intrinsically diverse and because personality, character, and intelligence are complex traits independent of specific genes. Even if some bizarre researcher or physician wanted to create "designer babies," he or she would not be able to do so. In fact, even cloned animals do not look like each other. We are not our genes. Our genes are just the house we live in. All that our genetic IVF technology is providing is a way for couples to avoid the tragedy of having children with fatal or disabling diseases.

CHAPTER 14

# Understanding and Preventing Miscarriage

## Chromosome Errors Cause Most Miscarriages

The ticking of your biological clock involves not only an increased incidence of infertility with the advancing years, but also a dramatic increase in miscarriage. More than 90 percent of miscarriages are caused by chromosomal and genetic errors in the embryo. We've already discussed in the previous chapter how we can prevent trisomy 21 (Down syndrome) pregnancies with PGD. The same PGD technique can be used to prevent recurrent miscarriage.

Women with recurrent miscarriage usually produce embryos that have an abnormal number of chromosomes. However, an occasional embryo from such patients will be normal. Rather than just allowing these otherwise fertile women to get pregnant spontaneously and miscarry over and over again, we can do IVF, obtain as many as fifteen or more embryos, and test them each before transfer back into the woman's uterus. The one or two embryos that are actually normal can be placed into her uterus so that she can then carry a normal, healthy full-term pregnancy, without the fear of one heartbreaking miscarriage after another.

There is a lot of confusion about miscarriage. In order to really understand miscarriage, you would have to perform a karyotype (i.e., analysis of chromosomes) on the products of conception immediately if there is an early sign on ultrasound of fetal demise. Waiting until the natural passing of the products of conception will make diagnosis impossible. Often, the fetal karyotype will show a normal 46XX, but this is simply caused by contamination with maternal cells. This occurs because the products of conception are passed so late after the fetal demise that the DNA of the fetus is completely degenerated, and the only living cells to grow and culture in the karyotype test are the mother's. That is why there has been a misconception over the previous decades that only 50 percent or less of miscarriages are caused by chromosomal error. Dr. Mary Ann Perle of New York University has shattered that myth. Detailed testing with an early D and C and careful dissection the moment the fetal heartbeat stops, before the tissue has had a chance to degenerate, demonstrates that most miscarriages are caused by chromosomal and genetic errors in the embryo itself, and not by problems in the uterus or in the woman's general system.

### *Screening Embryos for Chromosomal Errors*

A twenty-nine-year-old woman got pregnant four times over two and a half years and miscarried each time. She appeared to be fertile but "just couldn't hold" her pregnancy. On two of those occasions, the miscarried fetuses were chromosomally tested. One was monosomy X (only one X chromosome), and the other was a trisomy 17 and 18 (three copies of both chromosome 17 and 18). Clearly, this was a woman with a propensity for ovulating aneuploid eggs. After the pain and suffering of four consecutive miscarriages, she feared ever becoming pregnant again. So we decided to do IVF with PGD. We were able to stimulate her sufficiently to get seventeen eggs, fifteen of which fertilized. She made many beautiful-appearing embryos, but only two of them were chromosomally normal, and they were both 46XX girls. We replaced these two embryos into her uterus, she became pregnant, and delivered a healthy baby girl nine months later.

A thirty-two-year-old woman had a history of five previous miscarriages in her twenties, and despite her young age, she was simply afraid ever to get pregnant again. Out of thirty-seven embryos we obtained during IVF (administered not because she couldn't get pregnant, but rather to avoid miscarriage), only three were normal, two normal females and one normal male. After all these miscarriages and fear of ever getting pregnant again, she now had a healthy twin pregnancy, a normal boy and a normal girl.

A thirty-three-year-old woman with a history of cancer of the uterus wanted desperately to have a child. She was treated with high-dose progesterone, and her cancer was cured. It was important for her to have a child as soon as possible because of the risk of a recurrence of this uterine cancer, which would require a hysterectomy. In fact, she did become pregnant with her first IVF cycle, but this pregnancy resulted in miscarriage because of the usual problem of chromosomal abnormality. Despite a history of uterine cancer, the problem was not with her uterus, but with her embryos. In the next IVF cycle we performed PGD, and of twenty-three embryos only three were chromosomally normal. All three were boys. She became pregnant and delivered a healthy baby boy nine months later.

You might wonder why it would be that not all of those chromosomally normal embryos resulted in a pregnancy. For example, in the last patient discussed, we transferred three normal male embryos, but only one implanted and survived. The reason for this is that we cannot test for all of the chromosomes. We have to pick the chromosomes that are most commonly abnormal in miscarriage. This generally means the smaller chromosomes: 13, 15, 16, 18, 21, and 22, along with, of course, X and Y. Thus, when our testing shows that an embryo is normal chromosomally, there may still be larger chromosomes that we could not test (i.e., chromosomes 1 through 12) that are abnormal, and which would prevent implantation altogether.

Very often, PGD in older women who've had recurrent miscarriage is disappointing because most of the embryos are chromosomally abnormal and would not result in a viable pregnancy, or there may still be undetected errors in the untested, larger chromosomes. Thus, PGD does not increase the pregnancy rate, but it will dramatically reduce the risk of miscarriage in women who are otherwise highly predisposed to miscarriage. In the worst case, with PGD screening, women can at least know whether any of their eggs are still capable of producing a normal pregnancy, or if it is time for them to consider donor eggs.

### *Aneuploidy Versus Chaotic Mosaicism*

It should be clear by now that the majority of human eggs are abnormal. They are either chromosomally abnormal, having too few or too many copies of specific chromosomes, or developmentally abnormal in the way they progress from stage to stage. This problem with human embryos, which is not seen anywhere else in the animal kingdom, is caused, for the most part, by intrinsic problems in the egg, and these problems increase in severity and frequency with increasing age.

There is a fourfold increase in chromosomal aneuploidy that occurs from a woman's late twenties and early thirties until her late thirties and early forties. This fourfold increase in chromosomal abnormalities is simply related to the aging of the egg, and it is superimposed on a background incidence of chromosomal abnormalities seen in the human that is unprecedented in any other animal. The background rate of chromosomal abnormality unrelated to the wife's or husband's age is related either to an intrinsic defect in her eggs or to an intrinsic defect in his sperm.

With aneuploidy, the chromosomes get stuck in their tracks, so to speak, and an extra chromosome may be left behind in the egg via a process called nondisjunction. Thus, not all of the chromosomes move to their proper positions in the process of reducing the chromosome number from forty-six to twenty-three. With aneuploidy, almost every cell in the developing embryo suffers from having an incorrect number of a particular chromosome. Three copies of chromosome 21, which results in Down syndrome, or three copies of chromosome 16, which results in an early miscarriage, are classic examples of aneuploidy, where there are just one or two chromosomes in error, and they are uniformly in error in every cell of the embryo. The rest of the chromosomes of the aneuploid embryo are normal. Aneuploidy is a uniform problem in all the cells of the embryo and is specifically caused by the aging of the egg.

However, chromosomal abnormalities can be much more complex, involving more than just one chromosome, and can be different in different cells of the embryo. This is called mosaicism. Mosaicism can be caused by either an intrinsic egg problem or by a defect in the sperm. In this kind of problem there may be several different chromosomes that have only one copy, or three copies, rather than the normal two copies. Furthermore, which chromosomes have an abnormal number of copies may be different in different cells of the embryo. These are very abnormal embryos that would not ever be likely to implant, or else would lead to an extremely early miscarriage. This more complex kind of chromosomal error is not due to aging, and is caused by an intrinsic problem either in the egg, or in the sperm, unrelated to the biological clock.

The first couple who helped us discover the role of the sperm in normal embryo development was a twenty-five-year-old woman married to a twenty-eight-year-old man who were celebrating their fifth anniversary when they first saw me. He had no sperm in his ejaculate. We were, however, able to find a small number of sperm in his testicles using TESE, and we injected them into his wife's eggs in an IVF cycle. Twenty-three eggs (out of twenty-six) were fertilized and subjected to PGD.

| Embryo # | # Cells Examined | Sex Chromosomes | 13 | 15 | 16 | 17 | 18 | 21 | 22 | Diagnosis of Embryo |
|---|---|---|---|---|---|---|---|---|---|---|
| 4 | 1 | XY | 2 | 2 | 2 | 2 | 2 | 2 | 2 | Normal |
| 5 | 1 | XO | 2 | 1 | 1 | 1 | 2 | 1 | 2 | Complex abnormal (mosaic) |
| 6 | 1 | XY | 2 | 2 | 2 | 2 | 2 | 2 | 2 | Normal |
| 7 | 1 | 3X | 2 | 3 | 2 | 3 | 3 | 3 | 3 | Complex abnormal (mosaic) |
| 9 | 1 | XY | 0 | 2 | 2 | 2 | 2 | 2 | 2 | Nulisomy 13 |
| 9 | 2 | XY | 0 | 2 | 2 | 2 | 2 | 2 | 2 | Nulisomy 13 |
| 11 | 1 | XY | 3 | 3 | 1 | 2 | 2 | 3 | 3 | Complex abnormal (mosaic) |
| 15 | 1 | XX | 2 | 2 | 2 | 2 | 2 | 2 | 2 | Normal |
| 17 | 1 | XX | 2 | 3 | 2 | 2 | 1 | 1 | 1 | Complex abnormal (mosaic) |
| 22 | 1 | XX | 1 | 1 | 1 | 2 | 1 | 1 | 2 | Complex abnormal (mosaic) |
| 26 | 1 | XY | 1 | 2 | 1 | 2 | 0 | 0 | 0 | Complex abnormal (mosaic) |

**TABLE 14.1**

**Results of TESE-ICSI and PGD for a patient with azoospermia caused by chemotherapy and radiation. Severe spermatogenic defects result in a higher incidence of complex (mosaic) chromosomal errors not related to the wife's age. Simple errors (aneuploidy) involving only one chromosome (like trisomy 21) are related to the wife's age.**

From those twenty-three fertilized eggs, only three embryos were chromosomally normal, two boys and one girl (see table 14.1). We replaced all three of those chromosomally normal embryos into her uterus, and she delivered healthy twins nine months later, one boy and one girl.

The fascinating discovery stemming from this couple was that in such a young woman, in whom the only problem was the infertile male, you would not expect to find such a huge number of chromosomally abnormal embryos. The embryos exhibited a complex, chaotic array of errors that had to be occurring during the course of cell division in the developing embryo, rather than originating in a nondisjunction event in the egg prior to fertilization. Such a large number of embryos with chromosomal abnormalities in this young patient was more likely caused by the sperm than the egg.

These chaotic abnormalities had to develop out of an improper structural system for cell division in the early embryo caused by a sperm centrosome defect. The motor that directs the whole system for cell division comes from the sperm centrosome. This is the little circular structure at the neck of the sperm that joins the head and the tail, and helps propel the sperm tail and gives the sperm its movement. This centrosome of the sperm is also what becomes the centriole of the fertilized

| Embryo # | Sex Chromosomes | 13 | 15 | 16 | 17 | 18 | 21 | 22 | Diagnosis of Embryo |
|---|---|---|---|---|---|---|---|---|---|
| 2 | XX | 2 | 3 | 2 | 2 | 2 | 2 | 2 | Trisomy 15 |
| 9 | XX | 2 | 1 | 2 | 2 | 2 | 2 | 3 | Trisomy 22, Monosomy 15 |
| 10 | XY | 2 | 2 | 2 | 2 | 2 | 2 | 1 | Monosomy 22 |
| 11 | XX | 3 | 2 | 2 | 2 | 2 | 2 | 2 | Trisomy 13 |
| 12 | XX | 3 | 2 | 2 | 2 | 2 | 2 | 2 | Trisomy 13 |
| 14 | XY | 2 | — | 2 | 2 | 2 | 2 | 2 | Normal |
| 15 | XX | 2 | 2 | — | 2 | 2 | 2 | 2 | Normal |
| 17 | XX | 2 | 1 | 2 | 2 | 2 | 2 | 2 | Monosomy 15 |
| 19 | XY | 2 | 2 | 2 | 2 | 2 | 2 | 1 | Monosomy 22 |
| 20 | XX | 2 | 2 | 2 | 2 | 2 | 2 | 2 | Normal |
| 21 | X | 2 | 2 | 2 | 1 | 2 | 2 | 2 | Monosomy 17 |
| 22 | XX | 2 | 2 | 3 | 2 | 2 | 2 | 2 | Trisomy 16 |

**TABLE 14.2**

**Results of ICSI and PGD for azoospermic patient with a thirty-eight-year-old wife using normal donor sperm. In this case, errors in the embryo involve only one chromosome (aneuploidy) and are related not to a spermatogenic defect, but to the wife's age.**

egg, which controls cell division for every cell in your body. In fact, every single cell in your body (which all have to divide) derives its centriole from your father's sperm. Chromosomally chaotic embryos can also develop from an intrinsic problem in a particular woman's eggs, but even then it is not related to aging of the egg.

Table 14.2 depicts the results of a thirty-eight-year-old woman using normal donor sperm for IVF. Only three of the embryos from twenty-two fertilized eggs were chromosomally normal. All of the abnormal embryos, except for number nine, were simple aneuploidies in otherwise normal-appearing embryos. This is the type of chromosomal error that is found in the normal-appearing embryos of aging eggs.

The chromosomal defects associated with aging eggs result in normal-appearing embryos. Chromosomal abnormalities associated with severely deficient sperm result in abnormal-appearing embryos. But even when the sperm centrosome is normal, a certain percentage of eggs (unrelated to aging) will be chaotic mosaics, abnormal in appearance and intrinsic to that particular woman's eggs at any age.

A couple who demonstrated this dilemma came to us because the husband had moderately low sperm production. The wife was young (twenty-nine years old) and healthy. During their first ICSI cycle, we were able to obtain many eggs, and there was a consistently high fertilization rate. With more than twenty-five embryos examined by PGD in each of three separate ICSI/IVF cycles, every single embryo had some sort of complex, chaotic abnormality, with poor cell division. So we tried using donor sperm in two subsequent cycles, thinking that perhaps a defect in the sperm centrosome was causing this poor result. But after several cycles with donor sperm, we continued to obtain only large numbers of chromosomally chaotic, abnormal-appearing embryos.

After much soul-searching, we decided the problem was the wife's eggs (even though she was young and produced many eggs). So for the next IVF cycle, we used the husband's sperm rather than donor sperm, but now employed donor eggs. This was a relatively bold step to take in view of the fact that she was young and healthy, and had produced so many eggs in every IVF cycle. As soon as we switched to donor eggs, there were quite a few chromosomally normal embryos, and she became pregnant immediately with twins.

The type of egg defect she exhibited (chaotic mosaicism) was *not* related to her age. Two percent of even young women are infertile, and this is usually because of an intrinsic problem with their eggs that has nothing to do with their biological clock. These two exemplary cases demonstrate that repeatable defects in embryo development causing consistent failure to get pregnant with ICSI and IVF may be the result of a defect in the sperm (which might be expected in view of the very low sperm production rate), or may be due to a defect in the eggs (despite the wife being young and having many eggs).

What relates to the biological clock is the more simple chromosomal errors called aneuploidy, which increase dramatically with the woman's age and with the decrease in her ovarian reserve. The number of embryos that *appear* abnormal does not seem to increase with a woman's age or her biological clock. What increases with the age of her eggs is the number of normal-*appearing* embryos that are actually chromosomally abnormal. Miscarriage is caused, for the most part, by the more simple chromosomal errors (aneuploidy) that increase in frequency with the age of the woman, and that result in completely normal-appearing embryos.

### *Preventing Miscarriage Caused by Chromosomal Translocations*

Another cause of recurrent miscarriage in young women is a different type of chromosomal error called a translocation, which was mentioned in a previous chapter. To understand how translocations cause recurrent miscarriage, let's use the *Encyclopedia Britannica* analogy. We have twenty-three pairs of chromosomes. Let's say that each chromosome is one volume of an encyclopedia. Each volume will contain at least 150 million letters that form words. A gene mutation would represent a misspelling of a single word or, at most, several words. A translocation would represent several hundred misplaced pages of the encyclopedia that are missing from their normal position in one volume, and pasted into another volume. All of the words and all of the paragraphs are intact, but the pages have been mislocated to another volume of the encyclopedia.

Translocations are the cause of many miscarriages. With translocation, part of one chromosome has broken off and moved to another chromosome. In a balanced translocation, using the encyclopedia metaphor, all of the words and paragraphs, and all of the knowledge, is intact, but the order of appearance and organization has been modified. These balanced translocations are found in almost 2 percent of infertile couples (although in only 0.2 percent or less of the general population).

Everything seems to work fine in patients with these translocations, except when they try to have children. For example, if you have a set of encyclopedias in which a single volume is missing 250 pages, and those 250 pages are relocated to a completely different volume, you cannot line up each of those volumes with another set of encyclopedias. If you try to line up the volume that is missing 250 pages with the same volume of a normal set of encyclopedias, it simply cannot match up. Homologous, or "like," chromosomes must line up during meiosis when either the egg or the sperm reduces its chromosome number from forty-six to twenty-three. For normal reproduction to occur, like chromosomes must be able to find each other so they can prepare for equal separation into the egg and the polar body, or equal separation into two different sperm. This reproductive pairing up, or buddy system, is hampered by the presence of translocations.

Translocations are an integral part of chromosomal evolution and development of species. For example, the genes of most mammals are pretty much the same. We are 98.5 percent mouse and 99.9 percent chimpanzee. In fact, we are approximately 60 percent fruit fly and 40 percent worm. These percentages are calculated by figuring the percentages of strands of DNA in humans that are found identically in other animals. We are all so alike in our DNA that what separates one species from another is that its members are only able to reproduce with other members of the same species. That is the long-range cosmic purpose of chromosomal translocations.

For example, a normal human karyotype when compared to the karyotype of chimpanzees and gorillas contains four major chromosomal translocations. Human chromosome 2 is a Robertsonian translocation of chimpanzee chromosomes 12 and 13. That means that if you took the chimpanzee chromosomes 12 and 13, and stuck them together, you would have what appears to be a human chromosome 2.

In general, most mammals, from rodents to primates, have highly conserved, very similar genes, but these genes are located in different chromosomes and are in a different organizational pattern in the various species, which prevents any possibility of interbreeding. That is the definition of a species. The genes of various species are very similar or nearly identical, but the chromosomal locations for those genes are different. Thus, translocations are an inevitable part of species differentiation, preventing related species from reproducing with each other. But it is also a cause of infertility and miscarriage in human couples.

There are two reproductive problems caused by translocation. The chromosomal confusion, which occurs with large balanced translocations when they try to line up for meiosis, can result in deficient egg maturation or deficient sperm production. However, in cases where sperm production or egg maturation does manage to occur, at least 50 percent of the subsequent fertilized eggs will have what is called an unbalanced translocation.

Remember, balanced translocations are complete reorganizations of where the genes occur on your chromosomes, but they do not affect your health in any way. However, during the shuffling process of meiosis an imbalance can occur with too much or too little of a large chunk of chromosome going to either the egg or the sperm. It is as if a normal volume 13 of a set of encyclopedias has joined up with an abnormal volume 13 that contains 250 pages of volume 14. Remember, either an overdosage of genes or an underdosage of genes leads to severe birth defects or miscarriage. In couples with recurrent miscarriage, a common problem is that either the husband or the wife has this balanced chromosomal rearrangement, i.e., translocation. This leads to an unbalanced chromosomal rearrangement in the sperm or the egg, and subsequently in the offspring. Such a couple may have one miscarriage after another, or, if there is a translocation involving chromosome 21, they may have a Down syndrome child.

However, an alternative is IVF with PGD. A single cell from each embryo on day three can be removed and analyzed for the presence of an unbalanced translocation in the embryo, and only normal embryos would be transferred into the uterus. Some of the embryos from these patients will have balanced translocations identical to their parents', and some will have completely normal chromosomes with no translocations because they will have inherited only the normal chromosome from each parent. With PGD, the nonviable embryos with unbalanced translocations can be left in the petri dish, and only the normal embryo or embryos with balanced translocations will be transferred back to the woman.

### *PGD Errors*

In some cases, even if chromosomally normal embryos are transferred, the woman still miscarries. This occurs because of two factors. One is that we cannot yet test for all of the twenty-four chromosomes in a single cell. But another is the potential for error in diagnosis. You do not want to discard a healthy embryo (incorrectly thinking that it's abnormal), and you do not want to transfer back an abnormal embryo to the patient (incorrectly thinking that it is normal). Because of a potential error rate of as high as 5 percent in trying to determine the number of chromosomes from testing just a single cell with FISH, it is possible that an embryo that was classified as normal may in fact be abnormal. The risk in the other direction is that an embryo that is thought to be abnormal (and is therefore not transferred to the woman) may occasionally turn out to have been normal.

Possible causes of error are failure of the FISH probe to hybridize, or the possibility that two chromosomes could be so close together on the slide that they appear as just one signal. Thus, an abnormality diagnosed as monosomic (only one copy instead of two) could in truth be a normal embryo with the chromosomes too close together to differentiate. Whether a chromosome is considered one or two is measured almost arbitrarily by the distance between the two spots. If the distance is less than one chromosome in diameter, it is considered to be one chromosome even though it might be two, and if the distance is greater than one chromosome in diameter, then it is considered to be two.

Because of the potential for errors, one should not take the decision to do PGD lightly, nor should it be done routinely as a matter of course in IVF. Rather, it needs to be restricted to women who have a specific reason for avoiding miscarriage, or an intense fear or risk of having an aneuploid offspring such as a Down syndrome child. Women who simply fail to get pregnant, particularly older women, who have the poorest pregnancy rates with IVF, may choose to forego PGD unless there is a specific high risk of miscarriage based on previous history. These women want to avoid even the smallest risk of not transferring a normal embryo that might have been misdiagnosed as abnormal.

The Europeans have tried to solve the error issue by testing two cells from the eight-cell embryo, rather than just one. Presumably this would reduce the risk of error because the second biopsied cell would be able to verify or refute the results on the first cell. But that approach increases the risk that a normal embryo that should be transferred will be misdiagnosed as abnormal. For example, if you had only normal embryos, and you assume a 5 percent error rate, 95 percent of those normal embryos would be diagnosed as normal. Five percent would be diagnosed as abnormal (even though, in truth, this 5 percent are normal). Then, if you biopsied a second cell, once again 5 percent of the 95 percent of normal embryos that were diagnosed correctly as normal with the first cell would now be diagnosed incorrectly as abnormal. Thus, only 90 percent of normal embryos would still have a diagnosis of normal based on evaluating two cells instead of just one. Therefore, 10 percent of normal embryos would be discarded unnecessarily because of conflicting results in the two biopsied cells.

However, the benefit of checking two cells is that your chance of transferring an abnormal embryo that was diagnosed as normal would be only 0.25 percent (5 percent of 5 percent). So by biopsying two cells, the chance of transferring an abnormal embryo becomes almost infinitesimal, but you also risk not transferring 10 percent of otherwise healthy embryos. Therefore, in the United States, most doctors would only biopsy one cell, and take the 5 percent risk of transferring a chromosomally abnormal embryo.

There is, however, another problem with screening for aneuploidy even if the FISH technique were error-free. Many normal-appearing embryos are mosaics, meaning some of the cells in the embryo are chromosomally normal and some of the cells are abnormal. Thus, you might remove a cell from the embryo that is chromosomally normal, even though the rest of the embryo is abnormal. Conversely, you might remove an abnormal cell, and the rest of the embryo might be normal. Nonetheless, despite this 5 to 10 percent potential for error, large studies from pioneers in this field all verify that the miscarriage rate is very dramatically reduced by routine PGD.

Although PGD has been a real breakthrough for the vast majority of couples with recurrent miscarriages, there are a smaller number of miscarriages that are not caused by chromosomal errors. I will discuss those in the next sections of this chapter.

## Miscarriages Not Caused by Chromosome Errors

The vast majority of miscarriages are caused by chromosomal errors in the embryo. But not all of them are. There are a wide variety of theories and speculations about the various causes of miscarriage other than chromosomal abnormalities, with a great deal of far-ranging debate. The fact that eggs from young women transferred into older women result in a high pregnancy rate and a low miscarriage rate makes it fairly clear that the major problem is with the aging ovary. However, less commonly there are problems other than the aging ovary (or intrinsic genetic problems with the eggs) related either to the woman herself, or to the uterine environment into which the embryo is placed.

Several years ago, a young woman in her late twenties with a puzzling problem was referred to us by her employer. She already had one child and readily became pregnant four times after the birth of that first child, but each of those pregnancies ended in miscarriage within the first three months. This woman had no difficulty whatsoever getting pregnant, but she suffered from recurrent miscarriages only after the birth of her first, healthy child. Because her local doctors had failed to give her an adequate answer, I assumed this would be a very difficult case requiring PGD to determine the chromosomal constitution of her embryos. We planned IVF with PGD, but first we took a routine X-ray of her uterus to make sure that it was normal. For fertility specialists, this is a simple, routine request, almost like a blood count, urinalysis, or Pap smear in the yearly physical exam. We simply wouldn't do IVF without being certain the uterus is normal. When we performed a hysterosalpingogram (HSG), we found that the upper and lower walls of the uterus were stuck to each other, forming a so-called pillar. This had to have been caused by retained placental fragments during the delivery of the woman's first baby five years earlier. She had gone through all these miscarriages over the last five years with no chromosomal evaluation of her miscarriage (which is a common oversight), but also no evaluation of her uterus. With a relatively simple hysteroscopic operation to separate the scarred adhesions between the top wall and the bottom wall of her uterus, she became pregnant very quickly on her own, with no need for IVF, and had a healthy delivery.

### *Thrombophilia and Folic Acid*

Another possible cause of miscarriage not related to chromosomes or to the biological clock is thrombophilia. The most common form of thrombophilia is the MTHFR defect, which impairs folic acid metabolism. This defect is a bit controversial and often misrepresented. A large percentage of any normal population (10 percent) are genetic carriers of this defect. These carriers have only a mild reduction in their ability to metabolize folic acid, and these individuals are called heterozygotic MTHFR carriers. The MTHFR defect acts the same as other autosomal-recessive gene defects such as cystic fibrosis. If one of your two genes is normal and the other of the two genes is defective, you are a carrier but do not have the disease. If, however, you have a defect in *both* MTHFR genes (which would be the case in 1 out of every 400 women), you have a risk of hypercoagulability of the blood, an increased risk of heart disease later in life, and a higher risk of miscarriage. When both MTHFR genes are mutated (not just one), they are called "homozygous." This gene defect causes an increased level of the amino acid homocysteine in your blood because the MTHFR enzyme is necessary to process homocysteine in your body.

Taking folic acid along with vitamins $B_6$ and $B_{12}$ corrects this imbalance. Folic acid is abundantly present in dark-green leafy vegetables, several cereal grains, and citrus fruits. Therefore, women who eat lots of broccoli are very unlikely to have a problem even if they carry this gene defect. Some patients with MTHFR homozygous gene defects are fertile and have had no problem with miscarriages, and others with the same gene defect have had great difficulties. It is clear that heterozygous MTHFR defects cause no problem, and even homozygous defects only cause miscarriage late in pregnancy, if at all. The MTHFR defect is never the cause of early miscarriage or failure to get pregnant.

MTHFR is just one of several so-called thrombophilias, all of which can be screened for routinely with a blood sample. If such a screen is positive, you can simply take folic acid and vitamin B replacements and conscientiously change your diet. In some cases, your doctor may want to put you on tiny doses of aspirin to protect against the higher risk of clotting in the developing placenta.

However, some of these thrombophilias have been vastly exaggerated, and such diagnoses have often been abused and overused to the patient's detriment. Some thrombophilias have been alleged to be caused by so-called antiphospholipid syndrome, which causes the body's immune system to attack itself. In fact, there are labs and doctors who have made huge amounts of money pushing antiphospholipid defects as a cause of failure to get pregnant or maintain a pregnancy in many infertile women. In the 1990s, the American Society for Reproductive Medicine undertook a massive review of all of the studies evaluating treatment of this condition; they found the diagnosis to be irrelevant, and the treatment worthless.

With antiphospholipid syndrome, your immune system fails to recognize self from not-self. This is a relatively rare autoimmune disease whereby your body's immune system attacks your own body as though it were a foreign invader. These rare conditions are characterized by joint pains, fatigue, and, among other things, higher coagulability of the blood. Autoimmune diseases are slowly progressive and debilitating for the rare patients that have them. However, patients with severe autoimmune diseases are *not* infertile. They have no difficulty getting pregnant, but they simply have a higher rate of late miscarriage than a normal population. Therefore, their pregnancies are treated with aspirin and sometimes heparin (a much stronger and potentially dangerous anticoagulant) to protect the placental blood flow and allow the pregnancy to go to term.

Some years ago it was speculated that women who failed to get pregnant or women with recurrent miscarriage might have some sort of subtle, subclinical, undetected version of autoimmune disease. A huge battery of expensive tests were concocted to attempt to define these autoimmune diseases that were not clinically apparent in any way other than infertility. An extremely expensive form of treatment was then devised called intravenous immunoglobulin (IVIG) therapy, in which the patient's blood was sent to an out-of-town laboratory that developed antibodies to that patient's antibodies. The blood was then sent back to the infertility clinic and administered to the patient, supposedly to block her body's antibody attack on her uterus. These so-called IVIG infusions were extremely expensive and appeared, to some in the field, to be a money spinner that lacked merit. Carefully controlled studies and reviews of these studies have now been published in scientific journals demonstrating the complete lack of effectiveness of this expensive therapy.

Many years ago, we treated a woman in her late thirties with multiple IVF attempts, each one resulting either in failure to get pregnant or in an early miscarriage. On her own, she consulted an outside laboratory that we would have nothing to do with, and she had a detailed autoimmune evaluation costing several thousand dollars. It supposedly revealed that she had these so-called antiphospholipid antibodies, and she insisted on being treated with heparin, baby aspirin, and even IVIG infusions for her next IVF cycle. But when the chromosome test came back from her miscarried pregnancy, it demonstrated that the fetus had trisomy 16, a chromosomal error that was clearly incompatible with life, and this was the true cause of her miscarriage. She finally decided to try donor eggs from a younger woman, without any heparin, aspirin, IVIG, or any other antithrombophilia treatment, and this time she delivered a healthy baby girl without any problems. Slick marketing from one of these autoimmune thrombophilia labs had convinced her that her miscarriages, and her failure to get pregnant, were caused by her being immune to her own tissue, and they had recommended worthless treatment that was very profitable for them. But her problem was clearly her aging eggs, which were prone to chromosomal errors.

Another couple came to us from the East Coast because the husband had azoospermia, and a TESE attempt back home revealed no sperm in the testes. The couple wanted to try again to see whether there were just a few sperm that had somehow or other been missed in his previous TESE procedure at a different institution. We did find enough sperm in his testes (very few) to perform ICSI with her eighteen eggs. We transferred three beautiful-appearing embryos, and she became pregnant. However, she miscarried in the first three months. Devastated by this, she sought another opinion from a well-known infertility doctor on the East Coast. His routine testing for "thrombophilia screen" revealed a positive Leiden factor in her blood, which could have been implicated as a possible cause of miscarriage. In fact, this doctor told her he was *certain* this was the problem. He recommended doing her next IVF cycle taking heparin and baby aspirin. However, when the chromosomal testing (karyotyping) of her miscarried fetus came back a week later, it revealed trisomy 16, clearly a chromosomal error in the embryo and a very common cause of miscarriage. She then underwent another TESE-ICSI procedure with us, without using any heparin or anticoagulant therapy, and she became pregnant again, but this time she delivered a healthy baby boy.

Thus, even when it was thought that a subtle thrombophilia was found to be the cause of her miscarriage, the true cause was a chromosomal error originating in her eggs. Although we have to be aware of these thrombophilias, nutritional defects, or possible antibody causes for miscarriage, these are generally overstated conditions. The wholesale administration of aspirin and anticoagulation regimens to infertile women, or to women with recurrent miscarriages, is certainly ill-advised and, in most cases, not likely to solve the problem. Nonetheless, there is a great deal of controversy on this subject, and many patients will say to their doctor, "Why not try it if there's nothing to lose?"

Deficiencies in factor V Leiden are commonly found in up to 4 percent of the population, and further studies have failed to find any increased incidence of this defect in women with recurrent early miscarriage. However, other thrombophilias, such as protein C deficiency, have been shown to be increased in women with recurrent miscarriage. There is still great controversy and uncertainty surrounding the contribution of thrombophilia to recurrent miscarriage, and many infertility physicians do not even recommend routine testing for these defects.

Nonetheless, we do endorse treating MTHFR defects with vitamin supplementation. It was well established as early as 1992 in England that folic acid deficiency in the early embryo results in neural-tube defects, which are among the most common and heartbreaking congenital birth defects in children. One of the biggest fears of expectant mothers (completely unrelated to the biological clock or to the woman's aging) involves these neural-tube defects, which cause meningomyocele, hydrocephalus (enlarged head), or even anencephaly, when a child is born without a brain and dies immediately upon birth. Around 1992, it was discovered that putting women on folic acid vitamin supplements during early pregnancy dramatically reduced the incidence of these terrifying neural-tube defects. Since then, women who are attempting to get pregnant anywhere in the modern world are routinely placed on folic acid supplements to protect against these birth defects. If a woman has an MTHFR defect, she will merely need to be on higher doses of folic acid supplements, or on a diet even richer in folic acid. We see no problem associated with routinely administering this increased folic acid, vitamin $B_6$, vitamin $B_{12}$ regimen, since it is almost a routine part of proper pregnancy management in the current era. But it is not likely to solve the problem of recurrent miscarriage.

### *Cervical Incompetence*

Another cause of miscarriage unrelated to chromosomal abnormalities in the embryo is frequently seen in women who have already had a child with a traumatic delivery, or who have had treatment for cancer of the cervix. It is called cervical incompetence. I will give an extreme example of a thirty-six-year-old couple who had been trying to have children for several years after the wife's quite remarkable history of cancer. Several years before coming to see me, the wife had a Pap smear that identified an early cancer of the cervix that in the past would have been treated with hysterectomy. However, the woman knew she wanted to try to have a child, and she sought out a pioneer in cervical cancer in Toronto. This doctor performed a radical trachelectomy, removing only her cervix and saving the rest of her uterus. She still had her uterus, as well as a tiny opening from which she could menstruate and, hopefully, through which sperm could travel. But she was having a hard time getting pregnant.

Because of the rough surface of this little opening to her uterus, which bled easily when she underwent IVF attempts in her local community, and despite the transfer of perfectly good embryos, she did not become pregnant. We did nothing differently in our IVF cycle other than transfer her embryos through a small abdominal incision (using ZIFT) into the fallopian tubes, rather than transvaginally via what remained of her scarred cervical opening. Thus, there was no uterine irritation caused by our embryo transfer, and as we anticipated, she became pregnant quite easily.

However, three months later, she began to go into early labor, and the opening into her uterus began to enlarge, simply because she had no cervix left. Her obstetricians were extremely quick and resourceful. They put her in an upside-down position, took her to the operating room, and performed cervical cerclage, tightly stitching the opening to the uterus. She then remained on bed rest and took drugs to prevent contractions (called tocolytic agents), and she wound up delivering a healthy baby girl many months later by C-section. What her case dramatically demonstrates is the importance of the cervix (the muscular passageway into the uterus) in acting as a sphincter to prevent premature delivery and miscarriage.

There are more subtle versions of cervical incompetence. A thirty-five-year-old couple from a very remote area of the world managed to make their way to St. Louis after eight years of infertility. The woman had become pregnant and delivered a healthy daughter twenty years earlier with a different partner. However, she was now unable to get pregnant. Her husband turned out to have a low sperm count, and she had severe adhesions on her fallopian tubes, preventing egg pickup from the ovary. So we performed IVF, obtained excellent embryos, transferred two of them, and froze the extras for future pregnancies.

However, at the time of embryo transfer, we warned her that her cervix looked as if it had been damaged from her previous traumatic delivery and that in fourteen weeks she would need to have a cerclage operation to cinch up her incompetent cervix tight, so as to hold the pregnancy. This couple was low on funds and did not fully believe what we had told them; they decided she would carry her pregnancy back in her remote home community. At eighteen weeks, her cervix opened up and she lost the baby. After traveling halfway across the world with undaunted dedication to her goal of having a baby, this woman's perfectly normal pregnancy was lost because of a failure to stitch her previously damaged cervix at fourteen weeks.

The cervix can be damaged either by an aggressive Leep procedure to prevent cancer after a Pap smear comes back abnormal, or by the more unusual complete removal of the cervix because of cancer (trachelectomy). However, it can also be damaged by a traumatic, abrupt delivery, which, unbeknown to the patient, can lead to intrauterine scarring or to an incompetent cervix.

### *Uterine Abnormalities*

Miscarriage can also be caused by an inherent abnormality in the structure of the uterus. There are two basic types of congenital structural abnormalities of the uterus, and there are several subvarieties. One type of congenital abnormality is a double, or bicornuate, uterus, which

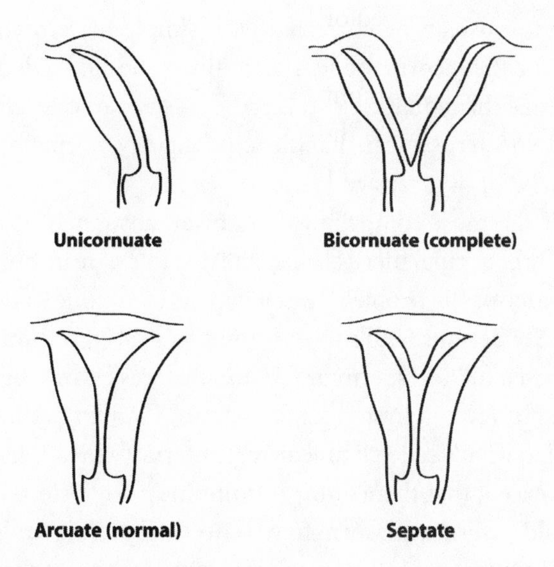


**FIGURE 14.1.** Variations in uterine structure.

simply means that instead of one uterus there are two, usually with a common cervical opening (see fig. 14.1). This is very similar to the uterine structure of most animals that have two uterine horns. At six weeks of fetal life, the Müllerian ducts are paired structures that fuse and develop into the uterus, the upper vagina, and the fallopian tubes. In most animals, the Müllerian ducts do not fuse, and so these animals have a double uterus normally. In humans, they fuse into one uterus and one upper vagina, but the fallopian tubes remain separate. Bicornuate uterus is simply caused by the failure of the original Müllerian ducts, at six weeks of fetal life, to fuse in the center and form a single uterus. Thus, a woman who has a bicornuate uterus really has a normal variation that is closer to most of the animal kingdom than the usual human single uterus. This bicornuate uterus may look abnormal and you may be told by your doctor that it is a problem, but it really isn't a problem.

The problem is with the so-called septate uterus, in which the two Müllerian ducts fuse partially but not completely (see fig. 14.1). In this case, there appear to be two uterine cavities, but they are enclosed within one common muscular uterine exterior. With this type of uterine abnormality, which is often confused with the bicornuate type, the uterus cannot expand the way it is supposed to in pregnancy, and there is definitely a higher incidence of miscarriage. This congenital problem of septate uterus can be corrected with simple hysteroscopic surgery. However, for the bicornuate uterus, nothing should be done because it simply means that you have two uteruses instead of one, and either one of those two uteruses can handle a pregnancy normally without an increased risk of miscarriage.

One of the most compelling cases of an absolutely absurd-looking congenitally abnormal uterus, which created lots of fears but in truth was not the source of the problem, was a patient who came to us in the early days of ICSI. Her husband's sperm count was severely diminished, with less than half a million sperm per cc, and this was clearly the cause of her infertility. However, a hysterosalpingogram X-ray in her local community revealed what's called a unicornuate uterus (which is like a bicornuate uterus except that there's only one uterine horn instead of two). This is a very oddly misshapen form in which a single cervix leads into half of a uterus. The doctors in her area were certain she could never carry a baby with such a strange-looking uterus. Yet this woman delivered healthy twin girls after her ICSI procedure, and the fact that she had this funny-looking unicornuate uterus had no negative impact on her ability to get pregnant or to carry the twin pregnancy fully to term.

Another compelling example of this phenomenon is a woman in her fifties who came to us from Europe because she and her husband required donor eggs. Her HSG, which had been performed many years ago in Europe, revealed a bizarre-looking type of bicornuate uterus in which she actually had two cervical openings and two completely independent uterine structures. However, she was not concerned about this because her doctors in Europe were very sophisticated and had explained to her that this would not present a problem for carrying a pregnancy. When we performed her IVF with donor eggs, we transferred two embryos into one of her two uteruses and one embryo into the other uterus, rather than putting all three into one of them. As it turned out, she carried a twin pregnancy that developed from the embryos implanted into one uterine cavity, and that single uterine cavity was quite sufficient. She delivered normal, healthy twins nine months later despite this odd-looking and apparently abnormal bicornuate uterus.

A fifty-two-year-old woman had come to our clinic in St. Louis fifteen times and had attempted to get pregnant for the previous eight years with fifteen cycles of IVF. Her perseverance was amazing. Finally, after many years, she agreed to use donor eggs. All along she was noted to have several large fibroid tumors, each three inches in diameter, within the muscle of her uterus. Her doctors at home were concerned that these large fibroids in her uterus might interfere with pregnancy, but they were just in the wall of the uterus and did not protrude inside the uterine cavity. So we ignored them, and she got pregnant (using donor eggs) and delivered healthy twins. Thus, in most cases, the embryo is still more important than the uterus.

In summary, miscarriage is not always caused by chromosomal abnormalities in the embryo, and can be related to structural problems in the uterus or cervix, or to systemic problems in the woman herself. But there are many uterine abnormalities that are simply wrinkles that don't adversely affect your ability to carry a child. Some systemic abnormalities are a potential cause of miscarriage, but they can usually be treated, and most don't even require treatment. The majority of miscarriages are caused by chromosomal abnormalities, and the risk of miscarriage in such cases can be lessened by performing a genetic analysis of the embryos (using FISH) prior to IVF transfer.

CHAPTER 15

# Reversing Vasectomy, Sperm Blockage, and Tubal Ligation

Microsurgery is extremely effective in restoring fertility to men when there is obstruction to sperm outflow, or to women whose tubes have been tied. There are three major types of obstruction to sperm outflow, the most common being vasectomy. The second most common type is blockage in the epididymis caused by infection, and the third is congenital blockage (which often involves complete absence of the vas deferens). In well over 90 percent of such cases, properly performed microsurgery should restore the man's fertility with no need for an IVF procedure. In the same respect, more than 90 percent of women whose tubes have been tied can also have more children by simply having their tubes reconnected with microsurgery.

## Vasectomy Reversal and Microsurgery

### *Why Do Men Want to Reverse Their Vasectomy?*

Vasectomy is one of the most common operations performed today in the United States, and it is the most popular method of birth control in the world. About twenty-five million American men have been vasectomized, and almost a quarter of a million more undergo this operation every year. Despite careful counseling and the warning that this procedure should be considered a permanent step, many men change their minds at a later date. A marriage can break up, and the man may remarry several years later.

Our lives and our families are held together by such thin threads that few of us can feel quite comfortable, at least while we are young, with the decision to be sterilized. One patient of mine had two healthy children, a wonderful wife, a beautiful home, and just about everything anyone could want out of life. When his third child, a boy, was born, it was an absolute culmination of all his desires. The patient waited several months to make sure the child would be healthy before having his vasectomy performed by a local urologist. One month after the operation, he and his wife noticed a lump on the four-month-old child's arm — it turned out to be a rare and incurable malignant tumor of the muscle. The child died four months later. The couple knew that having another child would not replace the one they lost, but they simply had to have another child.

I remember reading with extreme sadness a newspaper story about how the first baby born on New Year's in 1990 in St. Louis was found dead in his crib of sudden infant death syndrome (SIDS) a month after his birth. Death in childhood is extremely common. I have seen many hundreds of cases of couples who thought they had all the children they wanted, but then, when a child died, they wanted the husband's vasectomy reversed in order to have more. One man I operated on was actually a vasectomy counselor at a Planned Parenthood center and had warned more than ten thousand men about not having a vasectomy until they were certain they would never want more children no matter what tragedy or accident might befall their family. Then his nine-year-old son died after being hit by a car in his neighborhood while riding a bicycle. He immediately wanted his vasectomy reversed.

These tragedies happen when you least anticipate it. A rancher was shoeing his horse while his two-year-old was just standing around admiring everything his father did. The horse suddenly and unpredictably kicked and not another sound was heard. The patient told me how strange it seemed that one second his child was alive and the next he was dead, and that the child hadn't uttered a sound. He couldn't even believe it had happened, even though he was right there. Two months after his child died, he desperately sought reversal of his vasectomy.

There are many other reasons why vasectomy reversal is so commonly requested. I am an outdoors enthusiast, and I realized on a trip to the far Arctic, in one of the most remote regions of the world, just how intense is the human will to reverse a previous decision to be sterile. I was traveling in the barren region of the magnetic North Pole, thousands of miles from any populated area, on a three-man expedition consisting of myself and two Eskimos. Kalook, my guide, had no idea that I was an expert on vasectomy. He just knew I was a doctor of some sort. He looked sad on the third day of our trip as he stared at the floor of the igloo. He said to me, "I made a very bad thing last year." I asked what happened. He said, "The government sends a doctor to our camp every year, and last year he gave me a vasectomy." Kalook already had five children, quite enough according to the view of the government and the social worker who had advised him. But Kalook deeply regretted that he could not have any more. He said, "I am so sorry I did that; I would like to have more children." I started to laugh, patted Kalook on the back, and said to him, "My friend, you have come to the right igloo." For reasons that will become apparent by the end of this portion of the chapter, I could assure Kalook almost a 99 percent chance of having his fertility restored.

Several years ago, I reversed the vasectomy of a sixty-two-year-old man whose first wife had died and who was now remarried to a woman in her late thirties who had not been married before and had never had children. He already had five grown children, and the question arose: Why should this man in his sixties want to try to start a new family? The fact is, when this man arrived at my office, he didn't look his stated age — he looked barely over thirty-five. His father, who came with him, was in his eighties, and his grandfather, whom they left home to manage the ranch, was ninety-nine and leading a life that was certainly more active than mine. There was no question that despite his age and this unusual request, this man would be a great father, and that because of his genes he would possibly even outlive his younger wife. But two previous attempts to reverse his vasectomy had failed. As this section of the chapter unfolds, you'll understand why they failed and how we were able to perform a delicate operation repairing the fragile ductwork closer to the testicle (the epididymis) and thus restore this man's fertility. He has now begun a second family at almost sixty-five years of age.

The problem with cases like his is that pressure buildup from the vasectomy causes damage to the delicate ductwork closer to the testicle. When we bypassed the epididymal damage, his sperm count returned to normal levels within six months. We have performed many thousands of such successful operations on men whose first vasectomy reversal had failed despite what appeared to be an accurate reconnection of the vas. Therefore, most men with this problem now can once again father children.

### *The "Simple" Microsurgical Operation to Reconnect the Vas Deferens*

Though it is easy to perform a vasectomy (it takes only five minutes in the doctor's office), it is very difficult to reverse it because of the microscopic size of the inner canal that carries the sperm. The outer diameter of the vas deferens is fairly thick, about one eighth of an inch, and the tough outer muscular wall makes it feel like a copper wire through the scrotum. It is therefore an easy structure for the surgeon to identify and cut. But the diameter of the inner canal that carries the sperm is about one seventieth to one hundredth of an inch, or roughly the size of a pinpoint. This inner canal has a lining that is about three cells thick, approximately 1/2,000 of an inch. Vasectomy had always been considered a relatively permanent condition because of the obvious difficulty in surgically reconnecting such a delicate, tiny tube. With the microsurgical technique that we developed in the 1970s, this problem of reconnecting the vas deferens was solved, but the problem in getting high success rates goes far beyond this "simple" microsurgical reconnection. Just "reconnecting the vas" will give only a 25 percent success rate because pressure damage closer to the testicle, in the epididymis, prevents sperm from ever reaching the vasectomy site. Over 90 percent success rates can still be achieved with microsurgery to bypass epididymal damage, but this surgery is much more delicate than just reconnecting the vas.

But for the moment let's get back to the "simple" microsurgery for reconnecting the severed vas, since in some cases, this is all that is needed. In order to achieve a nonobstructed reconnection, it is necessary to stitch accurately, in two layers, the delicate inner lining in a leakproof fashion, using a thread invisible to the naked eye (see fig. 15.1). This surgery is performed under a microscope with very high magnification, using delicate instruments especially designed for this purpose.

This microsurgical technique for reconnecting the vas is equally successful in cases where previous attempts at vasectomy reversal have failed. In these circumstances, the scar tissue from the previous surgery may make the operation somewhat more difficult, but it should not interfere with obtaining an accurate reconnection. But if the failure of vasectomy reversal is instead caused by blockage in the epididymis, merely reconnecting the vas won't work.

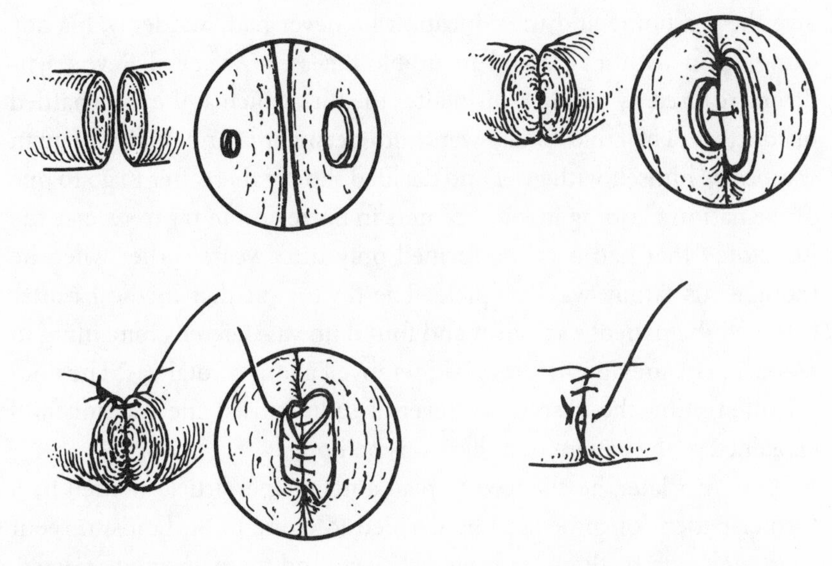

**FIGURE 15.1**

This rough overview illustration demonstrates the basic strategy of the microscopic two-layer reconnection of the vas deferens.

The use of a microscope alone does not ensure that an accurate reconnection will be achieved. The surgeon must spend a great deal of time practicing before he or she develops sufficient skill to do this sort of surgery with confidence. But even with very crude surgical techniques, some sperm can often be found in the ejaculate after the procedure. But if the amount and quality of sperm are poor, then pregnancy rates will still be very low.

Many patients are told that too large a segment of vas has been removed to allow a successful reconnection. They are told that their vasectomy cannot be reversed simply because the doctor who originally performed the vasectomy took out a huge piece of the vas rather than just severing it. Actually, the majority of urologists take out an unnecessarily large piece of vas when they perform a vasectomy, but this in no way reduces the chance of a successful reconnection. This is because men possess an enormous extra length of vas, far in excess of what is necessary for sperm to transit from the testicle into the ejaculate.

One of my earliest patients was a very hardworking Mexican immigrant from California who was raising three beautiful children (two girls and a boy), holding several jobs, and saving up enough money to give them a home and the education he never had. Suddenly, his boy came down with a rare and incurable illness, now called Reye's syndrome (caused by taking aspirin after the flu), which at the time baffled his doctors. The child finally went into deep coma and died. The man was beside himself with grief and decided shortly thereafter to go to one of the nation's leading medical centers in his region to try to reverse the vasectomy that had been performed only three years earlier when he thought his family was complete. The doctors at that medical center explored the patient's scrotum and found no vas deferens remaining to reattach. His previous doctors had removed all his scrotal vas. The doctor attempting the vasectomy reversal sadly closed the incision and explained to the patient that there was no hope.

One year later, he chanced to read a newspaper article written by a former patient of mine, and he decided to come to St. Louis to see if anything could be done. As expected, we found there was no vas deferens left in the scrotum, but by extending the incision into the abdomen we were still able to free up his vas enough to reconnect. The patient now has three more children.

I remember operating on one man in 1987 who had had simply the most incredible vasectomy I've ever seen in my life. The surgeon who performed his vasectomy must have been in a terrible mood that day. More than four inches of vas had been removed on both sides. This meant not only that the man's scrotal vas deferens was completely gone, but also that much of his abdominal vas deferens had been pulled out with it. It was really hard to believe. I've never seen another case quite that bad before or since. To reconnect that vas required a huge incision going all the way into the hernia region of the abdomen. Even so, we were able to sufficiently free up the remaining portion of the abdominal vas so that it could come down into the scrotum and thereby reestablish his fertility. So previous surgery, no matter how messy, with enormous scarring and segments of vas missing, should never be an impediment to obtaining a successful reversal of vasectomy in the proper surgical hands.

### *How Does Vasectomy Affect the Ducts of the Testicle?*

After vasectomy, the testicle continues to produce fluid and sperm, which accumulate and dilate the entire sperm ductal system. Fluid and sperm accumulate in the epididymis, the tiny, delicate, twenty-foot-long canal (coiled up into a length of only one inch) that carries sperm out of the testicle into the vas deferens. In this area, the sperm ductwork is only 1/300 inch in diameter, and the thickness of the wall of the epididymal duct is only 1/1,000 inch. This buildup of pressure is usually not felt by the patient because the duct is so tiny.

Eventually, the pressure builds up to a point where rupture or clogging occurs in the epididymis. This is the major culprit in restoring the man's fertility. It is what prevents patients from recovering normal fertility despite what might be a proper reconnection of the vas. The good news is that with extremely refined microsurgical techniques, the damage in this area can be repaired or bypassed, and the success rate for reversal of vasectomy can still be quite good.

Ironically, it is the sloppier vasectomies, the ones that result in sperm leakage at the vasectomy site, that are the easiest to reverse. This is because these patients have a persistent low-grade leakage of sperm from the cut end of the vas deferens. A small lump, called a sperm granuloma, forms at the cut end of the vas deferens. This lump, which can be felt through the scrotum, is a dynamic structure, with sperm constantly leaking into it and being reabsorbed sufficiently to prevent the pressure increase that would normally occur. Patients with such a lump at the vasectomy site do not require bypass of the much more delicate epididymis.

### *Length of Time Since Vasectomy*

We originally demonstrated in 1977 that the longer the period of time since vasectomy, the worse the chance for successful reversal (despite an anatomically perfect reconnection of the vas). In 1978, we discovered the cause of the problem. The answer, of course, was that the pressure buildup caused obstruction in the epididymal ductwork between the testicle and the vasectomy site. The longer the period of time since the vasectomy, the more fluid and the more pressure buildup. Thus, there is a greater likelihood for epididymal damage.

We then developed a more intricate microsurgical operation in which we could locate the points of epididymal blockage where normal sperm were present, and bypass them. One of the first patients we tried this new operation on was a man on whom I had performed a vas reconnection in 1974, fifteen years after his original vasectomy. He had no sperm in the vas fluid, and he remained sterile despite a perfect vas reconnection. Then, in 1979, I let him know that we thought we had discovered the cause of the problem, and I invited him to come to St. Louis for an attempt at bypassing the epididymal blockage. As it turned out, our concept was correct, and he now has three grown children and a very happy wife.

### *With Modern Vasectomies, Blowouts Occur Much Sooner*

It used to be that only a small percentage of the patients requesting vasectomy reversal within ten years had this epididymal problem. Unfortunately, the situation has gotten worse because of a change in the popular method for performing vasectomy. In the late 1970s, at the time of vasectomy reversal, almost 90 percent of our patients had normal sperm in the vas fluid, indicating no epididymal blockage; today, only about 20 percent do.

Blowouts and secondary blockages in the epididymis are now occurring very soon after vasectomy. The majority of patients I see whose vasectomies were done even less than ten years ago now have blowouts in the epididymis. To maintain a high success rate for vasectomy reversal in the new millennium will require epididymal bypass operation rather than just the simpler microsurgical reconnection of the vas, and this applies to men whose vasectomies were recent as well as men whose vasectomies were a relatively long period of time ago.

The reason for the increased and earlier epididymal damage from vasectomy is the popularity of the cautery technique for vasectomy and the emphasis on getting a leakproof seal of the cut ends of the vas at the time of vasectomy. Because of a fear that leakage at the vasectomy site could lead to an occasional unwanted pregnancy after vasectomy (as a result of recanalization caused by the leaking sperm), urologists are using either cautery or very carefully applied clips to create an absolutely watertight, leakproof, completely solid seal at the cut ends of the vas. Thus, there is a faster and more severe pressure buildup, leading to earlier epididymal damage.

In fact, I have recommended that if a vasectomy is being performed, the urologist should leave the cut end completely unsealed in order to avoid any pressure damage. I call this open-ended vasectomy (see fig. 15.2). The abdominal side of the vasectomy can be carefully sealed to avoid unwanted recanalization. This is our current approach for providing easily reversible sterilization, and I recommend it for all vasectomies.

### *How Is the Epididymal Blockage Bypassed?*

Under the operating microscope, you can microsurgically cut into the epididymal tubule, moving closer and closer to the testicle until

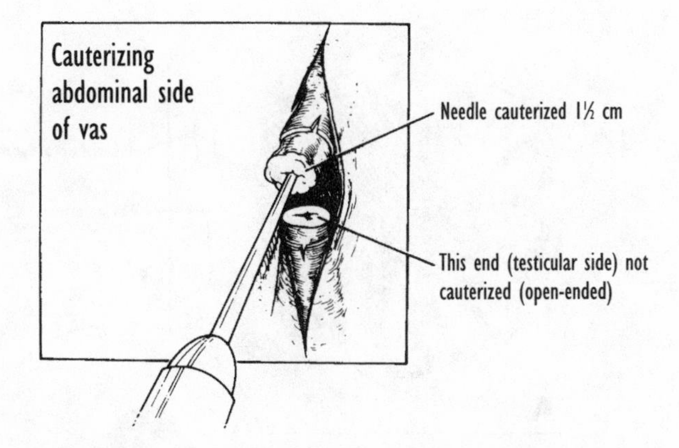


**FIGURE 15.2**

If the side of the vas draining fluid from the testicle is not cauterized and is allowed to leak, the epididymis suffers no pressure damage, and vasectomy reversal is much easier. This is the so-called open-ended vasectomy.

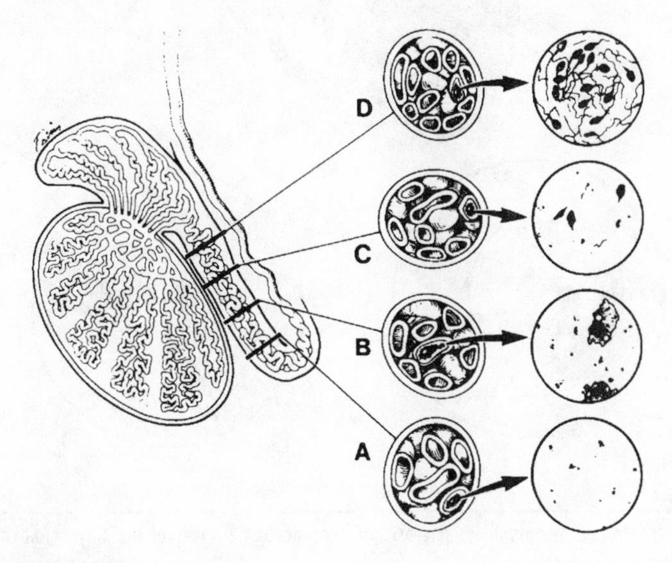


**FIGURE 15.3**

Microsurgically transecting the epididymis closer and closer to the testicle eventually gets beyond the areas of secondary blowouts and blockage to where the reconnection to the epididymis has to be performed.

there is suddenly a brisk outpouring of huge quantities of sperm under high pressure (see fig. 15.3). The epididymal tubule is so fragile (the epididymal wall is 1/1,000 of an inch) that it must be sewn to the inner lining of the vas with thread that is virtually invisible to the naked eye. An

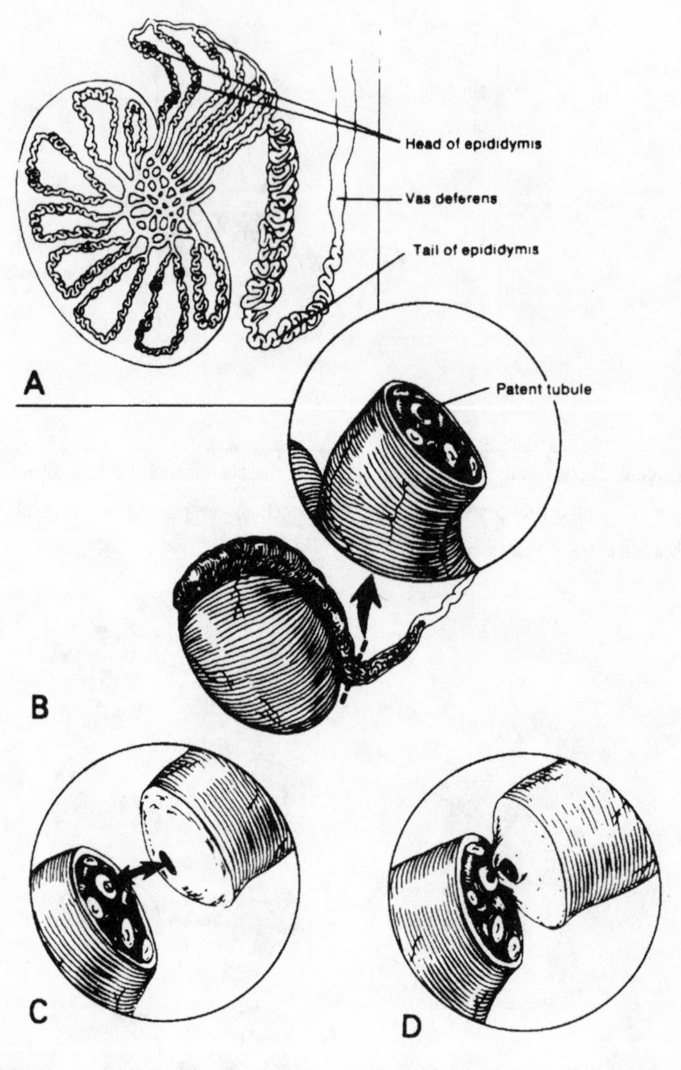


**FIGURE 15.4**

My original end-to-end technique for microscopic reconnection surgery of the tiny epididymal tubule to the vas.

absolutely perfect connection of that inner lining of the vas to the opening in the epididymal tubule is essential. As figures 15.4 and 15.5 illustrate, there are two equally good ways to do this, "end to end" or "end to side." If a sloppily performed attempt at reconnection is made, however, sperm will just leak out and result in scarring with either partial or total blockage.

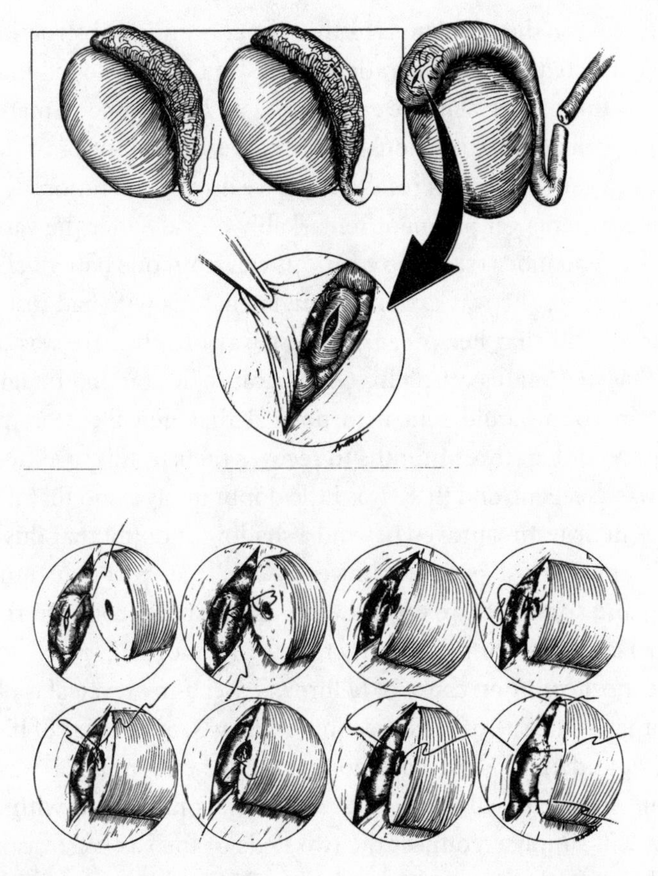

**FIGURE 15.5**

My new, refined end-to-side technique for bypassing epididymal blockage requiring less surgical dissection than the original technique.

### *Recovery of Fertility After Vasectomy Reversal*

Sperm counts do not return to normal immediately after vasectomy reversal. All of the old sperm that have been stored up over the years since the vasectomy have died of old age. This dead sperm material must be cleaned out after the vasectomy is reversed in order to make room for a fresh crop of sperm, which usually does not appear until at least three months later. Also, the dilated epididymal duct may require many months to recover its microscopic muscular ability to transport the sperm by the slow pumping action called peristalsis.

Usually, if the microsurgery is performed well, the patient is fertile within a year. On the other hand, if the sperm count is very low and the motility is poor, the problem is likely to be continuing obstruction. This can be corrected with re-operation. Since we first developed microsurgical vasectomy reversal in the early 1970s, we have found in many thousands of patients that previous failure of vasectomy reversal does not have any negative effect on results when we do a re-operation.

Some patients get pregnant remarkably quickly after the vasectomy reversal. I remember receiving a furious call from one patient six weeks after his surgery; he was extremely angry that his wife had just missed her period and that her pregnancy test was positive. He was actually afraid that maybe this wasn't his child because he couldn't imagine that his sperm count could return to normal that quickly. Most patients require more than three months to recover their fertility, yet his sperm count was excellent, and there was little doubt in my mind that it was his child. Genetic testing proved beyond a shadow of doubt that this indeed was his child. Most patients, however, don't get pregnant quite that quickly, and some require up to a year for the sperm count to rise to its maximal level, and for the motility to return to normal.

The most common cause of failure of vasectomy reversal is obstruction, either at the site of reconnection of the vas, or because of blowouts in the epididymis. Most commonly, when performing a vasectomy reversal, physicians who are not extremely comfortable with microsurgery will simply reconnect the two ends of the vas (vasovasostomy) regardless of whether there is blockage from blowouts in the epididymis. This simple reconnection of the vas will not result in success in at least 80 percent of cases because of this additional blockage in the epididymis. Failure to bypass this epididymal blockage will guarantee failure in the majority of surgeries attempting to reverse vasectomy. A proper microsurgical vasoepididymostomy should relieve all obstruction and result in a successful return of normal sperm count in most patients.

For more than twenty years it has been speculated that the reason for the low success rate after vasectomy reversal is that the man develops antibodies to his own sperm and that these sperm antibodies prevent him from impregnating his wife even though a successful reversal operation has been performed. This is foolish. I have re-operated on thousands of patients who have had a previous vasectomy reversal elsewhere and whose wives' failure to get pregnant had been blamed on "sperm antibodies." After re-operating, the sperm count and the motility improved in most of the men, and then the wives did get pregnant. In fact, there was no difference in the pregnancy rate of patients who had high sperm antibody levels and those who had no sperm antibody formation after vasectomy. Therefore, we think it is safe to say that persistent infertility after vasectomy reversal is not caused by sperm antibodies.

### *ICSI with Retrieved Sperm*

The technique for aspirating sperm from the male, and using that sperm for ICSI and IVF in the female, was actually invented by our group. This procedure involves direct aspiration of sperm from the husband combined with the injection of a single weak or nonmoving sperm into the cytoplasm of each of the wife's eggs. We routinely perform this procedure for patients who have congenital absence of the vas, or for those in whom there is no possibility of surgical repair. However, for anyone who has had a vasectomy, or even one or more previous failed vasectomy reversals, the simplest, most cost-effective approach through multiple cycles of IVF and sperm retrieval would still be to reconnect the ducts microsurgically. This involves no greater surgical discomfort than sperm aspiration and gives a 90 percent chance for a successful return of fertility. It is certainly more cost-effective and simpler to have a vasectomy reversal than to go through multiple cycles of IVF and sperm retrieval.

Nonetheless, at the time of your vasectomy reversal, epididymal sperm should be frozen and stored as a backup, in case the operation should fail. If sperm is frozen at the time of your surgery, there still remains the opportunity for doing ICSI at any time in the future without your ever having to go through another surgical procedure. ICSI with frozen retrieved sperm is thus best viewed as a backup procedure.

## Obstruction to Sperm Outflow in Patients Who Have Not Had a Vasectomy

Not all cases of obstruction are a result of vasectomy. In some cases, the man has actually been born with obstruction and has never had sperm in his ejaculate. In other cases, obstruction results from an infection, which leads to scarring. The obstruction is almost always in the epididymis (but there are occasional exceptions). With modern microsurgical innovations, identical to those described earlier in this chapter for vasectomy reversal, the outlook for correcting these obstructions is very good, but the surgery is delicate and intricate. However, when a man has no sperm in the ejaculate, how do doctors know if this is caused by an obstruction?

### *Testicle Biopsy*

The diagnosis of obstruction in the male should really be quite easy. However, it is sometimes approached in a confusing way, which can lead to an embarrassing situation for the urologist and a tragedy for the patient. Adherence to a few simple principles will avoid these difficulties and allow a proper decision to be made. If a patient has a testicle biopsy that shows normal spermatogenesis (sperm production) and if he is azoospermic (has no sperm at all in the ejaculate), then he must have an obstruction.

The only other necessary piece of information is whether or not the physician can palpate (feel) a vas deferens in the scrotum on physical examination. If the patient has congenital absence of the vas deferens, then a totally different surgical approach would be necessary, one that will be described later in the chapter. But if there is a normal, palpable vas deferens and a normal testicle biopsy in an azoospermic patient, you can be certain that there is epididymal obstruction and that microsurgery is the appropriate treatment.

All other data are irrelevant, including a normal FSH level. The FSH level will be normal in a patient who is azoospermic without obstruction if the early precursors of sperm production are present. A normal FSH does not in any way ensure normal spermatogenesis. In fact, the majority of patients with azoospermia and a normal FSH have maturation arrest (not obstruction).

It is true that if the FSH is elevated, there is inadequate sperm production, caused by a small number of sperm precursors. Such a patient does not need a testicle biopsy to make a diagnosis. But most men with low sperm counts or zero sperm will have an FSH in the normal range. This does not mean that they have normal sperm production, and it does not mean that their diagnosis is obstruction. For that to be determined, a testicle biopsy must be performed.

The testicle biopsy will facilitate the husband's treatment only if performed and read by a physician who really understands how the testicle works. The biopsy involves taking a tissue sample through a one-quarter-inch incision in the scrotum. The procedure should be brief, but it must be done expertly. If the tissue is not properly excised, or if it is placed in formaldehyde (the usual fixative for tissue specimens from almost anywhere else in the body), it will become distorted beyond recognition. The tissue must be placed in a gentler solution (either Bouin's or Zenker's). Though the biopsy is quite harmless, a man should not have to part with a portion of his testicle unless helpful information will be derived. Contrary to expectation, the biopsy should not be very painful. The patient should have minimal temporary discomfort, which is relieved by Tylenol. If the testicle biopsy shows normal sperm production and the sperm count is zero, this indicates obstruction to the outflow of sperm, and such obstruction can be corrected microsurgically.

### *Microsurgical Vasoepididymostomy*

There is no difference in the rate of return of fertility in sterile men whose epididymal blockage is caused by vasectomy, is the result of previous inflammation in the epididymis from infection or trauma, or is congenital. The surgical approach for obstruction is identical to what was described earlier for vasectomy reversal patients, and the results are the same.

Any male who survives smallpox as a child is left permanently sterile because of the epididymal inflammation and subsequent scarring that smallpox inevitably causes. Smallpox was endemic in the Middle East and India twenty to thirty years ago, and was one of the most common causes of sterility in India for many years. As soon as I see a patient from one of these areas with a typical scar on the tip of his nose, which unmistakably identifies him as having been a smallpox victim in childhood, I know that he is sterile from epididymal blockage, and I know that the blockage is located in the head of the epididymis, fairly close to the testicle.

Years ago, when our first smallpox patient came to St. Louis from Saudi Arabia, he was accompanied by his Egyptian physician and brother-in-law. They didn't really believe that his epididymal blockage could be corrected, because this patient had had an attempt at surgery eleven years earlier in London that had failed. Nonetheless, this gentleman wanted very badly to have a child and made sure his personal physician and brother-in-law were there to observe the entire operation. The patient's wife became pregnant six months later, after the sperm count went up to over fifty million per cc with good motility.

A similar type of pilgrimage to St. Louis began in sub-Saharan Africa. A patient with a history of severe schistosomiasis of the bladder came to see me, again because of azoospermia. In America, most people have never heard of schistosomiasis, but it's probably the most common public health problem in the entire world. It infests almost all of Egypt and Africa and is caused by a parasite that invades the skin when one goes swimming or even wading in water that harbors the schistosomes. The parasite can enter the liver or the bladder and cause extreme illness or death. When you survive a severe case of bladder schistosomiasis, you are left with epididymal obstruction. This patient from a small African village left St. Louis no longer sterile.

Even in the Western world, many cases of male sterility (complete azoospermia) are caused by epididymal obstruction, but obstruction is more likely to be caused by gonorrhea, chlamydia, other sexually transmitted diseases, childhood trauma to the testicles, or congenital birth defects. For the most part, this male sterility can be cured with microsurgery without having to resort to IVF and ICSI. But not always.

### *Congenital Absence of the Vas Deferens*

About 20 percent of men with obstruction to sperm outflow have congenital absence of the vas deferens. As in all men with obstruction, the testicle is producing normal sperm, but this type of obstruction cannot be surgically corrected. There is no testicular defect in these men, and that is why this condition has been so incredibly frustrating over the past forty years. Every kind of effort had been made in the past to figure out a way to harvest these trapped sperm and use them to inseminate and impregnate the woman, but before ICSI, they were all unsuccessful. It was out of that frustration that Dr. Devroey, Dr. Van Steirteghem, and I decided to embark upon a combination of ICSI and MESA (microsurgical epididymal sperm aspiration). This idea was originally scorned because if the sperm were not able to traverse the epididymis, so the theory went, they would not be motile and would therefore be unable to fertilize. That fear has now been laid aside.

In the normal, unobstructed state, sperm do not become motile until they have passed through the majority of the epididymis. With obstruction, the opposite is true. The sperm that have passed farthest through the epididymis are nearest the point of obstruction, and these sperm are usually dead because they have been around for the longest period of time. They have died of old age. Sperm closer to the testicle that have not traversed the epididymis have better motility. This is quite the opposite of what was predicted. Normally, sperm farthest from the testicle are the most motile and the most fertile because they have been matured by virtue of epididymal transit. But in the case of obstruction, sperm closest to the testicle are the most recently produced and, therefore, have the best motility. This observation is what led to our remarkable success with these previously hopeless cases.

Several of these early patients still keep in close communication with me. One of them has become a skiing partner of mine and is also a law professor who helps to figure out the legal and ethical ramifications of the new reproductive technologies. Another is a religious fundamentalist who prays for me every day on the other side of the world. A third is a policeman from another city who has made me an honorary member of the force, and whose wife became president of a support group for patients with congenital absence of the vas, recognizing that it is a much more common condition than had been previously thought. These are couples who previously had no hope at all for having children. As Professor Donald Coffey of Johns Hopkins has said, "Every pessimist in the history of the world has been proven to be wrong."

### *TESE-ICSI Versus Microsurgical Vasoepididymostomy*

The development of ICSI with epididymal and testicular sperm at our center in St. Louis and in Brussels has made possible the delivery of normal babies even to couples in whom the man has irreparable obstruction, congenital absence of the vas, absent epididymis, blockage of the rete testis, or massive damage to the vas from bilateral inguinal hernia repair. However, the next question is whether TESE with ICSI might be preferable in all cases to surgical correction of the obstruction. To restate this, should we forget about microsurgery to correct obstructive azoospermia in the majority of cases that are reconstructible and simply schedule the wife for ovarian hyperstimulation and egg retrieval, combined with surgical or needle aspiration of sperm from her partner?

The advantage to eliminating surgery is that at centers where there is no microsurgical expertise, couples would still have a chance for pregnancy. This argument is rather silly in that any center with enough sophistication to perform ICSI should be able to develop the sophistication to perform microsurgical vasoepididymostomy. Nonetheless, the major reason that vasoepididymostomy is sometimes abandoned in favor of TESE-ICSI is that the doctors at many centers lack the surgical skill to perform a microsurgical correction.

If asked, patients would much rather be fertile as a result of a single operation, and then conceive in bed, romantically, than have to go through IVF and sperm retrieval procedures to achieve just a 35 percent chance of a live birth every time they want to have a child. When we present these options to patients with obstructive azoospermia, they invariably prefer microsurgery to correct the problem, and the women overwhelmingly appreciate that we males do not simply, casually say, "Why should your husband have surgery when we can just perform IVF on you (involving three months of injections and invasive procedures)?"

We feel the best approach for the majority of husbands with obstructive azoospermia, whether caused by vasectomy or natural causes, is microsurgical reconstruction, which eliminates putting their wives through all the aggravation and invasive procedures that IVF entails. However, at the time of this surgery, sperm retrieved from the epididymis should be frozen so that it's available for a future ICSI procedure in the event that he turns out to be one of the few cases for whom the vasoepididymostomy fails.

## Reversal of Tubal Ligation

Female sterilization is the most popular method of birth control today for married women in their midthirties who have had all the children they want. But it need not be a permanent procedure. Tubal ligation is a simple outpatient surgical procedure, and in 95 percent of cases, it is easily reversible.

But reversal of tubal sterilization is easy only if the sterilization was performed properly. Janet was a nurse who had married very young because she did not know anything about birth control, became sexually active in her late teens, and figured she'd better get married to avoid having illegitimate children. Several years later, she found herself unhappily married to a husband she did not love, with no time to pursue a career in nursing. She had two small children and didn't want to complicate matters further by having more. Still knowing nothing about birth control, she opted for the "easy" route — sterilization. Five years later, she was happily remarried to a doctor, was an accomplished nurse, and, in a sense, had truly benefited from that interval in which she did not have to worry about getting pregnant. Now, however, she wanted more children, and she had heard about our success with reversing tubal sterilizations.

But when we looked inside her abdomen, we were horrified to discover that the doctor who sterilized her had completely destroyed the fimbriated end of each fallopian tube, which is needed to pick up the egg from the surface of the ovary. At the time of ovulation, the open end of the tube normally sweeps down around the ovary, the fimbria coming to life like octopus tentacles and literally grabbing the egg off of the surface. Without this egg-collecting mechanism, a woman cannot possibly get pregnant. So Janet's decision in the heat of youth to have a tubal ligation turned out to be a poor one, only because she chose the wrong doctor and was not well counseled. If performed properly, female sterilization can have a very high degree of reversibility.

In the United States alone, more than 25 percent of married women use sterilization as a permanent method of birth control. Among married women ages thirty-five to forty-four, almost 40 percent rely on tubal sterilization. Oral contraceptives, by comparison, are used by only 14 percent of married women.

In China, sixteen million female sterilizations and nine million male sterilizations are performed every year. In South Korea today, 25 percent of all married women have been sterilized, whereas in 1974, only 2 percent were sterilized. Even in Latin America, with its largely Catholic population, many countries have embraced this method of birth control. Panama, El Salvador, Costa Rica, the Dominican Republic, Barbados, Colombia, and Brazil have some of the highest rates of female sterilization in the world. This dramatic increase is the result of the introduction of laparoscopy, whereby a little telescope is placed through the belly button to burn or block the tubes with great simplicity and very little pain.

Sterilization is most commonly chosen by women who are over thirty years of age, married, have several children, and don't want any more. Women who are sterilized under the age of thirty usually come to regret it. Even women who have as many as three or four children before age thirty are very likely to want more. Furthermore, women who are unhappily married at the time of their sterilization are very likely to regret the procedure after they get divorced and remarried.

In developed countries such as the United States, the most common reason women regret the operation is divorce, remarriage, and the desire to have children in a new marriage. Less commonly, the unexpected death of a child can prompt regret and the desire for more children. In poor, developing countries, child death is the major reason for regretting sterilization. The chance of a child making it to young adulthood is low in these countries compared to the United States or Europe. Poor people in developing countries are very likely to lose one or more children from infectious disease or malnutrition.

In the United States, child death is not that uncommon either. The most dangerous period in anyone's life is the first year, particularly the first six months. Sudden infant death syndrome (SIDS) is probably more likely to claim your child's life than any other cause. Once your child has made it past his or her first year, it is relatively clear sailing from then on. In fact, the puzzling thing to me is why anyone should be at all confused or surprised by sudden infant death syndrome. Anyone who has ever listened to an infant breathe as it sleeps during the first three months of life has to wonder how such a fragile being could possibly survive.

Infants just don't breathe right. The infant pattern of breathing is based on oxygen deprivation. As we mature, the breathing center of the brain is regulated by the amount of carbon dioxide in our blood. This means that long before your oxygen level gets dangerously low, a buildup of carbon dioxide stimulates you to breathe more, so your body constantly maintains an oxygen level very safely above the minimum required for survival. But this carbon dioxide breathing center in the brain is not well developed in infants. Their breathing is stimulated purely by oxygen deprivation. When their oxygen level goes too low as they sleep, this stimulates them to start breathing again. After they have gotten their oxygen level back up to adequate levels, they just stop breathing until the oxygen level goes down again. It is absolutely amazing that more infants do not die of sudden infant death syndrome.

So how can a woman who is sterilized immediately after delivering her baby possibly feel assured that one year from now her baby will still be alive? Although population planners do not emphasize this issue in the United States (or, for that matter, in the developing world), infant death is still a major reason why women may later regret having had a "permanent" sterilization.

For example, Cynthia had her second baby in 1977. It was born with multiple birth defects, including congenital heart disease. Yet she had a tubal ligation performed right at the time of the Cesarean section for the clearly logical reason that all she ever wanted was two children, and she figured that raising a child with all of these birth defects was going to be very expensive. She assumed that sterilization was permanent and wanted it that way. Even when the little infant died six weeks later, the emotional ordeal of having a child with birth defects was so overwhelming that she was still quite satisfied with her decision to be sterilized, and she did not want to have any more children. But five years later she came to our office begging to have microsurgery to reverse her sterilization so she could once again try for a second child. Decisions made during the emotional strain of birth and delivery rarely hold up later.

Nancy had two children who were both quite healthy, but she and her husband were schoolteachers with limited income who wanted to provide the best they could for those two children. So she had her tubes tied right after delivery of her second child, an approach frequently used because tubes are so accessible immediately after childbirth, when the enlarged uterus is pushing them up toward the abdominal wall. With this sort of timing, the woman never has to worry about birth control after going home from the hospital. The problem is that her child died two months later of SIDS, and three months later, she was in our office hoping that her sterilization could be reversed.

Clearly, the women most likely to regret being sterilized are those who have the procedure performed under the age of thirty, who are now in an unhappy marriage, or who have the procedure performed within one year of having their last child. At present, sterilization is not commonly performed on single, young women or teenagers with a history of sexual promiscuity and who may already have had one or more abortions. This is because most doctors are quite rightly concerned that ten years later these women will be likely to regret their decision and want to have children. Nonetheless, a significant minority of women do get sterilized under these circumstances because they are just so desperate. These women may regret their decision later. But these are not necessarily women to whom a sterilization should be denied. Sterilization may very well be their best move, as long as it is performed in a way that can be easily reversed.

### *Comparison of Tubal Sterilization in the Female to Vasectomy in the Male*

The fallopian tube in the female works quite differently from the vas deferens in the male. The entire ductal system that transports sperm out of the testicle is a closed one, and blocking it by vasectomy causes pressure buildup. In the female tube, the system is open. The fallopian tube drains freely through the fimbria into the abdominal cavity. There is no pressure buildup caused by tubal ligation. Therefore, the amount of time that has passed since the tubal ligation is of no consequence to the restoration of fertility with tubal reversal. No effort need be made to leave one side of the tubal ligation open as with vasectomy, because the tube is open at the fimbriated end anyway.

However, the length of the fallopian tube that has been damaged or removed by the sterilization procedure (unlike with vasectomy) has a tremendous effect on the reversibility. No matter how much tube has been removed, a good microsurgical technique can reconnect it. The problem is that if so much tube has been destroyed that this results in too short a tube, the fimbriated end will not be able to reach the surface of the ovary to pick up the egg. Furthermore, because the tube nourishes the egg during the first two days of the embryo's life, if the wrong area of the tube is removed, subsequent fertility would be unlikely despite a good reconnection.

Women are generally less likely than men to regret their sterilization, change their minds, and come back later for a reversal. Whether it is fair or unfair, in our society women have the bigger role to play in child rearing and do the most work, so they have a much truer perception of what having another child involves. Furthermore, women become biologically incapable of reproducing when they get older whether their tubes are open or not. So a woman who has her sterilization at age thirty-seven is pretty much near the end of her reproductive career and usually has no designs on reversing this decision. Men at age thirty-three have about fifty more years of reproductive viability ahead of them, and if they should get remarried, particularly to a young woman, they are more likely to request a reversal of their sterilization.

Sterilization in a man is simpler, safer, and easier to perform than in a woman. Vasectomy can be performed under local anesthesia in a doctor's office in just a few minutes. There is no major risk to health. Tubal sterilization, even with the modern techniques, still involves penetrating the abdomen, risking damage to vital organs or blood vessels, and requires a general anesthetic in most cases. Even on an outpatient basis, female sterilization must be performed in a hospital setting, and this involves sophisticated instrumentation and ancillary personnel. The total cost of a tubal sterilization is about $2,000 or more, whereas a vasectomy costs between $250 and $600.

### *Methods of Blocking the Tubes*

Whether by minilap or by laparoscopy, there are four basic methods for occluding the tube. The classic method is to use a piece of surgical thread to tie off a loop of tube and cut out the section between the tie. A second approach is fimbriectomy, in which the entire fimbriated end of the tube is removed. This is a rarely used and terrible approach that makes the sterilization irreversible. As long as the fimbriated end is not removed, the tubal ligation can be reversed.

There are several methods for occluding the tube through the laparoscope. The most common method is simply to "burn" the tubes with an electrocoagulating current transmitted through a special forceps. It has been feared that this burning (cautery) might make the sterilization irreversible by destroying the uterine side of the tube. However, even these "difficult" cases can be reversed successfully with proper microsurgical technique, which I will explain later in the chapter.

The remaining laparoscopic methods involve physical occlusion of the tube rather than cautery. The Hulka clip (named after the gynecologist who invented it) reliably occludes the tube and damages only the tiniest portion. The Fallope ring is a small Silastic band with a special applicator that cinches around a doubled-up loop of the midportion of the tube. The Fallope ring also damages only a small portion of the tube, is easy to apply, and probably is the most commonly used of the easily reversible methods of tubal occlusion (see figs. 15.6 and 15.7).

Every method of occlusion must destroy some small segment of tube, which then scars down. As long as the fimbriated end of the tube is intact and as long as less than two thirds of the tube is destroyed, microsurgery can restore fertility back to what it would have been if the woman had never been sterilized. Simple, minimally destructive occlu-

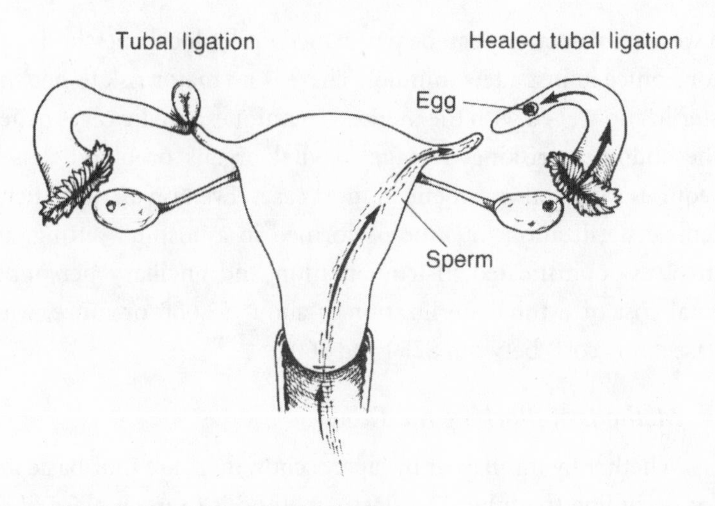


**FIGURE 15.6.** Tubal ligation and healed tubal ligation.

sion of the narrow isthmus region of the tube makes the most easily reversible sterilization, but that is not a requirement for reversibility.

Jennie was a twenty-seven-year-old housewife with a boy age three and a girl age six. She had her tubal ligation performed laparoscopically after the boy was about six months old, and she was relatively sure that he was healthy and growing normally. The doctor doing the sterilization wanted to make sure there was no unwanted pregnancy because this couple did not think they could afford any more children. So he burned the tubes with bipolar cautery all the way down to the uterus.

Three years later the little boy was riding with his father on a tractor on a calm, beautiful Sunday afternoon. He unexpectedly jumped off, and the big wheel ran right over him. He was dead instantly, and Jennie longed to have another child but was told that her tubes were just too badly burned to be repaired. Fortunately for her, we were able to reconnect the tubes to the microscopic openings coming out of the uterus (fig. 15.8). So, despite the difficulty, if less than two thirds of the tube is destroyed, tubal sterilization can still be reversed. Jennie has had two more children since then and has no intention of ever being sterilized again.

### *Reversal of Tubal Sterilization*

The major worry of the doctor performing your sterilization is that the operation might fail and you might get pregnant. For this doctors

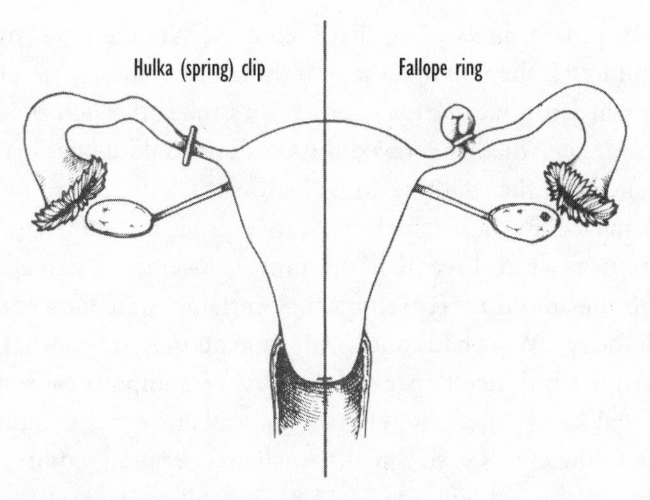


**FIGURE 15.7.** Hulka (spring) clip and Fallope ring.

can get sued. Generally, they are not worried about how to make the operation reversible. In fact, if you ask them to make it reversible, they may be afraid to perform the operation in the first place for fear you will sue them for sterilizing someone who should not have been sterilized.

There have been several lawsuits where women have sued the doctor on behalf of their child for "wrongful life." If you can believe it, the contention of such suits is that the child had a right not to exist because its mother had chosen sterilization. The failure of the sterilization resulted in the birth of a child whose right not to exist was denied. Fortunately, the courts have decided that such a lawsuit is absurd. But the courts have a funny way of compromise. If a "wrongful birth" occurs and the child is handicapped, then the doctor may be found liable for the entire cost of raising the child for the rest of his or her life over and above what it would cost to raise a normal child. Once again, the chaotic court system has clouded up the issues. Fortunately there are doctors who will discuss and consider your individual case according to your particular needs and do what is right regardless of the fear of an irrational lawsuit. But you can certainly see why they may lean heavily away from a reversible approach to sterilization.

Jan had three children and a happy marriage, and she had decided to have a sterilization three years before seeing me. Two years after the sterilization, Jan and her husband, Roger, knew they wanted a larger family and could afford more children. They had done such a good job of raising the three they already had that I felt quite sure there was room for more children if they wanted them. Yet when their local gynecologist, a well-known fertility expert, looked at Jan's tubes through the laparoscope to decide whether a reversal procedure could be performed, he sadly concluded that nothing could be done. The tubes had been "too badly damaged" by the original sterilization procedure. When we looked at his report, we realized that the fimbriae were not damaged, and although the ampullae were short, they certainly were long enough to nourish the egg. What had concerned her gynecologist was what looked like a technically difficult operation because of a unipolar cautery sterilization that had burned the tubes all the way down to the uterus. The opening to the uterus is so tiny that such an operation requires a great deal of microsurgical skill (see fig. 15.8). But still, virtually all such cases can be reconnected, and I knew there was enough healthy tubal length for pregnancy to occur. So Jan came to St. Louis so we could operate. Jan and Roger now have two more children.

Katie had a tubal sterilization performed in 1979, and a relatively inexperienced surgeon attempted a reversal three years later. The operation was poorly performed, and she wound up with total blockage on the right and partial blockage on the left. Two and a half years later, she got pregnant via the left tube. The sperm were able to find their way through the partial blockage to the egg, but unfortunately the egg was not able to move into the uterus two days later. This resulted in an ectopic pregnancy, which required emergency surgery. Thus, when I saw her in 1995, she only had one tube remaining and never dreamed that it

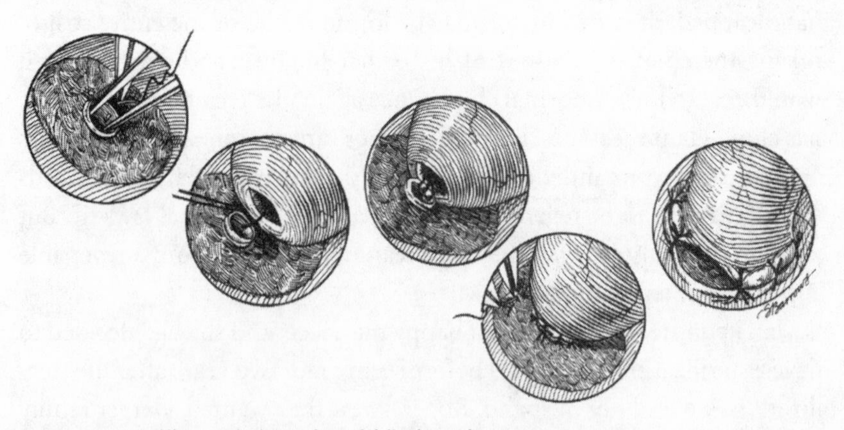

**FIGURE 15.8.** Microsurgical suturing of fallopian tube.

still would be possible to make her fertile. But when we operated we found a long, healthy tube that just needed to be reconnected properly, this time to the cornu, the tiny little opening coming out of the uterus. As long as there is enough tubal length, even on just one side, a technically difficult operation is not a problem. Katie was rendered fertile.

### *How the Type of Sterilization Affects the Technique for Reversal*

In the past, unipolar cauterization (burning) through the laparoscope has been the most common method of sterilization. This usually results in destruction of a fairly large segment of tube. Fortunately, the burn always seems to spread from the grasping forceps to the uterus, sparing the end of the tube leading toward the fimbria. It burns all of the isthmus right down to the uterus, and some of the ampulla. Thus, it is technically the most difficult type of sterilization to reverse. But because tubal length is often quite adequate, we still have an extremely high success rate with reversing this type of sterilization. But the technical difficulty of such a procedure usually overwhelms doctors who are not extremely experienced in microsurgery. For that reason, unipolar cautery is not an easily reversible sterilization.

The type of reconnection required after unipolar cautery is called ampullary-cornual, meaning that the large-diameter ampulla has to be reconnected to the tiny cornual opening of the uterus. To perform such an operation requires either making a tiny opening in the scarred ampulla so that openings of the same microscopic size can be connected, or cutting out the scar and tailoring this enlarged opening down to the tiny one-seventieth of an inch diameter that will allow it to match up with the tiny one-seventieth of an inch opening of the cornual end (see fig. 15.9). Bipolar cauterization (also performed through the laparoscope) allows the current to go down one tong of the forceps across the tissue to the other tong and never spreads anywhere but between those two points. Thus, the tube is burned wherever it happens to be grasped, and the burn does not spread in either direction. This type of cautery will damage very little tube, and if the tube is grasped in the narrow isthmus region, should result in the blocked ends of the tube being of relatively equal size and not very difficult to reconnect with microsurgery. The only catch here is that many doctors are so afraid that this bipolar cautery does not burn the tube adequately that they may burn the tube in several different places. This does not mean the sterili-

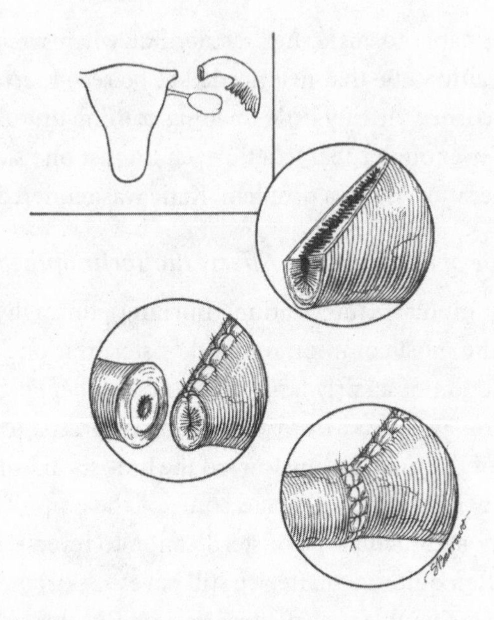

**FIGURE 15.9.** Ampullary-cornual reconnection.

zation is irreversible, only that more complex surgical techniques are required for the reversal.

The Fallope ring is a tiny Silastic band that looks like a very thick, round rubber band with an internal diameter of about one eighth of an inch. It comes loaded on a device that grasps the fallopian tube through the laparoscope or minilap and then pulls a loop of it up through the ring. Because the ring is so tight, the loop of fallopian tube loses its blood supply and disappears into scar tissue over the course of several weeks. Usually this procedure destroys very little tube, and it virtually always leaves enough tubal length for subsequent reversibility. Like the bipolar cautery, it usually doesn't damage the tube all the way down to the uterus, so a difficult cornual reconnection is not required. The only technical problem sometimes created by the Fallope ring and the classic tubal ligation is that often an area of isthmus and ampulla, rather than just isthmus alone, is destroyed. This means that to reconnect the tube requires surgically uniting the relatively large diameter of the ampulla to the somewhat smaller diameter of the isthmus. This is not a terribly difficult surgical problem and does not compare to the difficulty of reconnecting the ampulla to the cornual opening.

The easiest surgical reconnection is with lumens of the same diameter, and that is where the Hulka clip comes in. The Hulka clip never damages more than one fourth of an inch of tube. So if it is applied to the isthmus region, the reversal operation would simply involve reconnecting isthmus to isthmus, lumens of the same diameter.

To summarize, the Hulka clip, if applied to the narrow isthmus, damages the least amount of tube and is technically the easiest to reverse. Bipolar cauterization, as opposed to unipolar, should damage almost as little tissue as the Hulka clip, but many doctors are so fearful that they haven't really burned the tube adequately with the bipolar that they may burn it in several different locations. The Fallope ring, in my view, is just as reversible as the Hulka clip, and I advise patients that using the Fallope ring is virtually a completely reversible sterilization procedure. But because it may damage slightly more tube than the Hulka clip and may damage both ampulla and isthmus, the Fallope ring may present slight technical difficulties for less-experienced microsurgeons. Unipolar cautery, which is now much less popular, damages the most tube and creates a technical need for the most difficult reconnection procedure.

### *What Factors Affect Successful Sterilization Reversal?*

If we look at the success rates in various groups of patients on whom we performed a sterilization reversal, we get a clear picture of what factors affect reversibility. Virtually all our reversal patients have had a good connection, with perfectly open and normal tubes postoperatively. But despite near-perfect surgical results, not all our patients have gotten pregnant after reversal of tubal sterilization. Looking at the various categories of these patients helps us understand what makes the sterilization reversible and not reversible after a proper microsurgical reconnection.

When we first began doing microsurgical sterilization reversals for women in 1977, we decided that we would start with no preconceptions and offer the operation to absolutely any woman who requested it. At that time, there were many prejudicial misconceptions about what type of sterilization and what type of patient would be most easily reversed, about who could get pregnant, and who couldn't. We knew that none of these preconceptions was based on genuine observations of women undergoing truly meticulous, careful microsurgical techniques for reversal. Many doctors just assumed, for example, that reversal of a laparoscopic unipolar cautery sterilization was impossible to perform. Many assumed that if a woman had had a previous attempt at reversal that failed, there would be too much scarring to allow a subsequent reattempt at reversal to succeed. Many felt that women over thirty-five, or women whose sterilization was performed more than five years earlier, would have no chance for success, and these women were turned down. Of the many hundreds of women coming to us for sterilization reversal, we turned no one down based on any preconception, but we kept accurate, meticulous records of every aspect of their situation to see which patients were most likely to get pregnant.

The observations recorded for each patient were the age of the husband; the age of the wife; the sperm count of the husband; the number of previous children (if any); the duration of time since the sterilization was originally performed; the type of sterilization procedure performed (whether through laparoscopy, laparotomy, or minilaparotomy); whether unipolar or bipolar cautery, Fallope ring, Hulka clip, or ligation was used; the area of the tube that was destroyed; the areas of the tube that had to be reconnected; and, finally, the total length of tube remaining after the reconnection was achieved. Furthermore, we observed the character of the anatomic appearance of the ovaries, the quality of the menstrual cycle before and after the reversal surgery, and the amount of general scarring (adhesions) in the pelvis.

We hoped to find the answer to three specific questions: (1) What type of sterilization procedure is easiest to reconnect surgically? (2) Are there any types of sterilization procedures that are impossible to reconnect surgically? (3) Assuming a good reconnection is achieved, would anything else about the way the sterilization was originally performed stand in the way of getting pregnant now that the tubes were properly reconnected?

We found that the only things that affected whether these women got pregnant after sterilization reversal surgery were the *length of tube on the longer side* and her age. None of the other myriad factors we carefully and assiduously studied made any difference. As long as there was a fimbria left to pick up the egg, there was nothing else about the sterilization procedure that prevented pregnancy other than the length of tube that was left after the reconnection. In fact, the pregnancy rate over time was no different from what would occur based on age in a normal population of women.

The type of sterilization, whether through a laparoscope or a minilap, made no difference. Whether the tube was blocked by unipolar cautery, bipolar cautery, Fallope ring, Hulka clip, or ligation made no difference. The pregnancy rate was diminished only if the tube was less than one and a half inches long when the procedure was completed.

However, no woman can ever be guaranteed a pregnancy. For example, in a normal population of women who have already had children, about 15 percent are going to be relatively infertile. This number will clearly be higher for older women. Therefore, we cannot guarantee fertility to women who have more than one and a half inches of tube left after the sterilization reversal, but we can assure them that the sterilization procedure itself has had no effect on their fertility, and after the reversal, they should be just as fertile as they would have been at that stage in their life if they had never had sterilization.

### *How Difficult Is Tubal Reversal Surgery for the Patient?*

In the mid-1970s, when tubal microsurgery was first developed, it involved a major abdominal incision, a week in the hospital, and a six-week postoperative recovery. The actual microsurgery was delicate even then and posed no threat to the patient. It was just the surgical exposure that made it a very big operation. So whether or not to undergo the surgery was a formidable decision for any woman who was rethinking having more children.

Today, however, even the most intricate tubal microsurgery can be done as an outpatient procedure through a very small incision. The patient only needs to be out of work for a week and essentially needs no postoperative care. The surgery requires only a one-inch minilap incision just below the pubic hairline. A very unobtrusive plastic retractor allows us to get a microscopic view of any area we need to reconstruct through such an incision. We can even do an ovary transplant using this approach, and send the patient home on the same day or the next morning. Therefore, it is easier and more cost-effective for a woman to have her tubal ligation reversed than to undergo an IVF procedure.

We have seen many requests for reversal of sterilization by women whose husbands also need vasectomy reversal. If we weren't so certain about the return to normal fertility of women who have an adequate length of tube left, we would have difficulty suggesting that both the husband and the wife undergo surgery to try to have children.

Wanda and Bert were the first such couple I treated. Each had several children from previous marriages. They were now blissfully married to each other in a happy, stable relationship, and both they and their present children wanted them to have more kids. Wanda was told there was no hope for reversing her sterilization because it had been performed with unipolar cauterization with too much tubal destruction. As in all cases of female sterilization reversal, only two issues mattered: Could we technically accomplish a surgical reconnection? Was there enough tubal length? Despite the fact that the tube was burned all the way to the uterus, we were able to establish a beautiful ampullary-cornual reconnection. She had one two-inch-long tube that had no difficulty picking up the egg.

With confidence, we then suggested that Bert also go through vasectomy reversal surgery. Three months later, despite the dire predictions given by her regular doctors, Wanda became pregnant. In most of the cases we have seen where both the man and the woman had previously been sterilized in an earlier marriage, reversing the sterilization on both of them resulted in pregnancy. A more conventional approach for couples in which both the man and the woman have had a sterilization procedure is to perform ICSI on the wife's eggs using sperm retrieved from the husband's testicles or epididymis, rather than putting them both through a sterilization-reversal procedure. But I would disagree with that conventional view. I believe the argument still applies that if their sterility could be reversed with minimally invasive surgery, those couples would prefer getting pregnant naturally to undergoing possibly multiple cycles of IVF.

Some doctors have a negative view about women who change their minds and decide they want to have a sterilization reversed. This merely reflects a chauvinistic male attitude that does not admit to the vicissitudes of unpredictable problems that life presents. If your doctor takes that attitude when you ask about sterilization reversal, you might want to consider another doctor.

CHAPTER 16

# Donor Sperm

In the past, if the husband had no sperm in his ejaculate, the only solution was for the wife to have artificial insemination with donor sperm. Since we have developed the ICSI technique, there are now very few couples who would need to consider donor sperm, because the vast majority of previously hopeless cases of male infertility can now be treated successfully with ICSI. In most cases in which ICSI is not successful for dealing with male infertility, it is because of the wife's eggs, not the sperm. However, there are still a small number of cases in which no sperm at all can be found with TESE-ICSI, or in which the sperm are completely abnormal. Therefore, the need for donor sperm banks may have dwindled, but some couples will still have this need. The purpose of this chapter is to explain the process of using donor sperm for couples for whom there is no alternative.

In a sense, using donor sperm is really no different from adoption. It is simply a matter of adopting sperm. You're adopting the baby at a much earlier stage — prior to conception. Using the sperm of a well-selected anonymous donor is the most realistic and sensible solution for the few couples who simply have no sperm at all, even in the testes. The use of donor sperm or donor eggs (or even donor sperm and donor eggs) has tremendous advantages over classic adoption for parental bonding and child development, not to mention less cost.

## Is It My Baby?

There has always been a heated debate about where a child's personality and abilities come from, its environment or its genes. After counseling many hundreds of couples who have used donor sperm and having seen the results over the last thirty years, as well as having studied rather extensively the early childhood development research coming from the Harvard and the Ypsilanti early childhood projects, I have some definite views that could be of benefit to couples who are facing this issue of whether to use donor sperm (or donor eggs). It is obviously preferable emotionally to do whatever is possible to allow patients to have their own genetic baby using the husband's sperm. However, if such a solution is not at hand, the following observations should be seriously considered.

The divorce rate among couples who choose to elect donor sperm is less than 1 percent, even though the general divorce rate in our population is over 50 percent. This is not because the decision to have a baby by donor insemination in some way holds the marriage together. Rather, couples who wind up choosing this route have a solid relationship and a good basis of communicating with each other. Couples who have any flaws or weaknesses in their ability to communicate on tough issues usually won't choose donor insemination. Couples who do use donor insemination are a select group that have an extraordinarily solid marriage. They can deal with a potentially divisive issue and come to a common understanding that makes them both happy. So if a couple decides to use donor sperm, it is a very good sign that the marriage is going to remain solid.

Couples will frequently ask how the baby will do when its genes come half from the mother and half from some stranger. Very often they will say, "Well, at least if we go this route, as opposed to adoption, the baby will be one half ours." This outlook is a strong reason *not* to have donor insemination. My observation has been that when the husband and the wife both accept the baby as being 100 percent theirs, and take the view that the genetic contribution is of no significance, then the father-infant bonding is completely normal.

Although there is a controversial view held in some circles that a child's personality, intelligence, and athletic ability are basically genetically transmitted and that there is only a partial contribution from parental rearing, evidence from most donor sperm and donor egg couples, and from early childhood education projects, strongly refutes this commonly held genetic bias. In truth, the child's personality, intelligence, and even athletic skill (though not size, hair color, eye color, or body build) are overwhelmingly related to how he or she was raised in the first several years of life.

Children in the first year and a half of life are, in many respects, like parrots. They learn by copying what they see around them. A personality tends to emerge more clearly as a sense of individual identity around the age of a year and a half, when language skills first become readily apparent. The way in which a nongenetic offspring mimics his or her rearing father, regardless of genetic origin, is so striking that these parents are sometimes shocked and do double takes when a friendly neighbor (who knows nothing about the child's genetic origin) comments admiringly on how the child is the spitting image of his father. In couples who elect donor insemination, most of the time the father's bonding with the infant is no different than if it were his own "genetic" child.

The interesting thing is that the courts take a similar view in ruling on cases where a husband might allege that his wife got pregnant by having an affair with another man and that the child his wife bears is not really his. The courts define the father as the person who is living with the woman and are not terribly concerned about whose sperm fertilized the mother. (Of course, the courts have a different agenda in that their major concern is establishing a responsible father to handle financial arrangements for the child's future care.) Still, it is of interest that the official legal view does not contradict what the latest studies on early child development demonstrate.

It is true that we have all witnessed how a two-year-old's personality, intelligence, and skill level are quite predictive in many cases of how that child will eventually turn out as an adult, and this observation leads many to conclude unquestioningly that "it's just all genetic." That viewpoint is enhanced even further among natural parents (who have not required any infertility treatment) who are in one way or another unhappy with how their child has turned out. Even though it may be "their own genetic child," they blame the result on "genes," assuming that the child just had the bad luck of getting the parents' worst genes, because it takes away any possibility that they might have to blame themselves and their rearing efforts. There can be tremendous attractiveness in being able to allow genetics to shoulder the responsibility for how a child turns out. These erroneous "genetic" arguments can raise fear among couples who are considering donor sperm.

It is clear to me that in every case I have studied where parents have been unhappy with how their children turned out, the child's problems can be traced to the parents' dysfunction as parents and not to any genetic predetermination. When the final human genome sequence papers came out in *Science* and in *Nature,* the molecular geneticists who actually sequenced the entire human genome warned against two myths: determinism and reductionism. It was clear to them that who a person becomes is *not* in his or her genes.

Nonetheless, couples electing to use donor sperm prefer to make sure that the sperm comes from the healthiest, most intelligent possible source, and they might want to match up hair color, skin color, eye color, body build, etc. A good donor sperm program will pay close attention to these selective characteristics so that the couple may get as close a physical match to the husband as they'd like.

## How to Select the Donor

Artificial insemination was first successfully used in women by the famous physician John Hunter in England in the eighteenth century. In 1890, Dr. Robert Dickinson of New York was the first to use donor sperm for women whose husbands had untreatable infertility. This early use of artificial insemination with donor sperm was carried out in great secrecy. However, it became so popular by 1990 that more than thirty thousand babies were being born every year in the United States as a result of it. Patients are accepting it when there is no other solution, and most of the psychological, social, and legal fears about it have disappeared.

In 1964, Georgia was the first state to issue legislation that guaranteed that a child conceived in this manner would be considered legitimate. Oklahoma passed a similar law in 1967, as did Kansas in 1968, and all other states followed suit. Even prior to these legislative decrees, common law provided some protection for the legitimacy of such children. Unless it is proved that the husband had no access to the wife, any child born of her is considered to be his by the law. Whether or not the husband is the true father, he is the legal father of any child born to his wife while they are living together.

From a medical point of view, artificial insemination is extraordinarily simple. A sperm specimen obtained from the donor is drawn up into a syringe, and then either simply squirted into the vagina near the cervix or washed and placed with a catheter into the uterus. Since the sperm are only capable of fertilization for about forty-eight hours in the female reproductive tract, and since the egg is only capable of being fertilized within twelve hours of ovulation, the insemination must be timed appropriately just before ovulation. However, the pregnancy rate per cycle with donor sperm is much higher per attempt if it is used with IVF (60 percent) rather than with simple insemination (12 percent).

All donors have to be checked for the presence of hepatitis, AIDS, or venereal disease. Because of the possible six-month incubation time of the AIDS virus, frozen sperm is virtually always used today (as opposed to ten years ago), because it allows the donor to be observed for six months after the collection of the sperm, and have a repeat blood test for AIDS. Only if his blood test for AIDS is still negative six months after donating the sperm is his sperm used for donor insemination. Furthermore, the donor is screened for any history of genetic disease in his family. Even a history of diseases that are only partially genetically transmitted, such as diabetes, would generally rule him out as a sperm donor. The specimen is also carefully cultured for bacteria, such as gonorrhea or chlamydia, and the remainder of the sample is prepared for freezing and storage.

It has always been thought best for the sperm donor to be anonymous because problems could arise if the genetic father is known to the couple. With a greater openness in our society, and a better understanding of the relative lack of significance of genetic contribution as opposed to rearing, some physicians (though not the majority) are becoming more open to allowing selected couples to use sperm from donors they know. However, the vast majority of couples prefer anonymous sperm from a well-respected donor sperm bank rather than use a known sperm donor.

It is generally preferable to obtain donor sperm from a reputable sperm bank located in a region completely different from your own. Because of the requirement that anonymous donors' sperm be frozen in order to make certain that the donor doesn't become AIDS positive over the ensuing six months, before the sperm is used, and because of the meticulous detail that couples using donor insemination have a right to expect regarding the characteristics of the donor, many physicians are turning more and more to formally operated and carefully regulated frozen sperm banks. One of the very best sperm banks in the United States is the California Cryobank. It makes shipments of sperm all over the world and is presently the largest sperm bank in North America. It provides a detailed pedigree of every single donor, including race, hair color, eye color, skin color, body build, religious preference, nationality, degree of education, and even hobbies. In truth, all that really makes a difference is that there is no history of genetic disease; that the donor doesn't have hepatitis, AIDS, or venereal disease; and that he is a reasonable match of inherited appearance. The other issues, such as level of education achieved, hobbies, and interests, are simply a way of reassuring future recipients who might have lingering doubts about the possibility of any broad genetic transference of intellectual ability or personality.

There are so many cases of short parents having tall children that are genetically their own, of dark-haired parents having a redheaded child, that all of us are aware of the importance of recessive genes expressing themselves unpredictably in children that are genetically our own. In fact, even if there is a perfect matching of the donor to the recipient, the child may have a very different appearance because of these recessive genes.

The sperm bank should also make sure that no particular donor is overused. Population scientists have made it very clear that if a particular donor were to be used in more than ten different couples around the United States, there would be an ever-so-slight risk of a future unknown first-cousin marriage if the offspring of any of these families were to ever meet and get married. The temptation for a poorly organized sperm bank would be to use a particular donor over and over again and thereby avoid all of the expense related to the selection of new donors. Despite the increased cost, it is important that the sperm bank resist any such overuse of its donors, and that is why only the most reputable sources for sperm should be used.

There was a great deal of publicity in the early 1980s associated with the founding of the Nobel Prize Sperm Bank. This bank was started in the San Diego area by a very old, former Nobel Prize winner (who has subsequently died) who received his prize for inventing the transistor. It was his firm belief that intelligence was genetically transmitted and that the future of our society depended upon sperm from these most intelligent men being used for donor insemination. His sperm bank was never really taken very seriously, and never caught on. As one of my patients put it: "If genes do have anything to do with superintelligence and winning Nobel Prizes (which I don't believe they do), then we should be using the sperm from Nobel Prize winners' fathers, not from the Nobel winners themselves. By and large, the children of Nobel Prize winners are not any more distinguished than children born from parents with less illustrious minds."

The brain of modern man is really no different from the brain of Cro-Magnon man, who lived forty thousand years ago in caves and drew crude paintings on the wall. The human brain has been able to take us as far as we have come not because of inborn abilities, but rather because of its remarkable flexibility and capacity to learn. If I were born forty thousand years ago in a Cro-Magnon cave, I would not be a sophisticated microsurgeon or in vitro fertilization specialist. Nor would I have developed the complex language abilities that have allowed me to write this book. My brain would have developed in other directions appropriate to allowing me to figure out how to survive in an entirely different, more primitive world. If a genetically Cro-Magnon child were to be born today and reared by parents who encouraged the spark of curiosity, enthusiasm, and intellectual challenge, he or she would be just as likely to win a Nobel Prize as the child of anyone else born today.

## Frozen Sperm and Sperm Banks

All people dream from time to time about the possibility of immortality. Science-fiction novelists frequently toy with the idea of human beings being placed in a deep freeze just prior to the moment of death, to be revived perhaps two hundred years later, at which time science may have better treatments for illnesses and a way of prolonging life indefinitely. Life is, in a sense, a series of chemical events proceeding irreversibly toward death, and these chemical events cannot take place at –196 degrees Celsius. Thus, if an organism could be "safely" placed in a deep freeze, it could be preserved until a future century, and revived with subsequent warming.

Of course, freezing large animals would kill them immediately because of damage created by crystallization of water within their cells during the freezing process. However, it has been known since 1776 that human sperm are remarkably resistant to the damaging effects of freezing (because there is so little water in them). In that year, an Italian scientist exposed spermatozoa to freezing temperatures and noted that, after warming, some of them regained their motility. It was speculated then that frozen semen might be used not only in breeding the finest farm animals but also for saving the sperm of a man going off to war so that his wife might have a child from him even though he had already died on the battlefield. Although these crude, early studies established that sperm could survive freezing and thawing, the sperm were so terribly damaged that there was no possibility of practical application.

But in 1949, British scientists discovered, completely by accident, that if a relatively common chemical, glycerol, is added to the semen before it is frozen, the majority of the sperm survive freezing and thawing uneventfully. The researchers who made this discovery were so surprised to find live, healthy sperm in large concentrations after thawing that they had to go back to their laboratory shelf to find out which of the chemicals accidentally added to their sperm suspension was the one that protected the sperm against freezing. They finally discovered that it was glycerol. It took very little time after their remarkable discovery for frozen-sperm banks to find acceptance in the field of cattle breeding, and today, the vast majority of calves born in the world are the result of artificial insemination from frozen bull semen. In 1953, four years later, it was demonstrated that frozen and thawed human sperm could result in pregnancy and the delivery of normal babies. The first human sperm bank was established the next year.

With the advent of the ICSI technique, no matter how poorly sperm might thaw out after the freeze, they can be used quite successfully unless there is absolutely zero motility whatsoever, which is quite unusual. Therefore, although sperm of the majority of men do not freeze well enough for a subsequent pregnancy to occur with simple insemination, the sperm of almost all men will freeze adequately for subsequent pregnancy with ICSI.

Sperm freeze better than most other cells because there is so little cellular water content. The sperm head is basically an extremely compact, dense arrangement of DNA with much less water content than any other cell. Therefore, there is very little intracellular ice-crystal formation to damage it. Nonetheless, even sperm require some sort of cryoprotectant, in this case glycerol, whose function is to pull water out of the cell and to get inside it to act as a sort of antifreeze, preventing ice formation from any water still remaining inside. Subsequently, there was further improvement in cryoprotection by adding test yolk buffer to the glycerol and diluting the sperm 50 percent instead of 10 percent in the cryoprotectant.

There is no increased risk of birth abnormalities from frozen sperm. Whatever harm may come to sperm from freezing, either in the sperm's structure or ability to fertilize, there does not appear to be any increased risk of defective children. Extensive experience using both cattle and humans has now documented that frozen sperm from sperm banks is safe. Literally hundreds of thousands of normal pregnancies and births in humans using donor sperm have been reported in the scientific literature.

Perhaps the most exciting benefit for sperm-banking in the modern era is that because of the development of the ICSI technique we can freeze the sperm of anyone who is about to undergo a vasectomy, chemotherapy or radiation for cancer, or a sperm aspiration procedure, and who doesn't want to have multiple surgeries for future attempts at pregnancy. For all these conditions, we can freeze the man's sperm now, no matter how poor its quality, and offer a high chance of pregnancy once this sperm is thawed, if it used in conjunction with ICSI. Freezing of sperm has been attempted in the past with men who were about to undergo cancer chemotherapy, but it wasn't used very frequently because the chance for pregnancy from any one insemination would be very low. To have any kind of assurance, the patient might have to collect twenty or thirty samples of sperm to freeze prior to undergoing cancer treatment, and this would be too long a delay for his cancer treatment. Now, with ICSI, it is simply a matter of having one single sperm sample frozen and saved, and then the man can have whatever treatment he needs that may subsequently make him sterile, without the fear that he will not be able to have his own genetic child someday in the future.

## Insemination with Donor Sperm or ICSI with Donor Sperm

Not all infertility specialists agree, but I believe that if donor sperm is used, it should be used in conjunction with ICSI, not just insemination. There are several reasons for this. First, IVF with donor sperm gives a 60 percent pregnancy rate (or more) per cycle, while simple donor sperm insemination gives only a 12 percent pregnancy rate per cycle. You are thus five times more likely to get pregnant in any given donor sperm cycle using IVF. So in the long run, IVF is actually more cost-effective than artificial insemination. Second, the emotional impact of going through multiple unsuccessful donor sperm inseminations month after month can be daunting. If you don't get pregnant in one of the early donor sperm insemination cycles, you may even run out of that donor's frozen sperm sample, and then have to go through the trouble of selecting yet another donor. With IVF, you are more likely to get pregnant earlier, and with ICSI, you need never run out of that particular donor's sperm.

Most couples would prefer to have the same genetic origin for each of their children. With ICSI, just one single frozen specimen will be enough for you to have all subsequent children from the same donor. For each ICSI procedure, we just scrape a tiny chip off of the frozen pellet, leaving almost all of the rest of the sperm still frozen. One single donor sample can be used for hundreds of cycles. You do not have to worry that your original donor has disappeared or refuses to donate, or that the sperm bank might have exhausted all of that donor's deposits. Most patients confronted with the choice of insemination or ICSI with donor sperm agree fully that ICSI is the better choice.

CHAPTER 17

# Egg Donation and Gestational Surrogacy

## Surrogate Uterus (Your Mother Can Have Your Kids for You)

In 1980, I received a very sad letter from a twenty-five-year-old woman in the Bronx, New York, saying that when she had surgery for uterine fibroids, the doctor had to perform a hysterectomy, and she lost her uterus. Now she desperately wanted to have children. Unfortunately, at that time, I had to write to tell her there was no hope. I had predicted in my original book in 1979 that with the "new" IVF technology on the horizon, perhaps at some time in the future a woman without a uterus could have someone else carry her genetic child for her. Five years later that futuristic prediction became a reality.

In 1985, Dr. Wolf Utian and colleagues, from Cleveland, reported the first successful case in which a woman with no uterus was able to have her own genetic child. The story of that first case, reported in the *New England Journal of Medicine,* was absolutely spellbinding: A thirty-seven-year-old woman had become pregnant, but the uterus spontaneously ruptured at twenty-eight weeks of gestation, necessitating a Cesarean section and a hysterectomy. The baby girl subsequently died, and the woman was left childless and without a uterus. The couple, however, remained strongly committed to having their own genetic child, and the wife asked that an embryo of hers be transferred to the uterus of a friend who was interested and willing to carry the child as a surrogate. The friend was a healthy, married young mother of two. The reproductive cycles of the two women were synchronized (the reason for this will be explained later). The patient's eggs were incubated with sperm from the husband, and three days later, an eight-cell embryo was transferred to the uterus of her friend, who became the first human gestational surrogate. The surrogate became pregnant and nine months later delivered the healthy genetic baby of her ecstatic friend.

At the American Fertility Society meeting in 1986, a lady introduced herself to me and thanked me for the prediction that I made in my original book about gestational surrogacy. She told me it had prompted her to go to the IVF program in her community, where she requested IVF with a surrogate. And when I saw her at that meeting, her best friend was already pregnant with her genetic baby and ready to deliver and give it to her.

A few years later, I took care of a famous pair of sisters whose story appeared in *Good Housekeeping* magazine. Linda had gone through many failed attempts at IVF in other clinics. Her sister had already had several children without any problem and was quite willing to carry a baby for her. We were able to obtain six embryos from Linda's eggs and her husband's sperm. We put three embryos into Linda and three embryos into her sister. As it turned out, both sisters conceived, the surrogate with twins and Linda with a singleton. The twins were born in December, and the singleton was born in January of the subsequent year. Thus, triplet siblings were born safely, in different cities and in different years. The surrogate sister, of course, gladly gave the children back to their genetic parents. She has always had a very deep and close relationship, as a special kind of aunt, with the niece and nephew she carried for their mother.

We were approached by a twenty-nine-year-old woman who had had her uterus and both ovaries removed, and desperately wanted to have a child. Her husband had perfectly normal sperm, and they both wanted a baby by her husband's sperm. But who would provide the eggs and who would provide the uterus? In her family, one of her sisters was willing to donate an egg; the husband, of course, would provide his sperm; and another sister would allow the eggs and the sperm to be transferred to her so that she could carry the baby. This couple now has a beautiful daughter, with two special aunts, one who provided the eggs, and one who carried her. Thus, with an open attitude, and loving friends and family who are willing to help, virtually anybody can have a baby.

The laws in every state in the union clearly ensure that if the husband is living with his wife when she gets pregnant, whether the sperm came from him or not, he is the father of the child. The laws also ensure that if a woman carries her own genetic baby as a surrogate for another couple, she does not have to give it up involuntarily. Therefore, a surrogate for another couple must not be the egg donor. That is, to be a surrogate, a woman must not be the genetic mother. The laws are very consistent with what makes biological and psychological good sense. If the surrogate were also the egg donor, there would be a severe danger of psychological "bonding" conflicts, regardless of the original intent of the would-be parents and the surrogate. However, as long as the egg donor and the woman carrying the baby are different, we have never had a conflict.

One of our earliest surrogate cases was a twenty-seven-year-old woman who had a hysterectomy after experiencing severe bleeding during her previous pregnancy. The only way the doctors could save this young woman's life was to remove her uterus. Yet she had normal ovaries, and her husband had good sperm. What was the solution? As it turned out, her forty-eight-year-old mother was quite willing to serve as a surrogate uterus to carry her daughter's baby. Their menstrual cycles were synchronized with birth control pills so that day one of the mother's cycle occurred simultaneously with day one of the daughter's. The daughter was stimulated in the usual fashion for IVF, her eggs were fertilized with her husband's sperm, and her embryos were transferred into her mother's uterus. Astoundingly, the forty-eight-year-old mother became pregnant with her daughter's twins. Nine months later, she gave birth to two healthy grandchildren whom she then immediately turned over to her daughter and son-in-law.

Surrogate uterus pregnancies are here to stay; they are morally and ethically proper, and they offer an opportunity for a relative or a loved one to give the greatest gift possible to a woman without a uterus. One forty-year-old patient of ours had already gone through four cycles of IVF elsewhere and failed to get pregnant. All of her doctors recommended that she give up, but she refused. She had gone through fourteen years of infertility treatment for bilateral tubal infections and "clubbed" tubes. Women with blocked fallopian tubes caused by infection are known to have lower pregnancy rates with IVF. There are many theories to explain this, including the possibility of retained toxic fluid in the blocked tubes, or even that some permanent but subtle damage has been done to the uterus by the infection. This woman had her tubes removed just to make sure that the former was not a problem. Nonetheless, she failed to get pregnant with four IVF treatment cycles in another center and in her fifth IVF cycle with us. It was natural to attribute the fifth failure to her biological clock, since she was forty years old and pregnancy rates in forty-year-olds are quite low with IVF.

However, on the chance that her problem might be related to her history of tubal infection, her husband's cousin (who had already had five normal pregnancies and five children and whose husband was vasectomized so they could not have any more children) agreed, at age forty-two, to be a surrogate for this patient. Our forty-year-old patient had such a poor ovarian reserve by this time (after fourteen years of trying to have children, she was just about at the end of her biological clock) that we were only able to obtain two embryos. We transferred both of those embryos into her husband's cousin and warned them that the prognosis was extremely poor. Nonetheless, the cousin did become pregnant and delivered a healthy little baby girl nine months later. Despite the woman's vastly reduced ovarian reserve after so many years of unsuccessful treatment, the problem all along was simply that because of prior infection, her uterus was not receptive to implantation.

We've had many similar cases whereby the history of prior tubal disease has conferred a low pregnancy rate on couples, and after many failed attempts at pregnancy with IVF (to bypass the tubal blockage), resorting to a surrogate, who is usually a family member or close friend, solved the problem. Although removal of the fallopian tubes in these patients may improve their pregnancy rate with IVF, it often doesn't. If women who have diseased fallopian tubes don't get pregnant on their own with several cycles of IVF, using a surrogate is often a simple solution to the problem.

In some cases, it would be medically inadvisable for the patient to carry her own child, such as the Marfan's syndrome patient I discussed in detail in chapter 13. This was a woman who had a genetic disease that required her to have heart and blood vessel operations to protect her from sudden death, and who had to be on blood thinners because of these operations. A pregnancy for her would be fatal. Thus, when she got married, her mother came forward and offered to carry her babies for her. Not only was she able to safely have twins, which her mother carried (i.e., her mother carried her own grandchildren), but we were able to perform genetic diagnosis on those embryos to make sure that neither of these two babies would develop the same genetic disease that their mother had inherited from her father.

### *How Is It Done?*

Although the gestational surrogacy procedure is medically simple, I will outline the methods we use for synchronizing the cycles of the donor and recipient. This work had been going on for decades in cows before we applied it to humans. Embryos from highly prized cattle would be placed into the uterus of very-low-milk-producing cows, who would then give birth to prize heifers. Since embryos could be obtained every month, a prize cow could deliver twelve heifers a year via the uterus of surrogate cows rather than just one prize heifer a year. This vastly improved the efficiency of milk production around the world. Every time you go to the grocery store and notice how relatively inexpensive nature's most perfect food (milk) is, realize that it is partly because of these reproductive advances.

In humans, the synchronization is a little more difficult than in cows. Both women are placed on birth control pills. These pills, started at the beginning of the follicular cycle, put the women "on hold" and can be discontinued at the same time for both of them. The key factor in synchronizing the cycles of donor and recipient is that the recipient must start on progesterone injections one day after HCG is given to the donor. The purpose of synchronizing the donor and recipient is that the endometrial lining of the recipient must be at the stage of development in the monthly cycle where it is receptive to implantation of the embryo at its stage of development.

If you look at table 17.1, you will see our protocol for synchronization, whether it involves a surrogate uterus or an egg donor, two clinically opposite situations. For both of these situations, this synchronization schedule works the same. Both the donor and recipient are put on birth control pills to synchronize their cycles. The recipient also goes on Lupron so as to completely suppress her pituitary. On the first day that the donor receives gonadotropin, the recipient starts on Estrace (an oral, absorbable form of natural estrogen). The recipient's Estrace dose is six milligrams per day. Often, an estrogen patch is also used to guarantee the formation of an adequate uterine lining. The length of the artificial follicular phase during which the recipient is on Estrace and the patch is not important; the only significant factor is when she goes on progesterone. Whenever the donor receives HCG, which is often (but not always) on the tenth to twelfth day after gonadotropin has begun, the recipient starts on progesterone one day later.

TABLE 17.1

**Protocol for Synchronization of Cycles**

| | EGG DONOR'S PROTOCOL | RECIPIENT'S PROTOCOL |
|---|---|---|
| | Begin birth control pills daily between day one and day six of menses | Begin birth control pills daily between day one and day six of menses |
| | Last day of birth control pills | Last day of birth control pills |
| | Lupron 0.2 ml daily injections begin (must be on Lupron for fourteen days before gonadotropin begins) | Lupron 0.2 ml daily injections begin (must be on Lupron for a minimum of six days before beginning Estrace) |
| 1 | Lupron and gonadotropin | Lupron 0.2 ml, Estrace 6 mg, and patch |
| 2 | Lupron and gonadotropin | Lupron 0.2 ml, Estrace 6 mg, and patch |
| 3 | Lupron and gonadotropin | Lupron 0.2 ml, Estrace 6 mg, and patch |
| 4 | Lupron and gonadotropin | Lupron 0.2 ml, Estrace 6 mg, and patch |
| 5 | Lupron, ultrasound, estradiol, gonadotropin | Lupron 0.2 ml, Estrace 6 mg, and patch |
| 6 | Lupron, ultrasound, estradiol, gonadotropin | Lupron 0.2 ml, Estrace 6 mg, and patch |
| 7 | Lupron, ultrasound, estradiol, gonadotropin | Lupron 0.2 ml, Estrace 6 mg, and patch |
| 8 | Lupron, ultrasound, estradiol, gonadotropin | Lupron 0.2 ml, Estrace 6 mg, and patch |
| 9 | Lupron, ultrasound, estradiol, gonadotropin | Lupron 0.2 ml, Estrace 6 mg, and patch |
| 10 | Lupron, ultrasound, estradiol, gonadotropin | Lupron 0.2 ml, Estrace 6 mg, and patch |
| 11 | Lupron, ultrasound, estradiol, gonadotropin | Lupron 0.2 ml, Estrace 6 mg, and patch |
| 12 | Lupron, ultrasound, estradiol, HCG injection | Last day Lupron, continue Estrace 6 mg and patch. Begin progesterone injections the day after donor gets HCG. Continue Estrace 6 mg and patch. |

This always allows the synchronization to time out perfectly for embryo replacement into the recipient. Keep in mind that the donor-recipient synchronization is exactly the same whether this is a case where the recipient is a gestational surrogate carrying the baby for another woman or, in reverse, if it is a case where a donor is giving eggs to a patient who has no viable eggs of her own.

## Egg Donation (You Can Get Pregnant After Menopause)

While I have written that it is easier to get pregnant when you're younger than when you're older, and have urged women in their thirties not to delay high-tech treatment until it is too late, I'm going to turn around completely now and point out that if you do delay too long and you have run out of eggs and entered menopause, it is really not too late to have a baby. All that is needed is an egg donor, and then you can still carry your own baby in your late forties or fifties, or even sixties.

I recently saw a woman in her forties who first got pregnant seventeen years ago, and because she was not married, she had an abortion. She went on the birth control pill for ten years and finally fell in love and had a happy, stable marriage. She had been trying unsuccessfully to get pregnant in that marriage for six years. She had irregular, only occasional periods and was clearly about to go into menopause. We tried stimulating her with high doses of gonadotropin but were unable to get any eggs. When I delicately suggested the idea of giving up on her eggs and using a donor, she surprised me with her complete absence of anguish. She jumped up with excitement and told me immediately that she had in mind two or three very good friends who were in their early thirties who she felt would be happy to donate. Sometimes one can find close friends or younger sisters who are more than happy to donate an egg. However, in the majority of cases, we have to find and match egg donors for such patients.

Naturally, if you receive a donor egg, the genes of the baby will be a combination of your husband's genes and those of the woman who donates the egg, even though you will carry the baby for nine months and deliver it. What are the psychological consequences of your carrying a baby that is genetically not your own? This has been asked since 1983, when the first case of donor eggs was reported in Australia. Carrying the baby for nine months results in a solid, loving bond between the mother and the child, regardless of the genetic origin of the donated egg. This is not much different from the donor sperm situation discussed in chapter 16, except that donor eggs are even more favorable for bonding because the mother identifies with the baby (regardless of genetic origin) by carrying it. I would like to refer you back to the previous chapter, in which I talk about the issues of emotional bonding with the child, and about where the child's personality, intelligence, value system, and even athletic ability come from — genes or environment. Donor sperm is only occasionally used these days because of ICSI, and using donor sperm requires much deeper psychological preparation than using donor eggs. Donor eggs have *never* led to any problems, in our experience. I'd like to reiterate that nine months in the uterus results in solid bonding between mother and baby, even though the egg was not originally her own.

The medical world was initially shocked to hear about the first pregnancy using an embryo from a donor egg, which was achieved in a menopausal woman at Monash University in Melbourne, Australia, in 1983. Dr. Peter Lutjen, Dr. Alan Trounson, and their colleagues were the innovators of this idea. These brilliant reproductive scientists from Australia established what then seemed to be the impossible system of hormonal replacement for the menopausal woman that allowed her uterus to behave just like that of a woman in her twenties, permitting implantation of an embryo despite the fact that she had no ovaries to make the hormones that are normally necessary to sustain a pregnancy in the first three months.

Older women (late forties and fifties) have no difficulty getting pregnant so long as the donor eggs come from young women. The age of the uterus is not what is significant in the high pregnancy rate of these patients, but rather the fact that (1) the eggs come from healthy younger women, and (2) the recipient's only infertility problem is that she has run out of fertile eggs. With these two operative factors, pregnancy rate using IVF and donor eggs in menopausal women is over 50 percent, no different than what one would expect in younger women. The main determinant of pregnancy rate is the age of the woman from whom the eggs originate.

Women as old as sixty-three years of age have gotten pregnant quite easily with egg donation and have delivered healthy, happy babies. The oldest mother on record was reported by Dr. Richard Paulson in April of 1997. Dr. Paulson normally will not perform egg donation for women over fifty-five years of age, but this healthy-looking sixty-three-year-old woman successfully lied in order to get into the program. Although she was only two years away from being eligible for Medicare, she had no trouble conceiving and carrying the pregnancy normally because the eggs came, of course, from a younger woman.

Many of these older women getting pregnant with egg donation have multiple and often large fibroids in the uterus. These fibroids completely distort the uterine shape, and in prior decades, they were thought to be a cause of infertility. On the basis of the ease with which these women become pregnant with donor eggs and deliver healthy babies, it is now apparent that the vast majority of uterine fibroids, no matter how large, have no effect on a woman's fertility, and should not be overzealously operated upon. In fact, the only fibroids that should be removed for fertility are those occasional ones that protrude inside the cavity of the uterus. We have had many older patients with large uterine fibroids become pregnant with donor eggs and deliver healthy babies.

Many women in their late thirties and early forties who have run out of fertile eggs initially resist adamantly the suggestion of using donor eggs. They may insist on going through one unsuccessful IVF cycle after another, unwilling to even consider donor eggs. Eventually, years later, most of these women request donor eggs. Many of these women become like personal friends of the clinic because we come to know them so well. Despite years of negative feelings about the idea, all of them are overjoyed when they finally have a baby via donor eggs. We have had no unhappy experiences with this.

There are basically three different ways of organizing an egg donor program. One approach is with anonymous, shared egg donors. That means that younger women undergoing IVF who have extra eggs agree to give some of them to menopausal women who are on a waiting list. The recipients are placed on the appropriate estrogen and progesterone regimen to synchronize their cycles with the women who have the extra eggs to give.

The next approach is similar to that of running a sperm bank. The egg donor is paid a fee. The donor's cycle is synchronized to that of the recipient, just as with gestational surrogacy (see table 17.1). This can either be anonymous or with full disclosure. There are some possible ethical problems associated with this approach in that women are paid to undergo drug therapy and invasive follicle aspiration to donate eggs to someone they don't know and don't care about. In other words, they are taking a medical risk (however slight) simply for pay. However, with proper counseling, this has also turned out to be a very positive experience for both donor and recipient.

For example, a fifty-year-old patient from an Asian country needed egg donation. In addition, her husband required a TESE procedure to find the very few sperm that were being produced in his testicles. Obviously, finding an appropriately matched egg donor for her would have been very difficult using anonymous, shared oocytes from the pool of patients coming through an IVF center. However, using an agency dedicated to searching for young egg donors and doing appropriate screening and psychological evaluation, we were able to locate the perfect match for her. The recipient, of course, had to pay for all of the donor's expenses, plus legal and agency fees. But this cost was still far less than that incurred for adoption. These wonderful people are now happy parents despite being discouraged by their doctors at home from ever trying to have a baby, because she had no eggs and they thought he had no sperm.

A third approach is for patients to search among their younger friends or relatives for someone who is willing to donate an egg, to make all the legal arrangements privately with them, and then to go through a screening and counseling evaluation. This is a nonanonymous program, and no one is being paid — the gift is being made as an act of love.

Our first egg donation case, in the mideighties, prompted consternation by some administrators and "ethicists" who feared the future, but egg donation was endorsed enthusiastically by the patients, their doctors, their parents and grandparents, and even by the clergymen who represented the patients. A twenty-eight-year-old woman had lost both of her ovaries as a teenager because of surgery for benign ovarian cysts. Her twenty-four-year-old sister had always felt sorry and guilty that she would be able to have children, and her older sister would not. She and her family brought up the idea of egg donation, and despite some concern and trepidation, it felt right to me. This was the beginning of what has been one of the most personally and emotionally rewarding aspects of my medical practice. The sister with no ovaries conceived healthy twins who are now grown and happy young women, who might not exist today if we had reacted negatively to this unusual-sounding first request.

A year later, we were challenged once again to ponder the ethics of an even more complicated patient request. A forty-year-old woman, who was a very prominent lawyer, had run out of eggs and was married to an equally prominent lawyer who had no sperm. They were real experts on family law. They desperately wanted a child and preferred to preserve the genetic lines of their families. He had one younger sister, and she had one brother. Her brother offered to donate sperm, and his sister offered to donate eggs. Thus, the embryos generated by his brother-in-law's donated sperm and her sister-in-law's donated eggs allowed them to continue their family line, and still avoid consanguinity.

I was confronted years ago by a nurse who had gone through early menopause and was now forty-two years old and who strongly wanted to have a child with her husband, knowing full well that it would require donor eggs. Yet she was very intellectually bothered by the idea of bringing technology into the process of getting pregnant. She was a very deep and New Age spiritual person who feared the mingling of technology and conception. I remember telling her to read *Zen and the Art of Motorcycle Maintenance.* She was surprised that a conservative physician would have even read such a book, but our bond of trust as doctor and patient was immediately sealed. She and her husband now have a gorgeous and intelligent daughter, and it matters not to her or her husband that the conception was the result of technology.

The egg donor does not necessarily have to be young. Many years ago we saw a forty-three-year-old extremely successful businesswoman from the West Coast who had gone through several failed IVF cycles. She had a relatively good ovarian reserve for her age (eight eggs retrieved in previous unsuccessful IVF cycles in her home city). Her sister was forty-two years old and looked just like her. They suggested that we stimulate them both simultaneously for IVF and use all of the eggs retrieved, both from the patient and from her sister. She did not care which eggs resulted in the baby, hers or her sister's, and her husband did not care either. They just wanted to maximize their chance for pregnancy despite her age and her sister's age by using all of their combined eggs for her IVF cycle. As it turned out, we got eight eggs from her and nine eggs from her sister. She became pregnant and delivered a healthy baby. She has no idea if it came from her egg or her sister's egg, and she couldn't care less.

### *How Is It Done?*

We need to talk further about the technical aspects of (1) synchronizing the cycles of the donor and the recipient, and (2) giving the proper hormone replacement to recipients so that their uterus is prepared for implantation of the embryo and also to maintain the pregnancy until the placenta starts making its own hormones by eight to twelve weeks. Once again, you should look at table 17.1, because the protocol is virtually no different for surrogate uterus cases than for egg donation cases.

The difference is that in the surrogate uterus case, the recipient is not the patient but rather the helper, and in the egg donation case, the recipient is the patient and the donor is the helper. The only other difference in the protocol is that if the recipient is truly menopausal, she does not need to be placed on birth control pills or Lupron, because she is simply not making hormones at all. She would begin Estrace, however, on the same day that you see on the cycle chart (table 17.1) in this chapter. It is all timed with the same goal in mind — that the recipient's uterus is properly primed with estrogen, and that the recipient begins taking progesterone injections in addition to the estrogen one day after the donor receives her HCG injection. This ensures that the IVF transfer will be performed at the point in the cycle when the window of receptivity for egg implantation is open. Between day four and day six of progesterone replacement is when the day-three embryo must be placed into the uterus.

Even after it is clear that you are pregnant, you will have to stay on estrogen and progesterone supplements for up to twelve weeks longer, until the normal time in pregnancy when the placenta takes over the function of the ovary and produces all of its own self-sustaining estrogen and progesterone. This may require considerably less than twelve weeks, and the latest data indicate that by six weeks (contrary to our previous thinking) the placenta may be making enough estrogen and progesterone to sustain the pregnancy. This can be determined via weekly blood tests for estrogen and progesterone levels, and when the progesterone level begins to rise dramatically over what we know you're getting from replacement, then we know the placenta has taken over and hormone replacement is no longer needed. However, most infertility physicians, including me, feel better if you stay on the estrogen and progesterone for a full three months, just to be safe.

I thought nothing could shock me anymore until I came across a case that I have discussed in great detail with many physicians only for its theoretical interest. I do many operations for young boys and men with very high, undescended testicles. This surgery requires opening up the abdomen, dividing the blood vessels supplying these abdominal testicles, and reconnecting them microsurgically to the blood vessels closer to the scrotum. This is a so-called testicle autotransplant for men born with testicles inside the abdomen (where the ovaries are normally found in a woman). The goal is to transfer the testicles to the scrotum so that they can function properly. When I operated on one such patient many years ago, I was astounded to find an extraordinarily rare congenital abnormality. This man had a completely normal uterus, fallopian tubes, and upper vagina located within his abdomen. Nonetheless, he also had normal testicles, vas deferens, prostate gland, and penis typical of a normal genetic male. Of course, we brought the testicles down into the scrotum so that they would be able to function and make sperm normally. However, it would have been possible for this otherwise normal man to become pregnant. This particular case was the source for *Junior,* the famous Arnold Schwarzenegger movie about a man getting pregnant.

As the movie goes, he could have been placed on female hormones and used his sperm to fertilize, via ICSI, his wife's eggs. The resultant embryos could then be placed into his fallopian tubes, and he could become pregnant. Obviously, this would never be considered by us, but this rare case made for a great movie based on a true possibility.

The only reason I bring up this fascinating case is to point out that as long as there is a uterus, a woman can become pregnant despite having no ovary whatsoever. Also, as long as there is an ovary, even if she has no uterus, her eggs can be used to get a friend or relative pregnant with her baby. There are thus very few couples, no matter how severe their problem (if they have open minds), who can't have a healthy baby through the use of reproductive technology.

CHAPTER 18

# The Controversy over IVF, Cloning, and Stem Cells

We are all healthy carriers of at least ten (out of thousands of possible) lethal autosomal-recessive genetic diseases, like cystic fibrosis, Tay-Sachs, muscular dystrophy, etc. The reason so few of our offspring have these autosomal-recessive diseases is the very low chance that any two of us will be carriers of the same disease. Thus, our children will also be carriers of many different genetic diseases, but statistically they are very unlikely to marry someone who is a carrier of any of those same genetic diseases. But some do, and that is how genetically diseased children come to be born.

Now that the entire human gene sequence has been determined, young married couples can have their blood tested for all of the many hundreds or thousands of diseases for which they may be genetic carriers. This is already being done for Tay-Sachs disease for all Jewish married couples of Eastern European origin. If two people are carriers for the same genetic disease, the only safe way for them to have children will be to go through IVF and embryo biopsy regardless of whether or not they are infertile. My prediction is that as molecular biology methods become simpler and easier to perform, this approach will become the major arena for the future of disease prevention.

I don't see this ever becoming a problem of eugenics, i.e., of parents trying to have "super" genetic offspring. Here is the reason for my optimism: What we're discovering is that we can find all the various genes for basic bodily needs that, if defective, will result in disease. But claims for finding genes that affect levels of intelligence, personality, or even athletic ability are simply a fantasy. The concept of the existence of such genes is not borne out at all by our extensive experience with genetics, or with egg or sperm donation. We can find many specific genes whose absence produces a specific terrible disease, but no specific genes for intelligence, character, or athleticism. Our genes provide us with a physical home, but our genes are not what we really are.

We have observed that children who are born to infertile couples are much more competent physically, mentally, and emotionally than the norm, undoubtedly a consequence of the fact that they were wanted so very much. They are not the casual result of a moment of infatuated romance. We have observed carefully, with follow-up interviewing, often many years later, thousands of offspring from our infertile patients. The findings are consistent and obvious. The development of competent children who will become competent adults appears to relate to their emotional and physical interaction with everybody in their immediate environment during the first several years of life. This early cognitive imprinting is really what helps develop who we are. With the exception of specific genetic diseases, genes have very little to do with who we are and what we become. If genes really have little to do with who we are and what we become, then why has there been such extensive coverage in the press over the possibility of cloning?

## Cloning

### *Exposing the Hype*

The world was changed greatly on February 27, 1997, when a historic scientific paper by Dr. Ian Wilmut and Dr. Keith Campbell, from Scotland, appeared in the prestigious scientific journal *Nature.* Dr. Wilmut was able to take an adult cell from the mammary gland of a sheep, inject it into an enucleated egg of another sheep, and produce a genetically identical copy of the "donor" adult sheep, i.e., a clone (see fig. 18.1). Until this time, cloning was only considered a science-fiction speculation, the basis of some humorous movies, as well as the bloodcurdling movie *The Boys from Brazil,* in which the archvillain, Adolf Hitler, was cloned. However, nobody really took cloning seriously until Professor Wilmut's extraordinary paper in 1997. There has been enormous and frankly misleading hype about both cloning and stem cells (inextricably related) from scientists looking for funding, politicians looking for votes, and journalists looking for copy. In this chapter I will try to clarify the confusion for you and set things straight.

The genetic material in each one of our ten trillion cells is identical

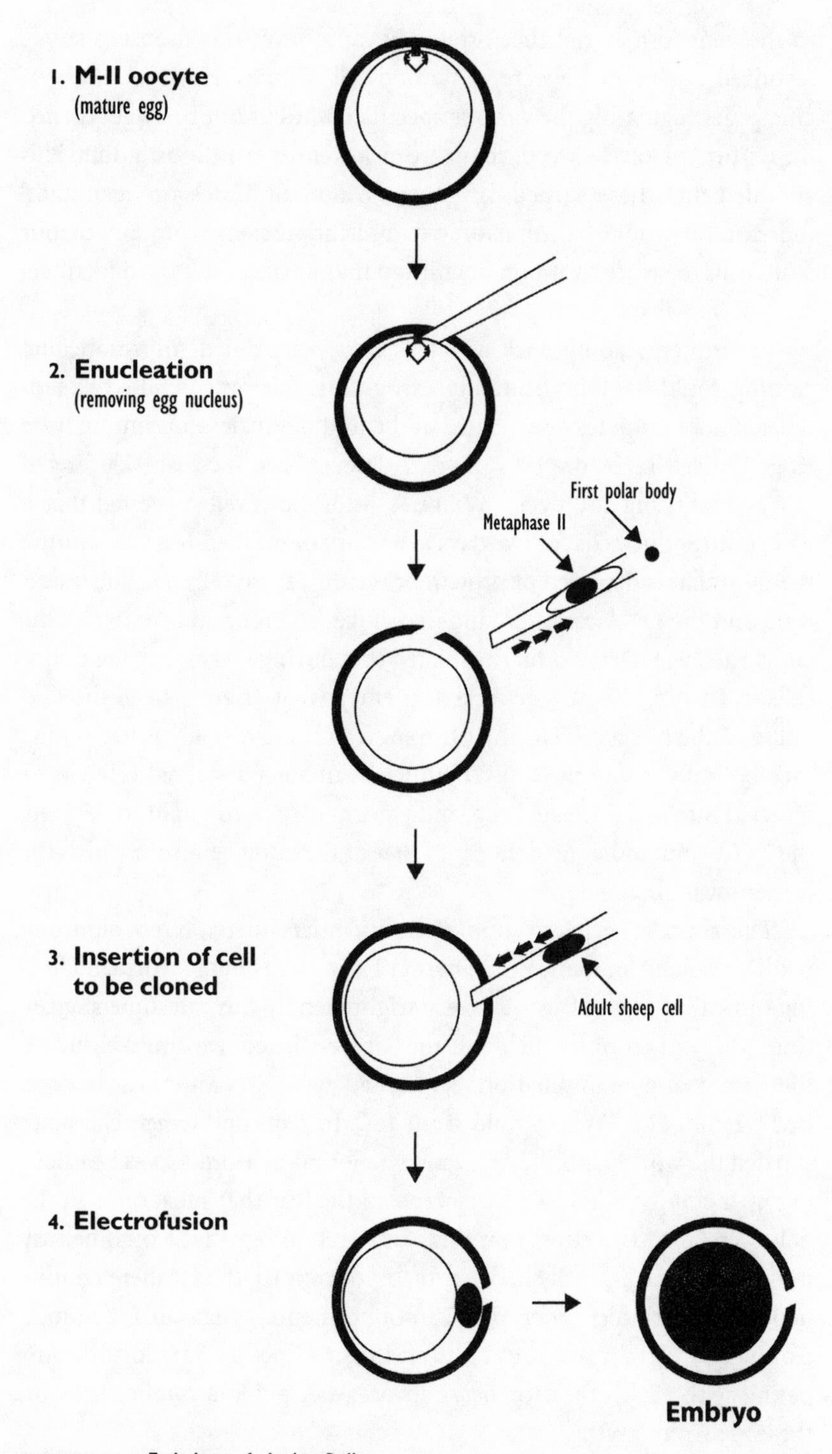


FIGURE 18.1. Technique of cloning Dolly.

to the genetic material that originally came from our mother's single fertilized egg when we were just a one-cell embryo. However, the specific genes regulating the various specific tissues of our body get turned on or turned off as we develop from an embryo into an adult. It is assumed that these turned-off genes do not turn back on again, and therefore, it would be impossible to use the nucleus from any of our adult cells to create a totipotent embryo that would result in an identical copy of ourselves.

Experiments going back as far as fifty years did demonstrate that cloning could be done from adult frogs, but this only resulted in tadpoles. Those tadpoles always died and could never develop into mature frogs. Otherwise, before 1997, there had never been successful cloning of any animal using adult cells. Wilmut's study, however, suggested that if you culture adult cells for five days in a "starvation" medium (i.e., culture medium that is deprived of protein or serum), these cells become quiescent, and the DNA can then undergo epigenetic reprogramming by the enucleated egg. Dr. Wilmut postulated that during starvation, the donor cells exit from the growth cycle and enter what scientists call the G-0 phase of the cell cycle. During this phase, nothing actually is happening metabolically inside the cell. The nucleus of such a starved cell can be inserted into an enucleated egg, and a normal embryo ought to develop, the DNA content being identical to that of the adult cell from which the nucleus was obtained.

This concept seems so simple, and the microinjection techniques so readily available in many of the best IVF programs in the world, including ours, that most of us were very frightened by this awesome suggestion. Many of us in the field felt that, if we wished, we could easily do these very same manipulations on human eggs with adult human cells. But we thought, "Who would want to?" In fact, one fringe character startled the world with the announcement that he would soon be opening up a cloning clinic. This exacerbated the fear that most of us in the field were already feeling, that this was a technology that would be easy to institute, and ethically had terrible implications. In fact there continued to be periodic apocryphal announcements of successful human cloning, by certain religious cults and fringe doctors ferociously competing with each other for news coverage. A gullible public feeds on these recurrent myths.

Yet in Dr. Campbell and Dr. Wilmut's original paper in 1997, the clone, Dolly, was the only successfully cloned lamb out of 277 attempts. Everyone thought they had found the key to making cloning work, that it would just be a matter of time before the procedure became more efficient, and that greater and greater numbers of sheep and other animals would be cloned. However, the fact remains that although cloning has been extended to cows, mice, pigs, cats, and other animals, literally *thousands* of cloning attempts have to be made in any experimental species ever studied before even *one* viable clone is born. There are high rates of miscarriage, as well as stillbirths, in those animals that do become pregnant. Furthermore, most of the few live births die in the first week of life from a variety of congenital abnormalities. Even the health of Dolly is in question, since she died from a severe lung disease at only six years of age, which is very young for a sheep (and in fact that was the age of the adult whose cells were used in the experiment to actually make Dolly). Her adult donor lived a normal life span even though Dolly herself did not. In all animals in whom cloning has ever been attempted, the success rates have been dismal, and the abnormalities extensive. Thus, no legitimate scientists can really imagine any attempt, or any reason for an attempt, to clone humans.

However, this has not stopped publicity seekers and entrepreneurs from engaging in one wild and unsupported announcement after another, claims that the press, until recently, has been only too ready to uncritically proliferate. In fact, one bioethicist who is actually procloning calls this the "media manipulation fraud of the century." Scientists know that any attempt at reproductive cloning of humans would result in a vast amount of pain and suffering because of fetal abnormalities, miscarriages, and only the remotest chance it would be successful in a rare case. It is therefore a clear matter of understanding among all scientists and doctors that this would be completely unacceptable human experimentation, based on all the preliminary data on failure and fetal abnormalities found in cloning experiments in animals.

Reproductive cloning is not what scientists are interested in anyway. Scientists are interested in the possibility of using cloning technology, as well as stem cells, to cure diseases of cellular insufficiency, such as diabetes, Parkinson's, bone-marrow deficiencies, and even certain forms of Alzheimer's-type senile dementia.

Most people find it unthinkable that an individual would want to see him- or herself reflected in another human being who is an identical copy. But in truth, if cloning were ever to be performed in humans, it would not result in the replication of an identical human being, but rather the delayed birth of an identical twin. Each human being is unique and different despite genetic similarity. The possibility of cloning humans, were it ever to be safe and medically reasonable, is as frightening to society as was Charles Darwin, who forced his contemporaries to take a completely new look at the creation of humans. In reality, Darwin did not threaten religion at all, and the technology of cloning stem cells would not threaten humanity. As Ian Wilmut said in 1997, "It doesn't have anything to do with creating copies of human beings. . . . I just want to understand things." The search for truth and the development of medical technology has never been a threat to our essential humanity, nor to our deepest religious convictions.

It was ludicrous to scientists and physicians that the national bioethics advisory committee hearing in December 2000 invited quacks and cultists to stir up absurd hype about cloning. It was a circus (paid for with taxpayer dollars) of a debate between scientists who really understood cloning and stem cell technology, and religious cult leaders and radical publicity seekers pretending to be on an equal intellectual level. It was like an unruly courtroom, but with no rules of evidence. The religious cult leaders talked about a man whose son was killed and who wanted the tissue of his son cloned so he could have his son back. Another was a retired physicist, who had no experience in either IVF or cloning technology, who was using this as a way of gaining recognition that he never had in his own field. Another was a European fringe fertility physician wishing to gain publicity to bring more patients to his clinic.

Why were political authorities so willing to sponsor, at taxpayers' expense, such a silly debate between legitimate scientists on one hand and cultists on the other? My guess is that it's not because politicians are that concerned about the obvious unacceptability of such a dangerous procedure medically, with all the suffering and misery that would result in abnormal births and miscarriages, or the false promises of immortalization and bringing back a dead son. In fact, the delayed birth of an identical twin (which is all that cloning really would be) is not equivalent to the danger of proliferation of nuclear weapons or biological warfare. It is not akin to the specter of widespread terrorism, which is readily possible in a complex society where weapons of mass destruction are so incredibly cheap and polarized hatred so ever present. The reason for the fear of cloning is not the fear of bad results. The fear is that cloning might work, requiring us to become philosophically introspective and possibly changing our vision of who we are.

In view of the emotional powder keg that cloning and stem cell technology has become, I'll try now to give you an objective rundown of how this science has progressed in the last half century, since the first frog was cloned in 1952. I will demonstrate how the technology we are currently applying cannot lead to "designer babies," but how the technology can someday help cure devastating diseases. Furthermore, if you are an infertility patient who requires IVF, you will need to understand this technology so that you can be aware of the possible implications of your having extra embryos frozen and saved for you as a result of your IVF procedure.

### *How Cloning Developed*

Embryo reconstruction by the transfer of a donor nucleus from an adult to an enucleated egg was first proposed in 1938 by a scientist named Spemann. He wondered whether the nuclei of cells change during the development of an early embryo when what start out as uniform-appearing cells differentiate into an enormous variety of different types of cells. The point of Spemann's suggested study in 1938 was to transfer the nuclei of cells at increasingly advanced stages of an embryo to determine at what stage the potential of the cells to develop into differentiating tissues becomes restricted. This experiment was actually first accomplished in 1952 by Briggs, King, and Martin, who used frogs. Their studies (strictly limited to frogs) were not used to clone an adult frog into another adult frog. That was impossible, and the notion that frogs could be cloned in that way became a popular myth. However, what they did demonstrate is that you could clone a normal fertile adult frog by injecting the nucleus of an early frog embryo (at the blastocyst stage) into a frog egg. That egg would develop into a completely normal adult frog, which was an identical clone of the adult produced by the embryo from which the donor cell was obtained.

In other words, you could not take cells from an adult frog, inject them into an enucleated frog egg, and have, as a result, a healthy cloned adult frog. However, you could take the cell from a very early frog embryo and use the nucleus of that cell to make a clone of that embryo.

The nuclei from later-stage embryos (or from an adult) proved to have no developmental potential. Thus, it was believed by legitimate scientists working in the field that although cells of early embryos are totipotential and could be used for cloning, any cells from later-stage embryos, or adults, were considered so differentiated that their nuclei could not possibly be used to clone a new individual.

However, in 1975 it was finally shown, again only in frogs, that a nucleus transferred from an adult skin cell could be injected into an egg and result in what appeared to be normal embryo development. But this embryo completely arrested at the juvenile tadpole stage and never grew into an adult frog. Frogs were popular for these studies because their eggs were so big, and they were much simpler reproductively than mammals, like mice and sheep. Thus, the thinking until the latter 1990s, the era of Dolly, was that frogs were peculiar in the animal kingdom in that they could be successfully cloned from embryo cells and even occasionally from adult cells, but those adult-cell clones would never result in a viable offspring that could grow into a normal adult. But none of these even moderately successful cloning experiments in frogs could be repeated in higher animals. In the mid-1980s it was widely held by leading scientists that the cloning of mammals (such as mice, dogs, cattle, or humans) by simple nuclear transfer was biologically impossible.

McGrath and Solter, of the renowned Wistar Institute in Philadelphia, stated in 1984, "It is now possible to address the question of why nuclei of early mouse embryos are unable to support development while nuclei from much older amphibian [frog] embryos are able to do so." Early embryo development from fertilization of the egg, up to the eight-cell stage (day three), is independent of the genes of the embryo and completely dependent upon the genes of the egg (from the mother). Genes of the embryo do not take over until the embryo is eight cells. Up until that time, embryo development is being directed by the genes coming from the mother. It was believed in 1984 that frogs and lower animals were different. But that is not true. We now know that the transfer from maternal genome to embryonic genome occurs at the eight-cell stage in humans as well as in most mammalian and lower species, and that frogs were actually easier animals to work with in the early days only because the eggs were so big compared to the eggs of mammals. In fact, the same problems are incurred in cloning frogs as in all other animals, and not a single adult frog has ever been developed from an adult frog cell. Thus, there was no reported cloning of an adult from another adult in any amphibians, reptiles, or mammals prior to the paper on Dolly in 1997.

In that initial experiment, it required 277 nuclear transfers to have a birth of a single normal cloned lamb (from an adult cell) that matured into an apparently normal adult. In contrast, four live lambs resulted from nuclei of embryo cells that were injected into 385 eggs, and two lambs were born from injection of fetal fibroblast cells into enucleated eggs. Thus, very similar to the study in frogs, success rates with cloning were always extremely low, with many abnormal embryos, many miscarriages, many stillbirths, and only a few live, apparently healthy animals. But the success rate was slightly higher (although still dismal) when either fetal or embryo cells were used as the nuclear source, rather than cells from adult animals.

All cells in your body have what's called a cell cycle. A cell goes from what is called the G-0/G-1 in the early phase (resting), just after cell division, to then synthesizing protein, usually over the course of twelve to twenty-six hours. It is in the early resting phase just after cell division that cloning is possible. Then it once again divides its DNA and replicates itself. After a certain number of divisions, most cells die and cannot divide any further. Stem cells are cells that are continuously replicating, almost eternally, so as to maintain a continued supply of whatever tissue cells are needed. Some types of tissue are rapidly turning over new cells on a daily basis, such as your stomach and intestines, your skin, and your blood cells. These tissues are in a continuous state of wear-and-tear usage and require a great deal of rejuvenation. A good example of this cell turnover is the "healing" that occurs when you have a cut on your hand, or a surgical incision. Fibroblasts and angioblasts move into the open area of a cut, proliferate rapidly, and ultimately form a mature scar that binds together the divided sides of the wound. In a similar manner, the red blood cells that are constantly supplying oxygen to all parts of your body are continuously being broken down and replaced by new red blood cells coming from your bone marrow. The same is true of your white blood cells, which fight infection. Your skin is always wearing down and is being replaced by new cells underneath the skin's surface. The wear and tear occurring in your intestines, as your food travels through, requires frequent replacement of the lining cells of the intestine in the same fashion.

Other cells of the body replicate much more slowly, or don't appear to replicate at all. It is these slowly replicating or nonreplicating cells that a team of doctors from Honolulu utilized to go beyond the early Dolly experiments by cloning mice, the most respected of all experimental animals for understanding mammalian biology and human disease. Dr. Yanagimachi's team in Honolulu had decided that understanding the mystery of healthy and unhealthy embryo development required that cloning be achievable in the mouse model. The mouse, with its rapid reproductive cycle (twenty days), can result in so many generations in such a short time that it is the standard animal for trying to study and understand human disease, much more so than the sheep or any other domestic livestock animal. Yanagimachi decided to try to clone mice not by starving cells into quiescence (the Wilmut approach), but rather by starting with cells that are intrinsically quiescent, i.e., that exhibit little cellular turnover or replication in the adult.

### *The Biology of Cloning*

Despite the high profile of nuclear transfer in mammals, the basic cell biology in this cloning process is not well understood. Initially, it was believed that as early embryo cells develop and begin to differentiate into various types of tissue, the totipotency of the nucleus is lost forever. Nonetheless, the occasional cloning success shows that some differentiated cells can regain their totipotency, and their nuclei can repeat all the developmental events initiated in the fertilized egg. This works better with the nuclei of embryo or fetal cells, in that a greater number of healthy, live offspring are produced by nuclear transfer involving embryo or fetal cells than adult cells. It makes sense: These "younger" nuclei are likely to be less differentiated. But what is actually happening to dedifferentiate any of these cells, whether embryonic or adult, is very poorly understood. The original and incorrect thinking was that adult cells that no longer divide, such as neurons (your brain cells or nerve cells), would be poor candidates for use in cloning, whereas cells that continually divide (such as your skin cells) would be good candidates. But the studies of Dolly show that the opposite is true. Forcing cells to be quiescent, to stop their metabolism, and to slow down, by reducing the protein content of the culture medium, seems to enhance the possibility of nuclear reprogramming.

Therefore, when the Honolulu group decided to use mice, they chose nuclei from adult cells that have intrinsically very low, if any, turnover, without "forcing them to slow down by nutritional deprivation." The three adult cells they studied were Sertoli cells (the supporting cells of the testicular tubules), neurons (brain cells), and cumulus cells (the cells that surround and nourish the ovulated egg). These three types of adult cells (like the adult cells in the Dolly experiment that went into the G-0/G-1 cycle phase via culture in a protein-deficient medium) are known always to be in the G-0 phase in the normal adult. All of these cells were used immediately for injecting adult nuclei into enucleated eggs of mice, with no prior in vitro culturing or any other prior manipulation.

In July 1998, approximately a year and a half after Wilmut's historical paper, Yanagimachi's group published their results in *Nature* (see fig. 18.2). Using adult Sertoli cells from the testes, they were able to get embryos to develop 40 percent of the time, but less than 1 percent developed into a fetus and none of them survived. Using neurons from the adult brain, they were able to obtain cloned embryos approximately 20 percent of the time, but again, less than 1 percent developed to a fetus and none survived. Using the nucleus from cumulus-cells, i.e., the cells that surround the mature ovulated egg and nourish it (the female counterpart to the male testicular Sertoli cell), out of a total of eight hundred cloned embryos that resulted from an adult cumulus-cell injection, only seventeen fetuses developed, and ten females survived to birth and were apparently healthy. This means that only about 1 percent of normal-appearing cloned embryos in these mouse studies using a specific type of adult cell (the cumulus cell) survived into normal adulthood. Similarly, in a third study, Yanagimachi reported that 5 out of almost 300 such embryos developed into normal females, again slightly over 1 percent.

These few healthy-appearing cloned mice were in turn cloned with the same technique for six further generations, always using the cumulus cell as the adult nucleus. The success rate declined with each subsequent generation. In one of the strains of mice, in fact, they could not clone beyond the fourth generation, and in the other strains studied, the success rate dramatically declined with each generation until in the sixth generation there was only 1 out of 1,000 that developed into a healthy live mouse.

The most fascinating but understated aspect of this monumental study of mouse cloning in Honolulu was that they could only clone females. In fact, up to that point it was absolutely impossible to clone

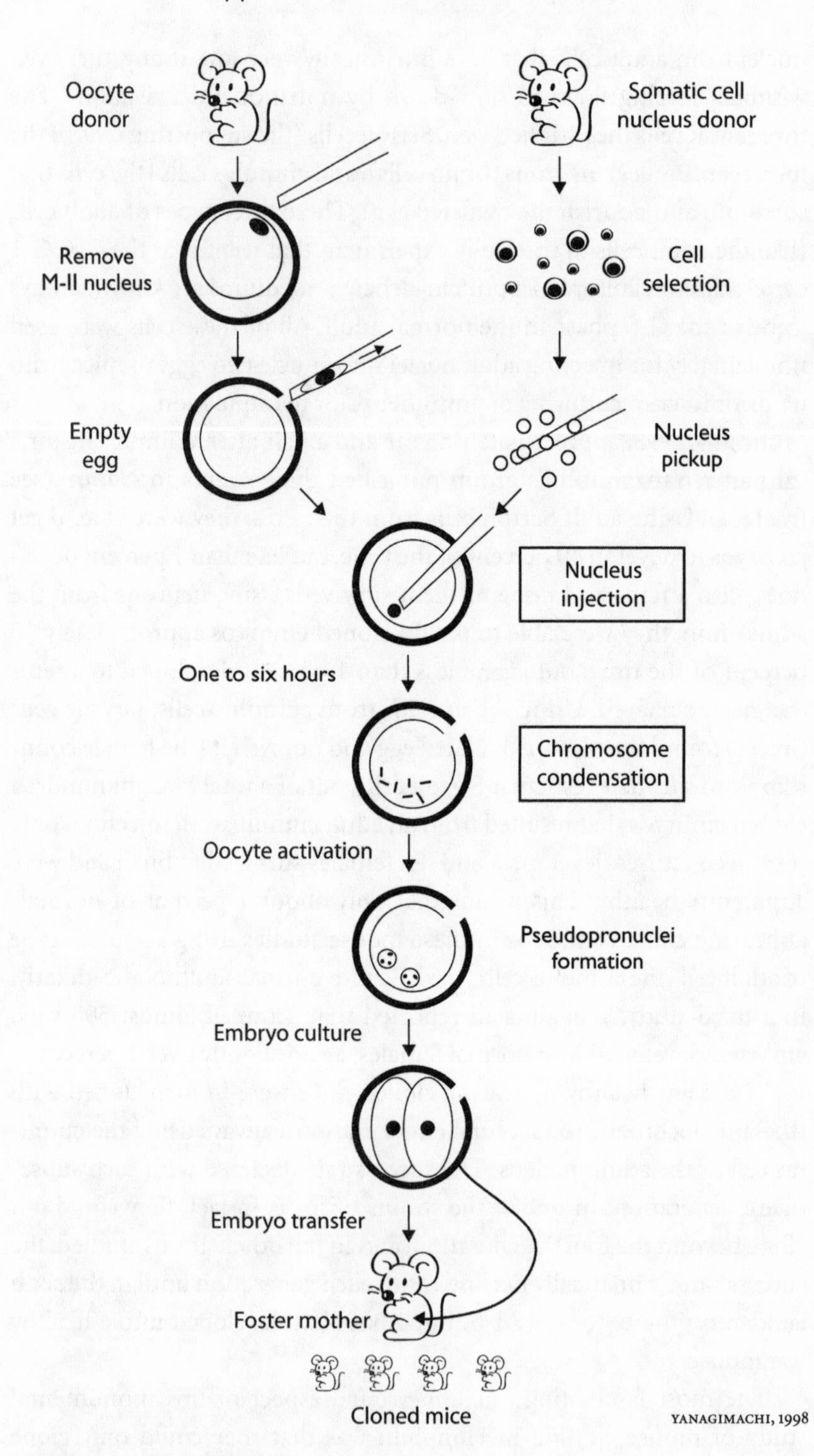


**FIGURE 18.2.** Cloning of mouse.

males. Dolly was, of course, a female, and the only adult cells that seemed capable of reprogramming in Wilmut and Campbell's study were cells that originated from the female reproductive tract. Remember, even Dolly came from the breast cells of a pregnant ewe.

Up until the end of 1999, none of the cloning experiments using adult somatic cells either in the sheep, the mouse, or the cow had utilized adult male cells. All of the cells that were successful in cloning, such as mammary gland cells, cumulus cells, or ovuductal cells, came from the female reproductive system, raising the question of whether males could be cloned at all from adult cells. This was accomplished with great difficulty by an amazing tour de force, once again by the Honolulu group. Yanagimachi's team used the same technique for enucleation of metaphase-II eggs that he had already described, and the only difference now was that instead of trying neurons, Sertoli cells, or cumulus cells, he used cells that were cut from the tail tips of the mice, dispersed and cultured for one week under standard conditions, and then cultured for three to five days in a protein-poor medium. Just like in the Dolly study, he starved these cells into quiescence. Although roughly half of these injected eggs developed into embryos, only 3 out of 274 (1 percent) developed to full delivery, but two of those three died within one hour of birth. The one remaining male mouse baby developed into a normal, fertile adult male. Out of more than seven hundred cloning attempts using male mouse tail-tip cells, one male (0.14 percent) was obtained. Although there were many pregnancies, there was a high rate of abortion throughout the pregnancy, a high stillbirth rate, and frequent perinatal deaths, indicating that nuclear reprogramming in the vast majority of cases was not normal.

The Honolulu team (as well as Wilmut) had shown that contrary to the previous dogma, mammals could be reproductively cloned from adult somatic cells, but the extremely low success rate, as well as the failure to achieve this with the use of most adult cells, nonetheless indicated that there were many regulatory differentiating factors and developmental checkpoints about which we hadn't a clue. We still did not understand very well what causes a cell to differentiate and to dedifferentiate or how to control it. There had to be myriad other processes occurring that we did not understand which led to poor embryo development, miscarriage, and stillbirths. The actual success rate for reproductive cloning is so low as to make it preposterous, from a medical point of view, to even conceive of doing this in humans, regardless of one's ethical views about the morality or immorality of DNA replication in a subsequent individual.

Thus, the proper scientific message to take home from the cloning experiments in animals is that we need to learn much more about DNA in adult cells. Through such basic knowledge, perhaps we will eventually understand DNA replication, both abnormal and normal, enough to deal better with cancer, aging, degenerative diseases, and various genetic illnesses. But the notion that it would be easy to perform cloning, at least at the time of this writing, remains naive.

However, there is one aspect to cloning that is much more exciting than the absurd goal of trying to create a genetic copy of an adult animal. That is the concept of therapeutic cloning, which is inextricably tied to the issue of stem cells. I will conclude this chapter with a section on stem cells so that you can understand the full circle we're now traversing. With PGD via IVF you can avoid the transfer of a genetically diseased or defective embryo. You can select out the few embryos that are actually healthy and thereby dramatically reduce the risk of having a severely handicapped child, something all mothers fear. PGD simply means picking the healthy embryos for replacement, and not replacing the diseased ones. Using stem cell technology, the possibility exists for actually curing, with gene therapy, a person or embryo that already has a genetic disease.

## Stem Cells

You have undoubtedly heard a lot about stem cells, and are aware of the political furor, but you probably don't really understand (nor do most people who argue about stem cells) what they are all about. In the rest of this chapter, I will try to explain this in a simple way. First, since 1981, when stem cells were first cultured in mice, they have been critical for studying (in mice) human genetic diseases. Second, stem cells play an integral role in the future for curing genetic diseases. The concept of using stem cells, whether adult or embryonic, to cure disease, by trying to get undifferentiated pluripotent cells to differentiate into healthy replacement tissue, is the exact opposite of cloning. With cloning, differentiated adult tissue cells are made to become totipotential, or undifferentiated, so that their DNA can direct, all over again, development of a new embryo. In other words, cloning and stem cells go hand in hand but function in reverse directions.

The stem cell revolution actually began quietly in 1981 with a relatively unobtrusive paper by Evans and Kaufman, from Cambridge, England, in the journal *Nature.* The title of the paper was "Establishment in Culture of Pluripotential Cells from Mouse Embryos." They utilized techniques that were originally used in 1975 at the Wistar Institute in Philadelphia, developed, ironically, by the same doctors who had stated categorically that mammals could never be cloned. Evans and Kaufman used early embryos from mice to culture indefinitely from them cells that were virtually immortal and could differentiate at any time into nonembryonic adult tissue.

Normally, during the first five days after fertilization, the embryo divides into two cells, four cells, eight cells, sixteen cells, etc., and eventually becomes a ball of cells called the morula on day four. By day five, this ball of cells has formed a liquid-interior cystlike structure, and is called a blastocyst. The blastocyst consists of a circumferential perimeter of cells called the trophectoderm (which will eventually become the placenta of the pregnancy), and a small glob of cells stuck to the inside of this wall, which is called the inner cell mass, or ICM. The ICM cells will go on to develop into the embryo proper, and the outer trophectoderm cells will develop into the placenta. The placenta works perfectly fine even if there are all kinds of chromosomal abnormalities in the cells, but the inner cell mass must be chromosomally normal in order to develop into a viable fetus.

Evans and Kaufman took the ICM cells from mouse embryos (blastocysts) and did what no one else had been able to do in the past. They maintained them in their undifferentiated stage of development in a culture system that allowed a perpetual replication of these cells without letting them differentiate into adult cells (see fig. 18.3). A "stem cell" is simply a type of cell that can replicate indefinitely and not develop the characteristics of any specific tissue. Its only job is to replicate over and over again, shedding off daughter cells that can differentiate into specific tissue. Previous attempts to obtain cultures of these pluripotential cells directly from the mouse embryo had been unsuccessful, even though there was always a very transient appearance in culture of healthy stem cells. Whenever attempts had been made to obtain immortal pluripotential stem cell lines from the mouse embryo inner cell mass, the embryonic cells would automatically skip the stem cell stage and differentiate into mature but disorganized adult tissue or into tumors.

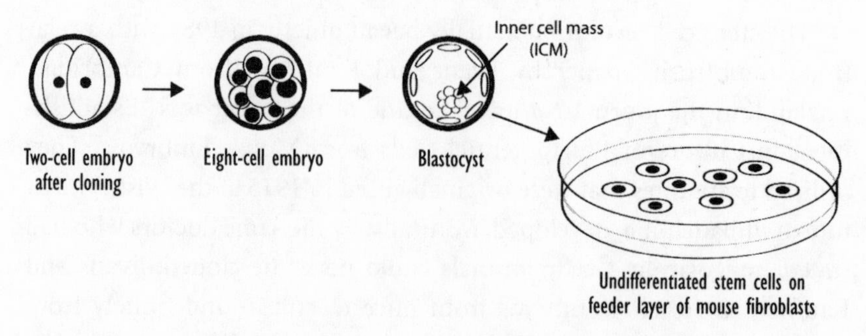


**FIGURE 18.3.** Production of stem cells from inner cell mass of cloned mouse embryo.

There is still a very poor understanding of why Evans and Kaufman were successful, but they found out that ICM cells obtained from the early mouse embryo had to be cultured on a monolayer of mouse scar-tissue cells (i.e., fibroblasts) in order to become immortal stem cells. These mouse scar-tissue cells had to be treated with a poison called mitomycin so that they could not proliferate themselves but could produce some sort of unknown byproducts that inhibit the differentiation of the ICM cells. As soon as these stem cells were removed from this so-called feeder layer of mouse embryonic fibroblasts, they would automatically differentiate in a disorganized way into a variety of cell types. If injected into mouse tissue, they developed into tumors called teratomas. For more than twenty years no one has really understood this obscure finding. It had been hoped that a substance called leukemia-inhibiting factor (LIF) was the magic ingredient that prevented these ICM cells from developing into differentiated adult tissue and that allowed them to eternally replicate as stem cells, but this was later shown not to be valid. Stem cells derived from embryos stop being stem cells (and will usually differentiate into tumors with a variety of tissue types) if they are not inhibited from doing so by being cultured on a layer of mouse fibroblasts, and no one can explain why.

### *Knockout Mice*

The major use of stem cells has been to study human genetic disease in the mouse. Over 98 percent of human genes are represented by very similar homologous genes in the mouse. Some molecular biologists have jokingly said that we are more than 98 percent mouse, as well as about 40 percent earthworm. This is because throughout the animal kingdom the basic genes necessary for life are replicated in every organism. Our basic system as mammals was built upon earlier reptilian and amphibian gene structures, with only relatively minor modifications resulting in mammals and, ultimately, primates and human beings. Thus, almost any gene that has been identified as defective in a specific human disease has a counterpart in the mouse and, indeed, in most animals. The discovery of the technique for growing mouse embryonic stem cells led to technology called the "knockout mouse."

This is the way the knockout mouse works. If a scientist believes he or she has identified a possible candidate gene for a human disease, the disease-causing mutation for this particular gene can be cultured with mouse stem cells. Some of the mouse stem cells will pick up this mutated gene by a process called homologous recombination, and thus will carry this same gene defect. These mouse stem cells can then be injected into the blastocyst cavity of a normal mouse, where they become a part of the early inner cell mass of this mouse embryo, which can then develop into an adult mouse that has that gene defect. If the adult knockout mouse with this specific gene defect has the comparable human disease, then you have absolute proof that you've identified the specific genetic cause for the disease. The assay system of the knockout mouse, achievable only through this stem cell technology discovered by Evans and Kaufman in 1981, has saved countless lives already by allowing molecular biologists to define specific genes causing a variety of human illnesses.

### *Use of Stem Cells to Cure Human Disease*

Remember that normally, these embryonic stem cells (ES cells) form mixed-tissue tumors if they are not suppressed by being cultured in mitomycin-arrested, or irradiated, mouse-fibroblast feeder layers. Even human embryonic stem cells must be grown on these feeder layers of mouse cells, or else they simply differentiate (in an undirected, chaotic fashion) into mixed-tissue tumors. It is not as though you can simply take these embryonic stem cells and grow them into whatever replacement tissue you want, such as substantia nigra brain cells to cure Muhammad Ali's Parkinson's disease, or spinal-cord cells to cure quadriplegia, or pancreatic islet cells to cure insulin-requiring diabetes. We have no idea at the present moment how to direct these undifferentiated stem cells into truly organized tissue for curing human disease. Furthermore, there is every reason to suspect that if simply replaced back in humans, or allowed to grow in routine culture, they would do nothing but produce tumors.

When taken off of their feeder layers, ES cells will differentiate spontaneously into a multitude of cell types in a random, uncontrolled fashion. If you were to inject these ES cells into a mouse whose immune system is compromised, they would develop into mixed-tissue tumors called teratomas, representing all the different embryonic tissue types, but still not in a predictable fashion. There is only one way that ES cells can be used, even in the mouse, for gene therapy or tissue replacement, and that was alluded to when I briefly explained the use of the knockout mouse.

Remember, these ES cells thus far cannot be magically formed into a kidney, a heart, brain cells, or pancreatic cells, or fix a severed spinal cord. The only way that the stem cells can achieve their totipotential development is by injecting them into an existing blastocyst, where they mingle with the ICM cells within that blastocyst and become an integral part of that developing embryo (see fig. 18.4). The ES cells injected into the blastocyst cavity will find their way into every cell lineage in the adult that develops from that embryo — into every cell, into every tissue, into every organ of the body, and even into its sperm and eggs.

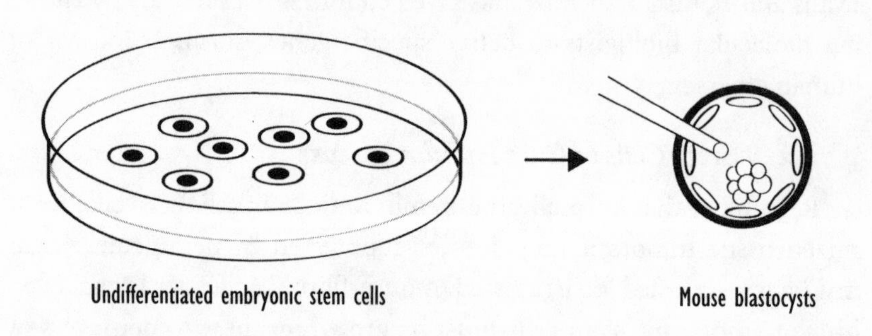


**FIGURE 18.4**

Cloned stem cells in which a gene defect has been repaired are injected into new mouse blastocysts.

So now you're probably scratching your head, wondering what good this does and how this can help us cure human disease. Stem cells can be used to correct disease-causing defective genes in much the same way as the mouse experiment in which they are used to create so-called knock-out mice. First, let me warn you that the only way stem cells can be of any benefit is by deriving them from an embryo cloned from the individual who has the disease you wish to cure. The ultimate goal would be to develop tissue that will not be rejected by the immune system of the person whose sickness you are trying to cure. Thus, stem cell therapy, if ever to work, is always going to be intricately associated with the concept of therapeutic, though not reproductive, cloning. With all the excitement and talk about the need for funding for stem cell research, scientists should be much clearer on this point because of the huge moral implications of using embryonic stem cell research for curing disease.

In fact, adult stem cells have already been used successfully for decades in humans to cure cancer. You can wipe out many widespread cancers by giving otherwise lethal doses of chemotherapy and radiation. These doses would be lethal because they destroy the blood-producing cells in your bone marrow that make your blood cells, and that control your immune system. For decades, oncologists have been able to solve this by replacing your destroyed bone marrow with bone marrow stem cells from a donor. These infused stem cells repopulate the cancer victim's body and accomplish two ends: (1) They replace the bone marrow stem cells of the patient that were destroyed by the massive doses of radiation and chemotherapy, and (2) they provide immune cells from a different person, the donor, that will attack any residual surviving cancer cells.

This long-established and successful form of adult stem cell therapy is often confused with the hype about embryonic stem cells. Embryonic stem cell therapy is just an illusion that will probably require years of basic animal research before it might (or might not) ever become a reality. The reason is that all cells in your body have some adult stem cells that are responsible for tissue renewal. Aside from the bone marrow, which is composed of just disorganized cells, most of the tissue of your body is extremely organized in an intricate fashion. We have no idea how either adult stem cells, or even embryonic cells, accomplish this organization. That is why if you try to infuse embryonic stem cells into animals, you just get mixed-tissue tumors. To try such infusions in humans would be absurd.

Stem cell therapy will work in only two possible ways: (1) an embryo from a diseased individual would have to be cloned to make stem cells. These stem cells would then have to be injected into blastocysts derived from standard IVF, which would then grow into healthy babies that could donate immune-compatible tissue to the diseased individual; or (2) adult stem cells (in contrast to embryonic stem cells) from the sick patient would have to be injected into blastocysts that would then develop into a baby whose tissue is compatible with that of the patient. The latter approach has fewer ethically explosive implications because no cloning is involved and no embryos are destroyed. These are the only two ways, at present, in which stem cells can be used for tissue replacement. Those who are morally against cloning embryos which will then be destroyed would prefer using adult stem cells as opposed to embryonic stem cells. But in either case, human IVF would be required, and in either case, a baby is being created just for the purpose of providing replacement tissue. The idea of using stem cells just to form into tissue-replacement cells is otherwise just far-fetched hype. In fact, we need much more animal research before even dreaming of doing intelligent research with human embryonic stem cells.

Korean stem cell researchers, however, have taken us a step closer to this goal. They have proven that even though creating a live cloned animal from adult cells is a rare event (almost all, if not all, cloned animals are abnormal, and most never even make it to birth), cloned stem cell lines from adults can be made relatively efficiently. It is even possible that new stem cell lines can be made for each new patient by injecting his nuclei into existing stem cells, which would completely avoid destroying embryos. The question is how these cloned stem cell lines might be used to cure the disease of the adults from whom they were derived.

Combining therapeutic cloning with gene therapy is the new frontier in treating genetic disorders, but overzealous and misapplied use in humans could be tragic. The dangerous nature of such an idea was borne out in 2001 when brain cells donated from aborted fetuses were transplanted into Parkinson's patients. The researchers hoped that these fetal cells (which would have otherwise gone to no use) could substitute for the deficient number of dopamine-secreting cells in the Parkinson's patient. Although these cells were not specifically derived from cloned cells of the sick patients, and immune problems would have to be treated with antirejection medicines, the immune problems did not turn out to be the reason these experiments in humans failed utterly. In about 15 percent of the patients, the transplanted dopamine-secreting cells grew very well, and they were not rejected by the patient's immune system. In those cases, however, there ensued an uncontrolled oversecretion of dopamine, so that the Parkinson's patients were completely unable to control their movements. They writhed with constant, jerky tremors that were much worse than those caused by the original Parkinson's disease. These same side affects can be caused by an overdose of the Parkinson's drug L-dopa, but at least the dose can be reduced. But in this situation there was no way to remove or deactivate the transplanted cells.

This was a severe blow to what had been considered a highly promising approach for treating Parkinson's disease, Alzheimer's, and other neurodegenerative diseases. The same problem will come up with any effort to use embryonic stem cells to create tissue in a dish and then use that replacement tissue to cure disease. It is the organization of these differentiated cells in the brain, or in the heart, or wherever the tissue replacement has to be done, that is so complicated and completely beyond our current understanding. Simply injecting these differentiated replacement cells into an organ is not going to ensure any sort of proper organized development. The uncontrollable movements in the Parkinson's patients mentioned above was reported to be "absolutely devastating." They chewed constantly, their fingers went up and down, their wrists flexed and distended, and they jerked their heads and flung their arms out in a completely uncontrollable way. Despite prior ad hoc reports of spectacular results and miraculous cures, this careful NIH-funded study demonstrated just how far we are from any cure for these patients. Furthermore, in those who did not have this disastrous side affect of oversecretion of dopamine, there was no improvement whatsoever compared to control Parkinson's patients. So the problem is not only with the generation of tissue that can be used for replacement in disease, but rather with the organization of that tissue in a properly functioning fashion.

However, stem cell and cloning technology could possibly be the most likely avenue to curing genetically lethal hematologic diseases caused by gene mutations in children or adults who would otherwise die. In chapter 13 we talked about a little girl who was dying of a condition called Fanconi's anemia, in which she could not make blood cells. Her parents underwent IVF (with PGD) to have another baby not only to make sure that the next baby did not have the mutated Fanconi genes, but also to ensure that the new baby would be a good HLA tissue match for their dying daughter. They gave birth to a healthy baby without

Fanconi's disease who was a perfect tissue match for their dying daughter just in time for the doctors to perform a bone-marrow transplant to save their daughter's life. Therapeutic cloning and stem cell technology have now been shown in mice to be able to accomplish a similar result for a limitless variety of genetic diseases.

Let me close this section by summarizing an amazing study from Rudolf Jaenisch's lab at the Whitehead Institute at MIT (which is right next door to David Page's lab, where our male-infertility genomics are performed). First published in 2002 in *Cell,* this landmark mouse study will be the model for all successful human gene therapy in the future. The Boston researchers took immune-deficient mice called RAG 2 and cloned them by injecting tail-tip donor cells into enucleated donor eggs using the Honolulu technique. These cloned embryos were then cultured to blastocyst stage, and the ICM cells moved into cultures of mouse embryonic fibroblasts to make embryonic stem cells that were genetically identical to the immune-deficient adult mice. These embryonic stem cells derived from nuclear transfer behaved like all embryonic stem cells in that when they were injected into another embryo they penetrated into every cell tissue type of that developing embryo. Remember, injecting stem cells into an adult is problematic, but when they are injected into a blastocyst, they develop normally. Gene defects can be repaired or created in these embryonic stem cells by culturing them in the presence of appropriate genes using homologous recombination, a process that automatically occurs within the stem cell culture. That is the basis of all knockout mouse studies.

The genetic defect of the RAG 2 mice embryonic stem cells was "repaired" by culture with a normal gene. These genetically repaired embryonic stem cells were then transferred into otherwise normal blastocysts that did not have an inner cell mass. (Actually, this is a rather complex process developed at the Whitehead Institute called tetraploid embryo complementation, for which I am only giving a vastly simplified description.) All of the cells of this embryo were entirely derived from the repaired embryonic stem cells. Thus, viable, healthy, fertile mice, genetically identical to the immune-deficient mouse but having the proper gene to correct that immune deficiency, were born. These mice that were derived from the repaired embryonic stem cells were then used as otherwise genetically identical tissue donors for the original diseased mice, resulting in a complete cure of their immune deficiency.

Thus, unlike PGD, in which an embryo can be selected and will result in a baby that can be a reasonable tissue match to cure a dying child, an absolutely identical tissue match in these mice could be created, in which the specific gene defect has been repaired.

Once these researchers proved that the genetically repaired stem cells could result in a genetically normal mouse that is otherwise a clone of the diseased mouse, they went a step further. They tried to get these stem cells to differentiate in vitro into blood-producing cells, and to skip the step of making a new mouse that could be used as a donor. However, these cells were able to colonize the bone marrow of the diseased mouse only slightly. Thus, therapy using this approach is still a long way off.

No legitimate scientist or physician has any interest in cloning human beings or in destroying life. But the knockout mouse technology and stem cells developed in the 1980s, along with modern IVF, carry great hope for the cure of human genetic disease. The infertile couple going through IVF may be confused by all the hype in the press over unused frozen embryos and the need for stem cell research. In fact, there are very few unused frozen human embryos, and we lack the basic understanding of cell differentiation and dedifferentiation that would be required for stem cell therapy or therapeutic cloning. Thus, regardless of any political or religious debate, what is most needed to bring relief to human disease via stem cells is basic research in animal models such as the mouse. For the infertile couple, the misleading hype that their embryos may be used to help paraplegics walk again is regrettable. But IVF, which has completely weathered more than twenty-five years of moral debate, is clearly an established therapy and will continue to bring joy and family into countless modern lives.

# Index

# About the Author

Sherman Silber, M.D. is an internationally renowned pioneer in infertility treatment and is considered one of the world's leading authorities on IVF, sperm retrieval, ICSI, vasectomy reversal, tubal ligation reversal, egg and embryo freezing, and the reproductive biological clock. He has contributed major scientific breakthroughs to our understanding of sperm production, and the successful treatment of the severest forms of male and female sterility. He performed the world's first microsurgical vasectomy reversal, as well as the first testicle transplant and the world's first ovary transplant. He developed, along with his Brussels colleagues, the TESE-ICSI technique, achieving normal pregnancy rates in otherwise hopelessly sterile men. Dr. Silber is the medical director of the Infertility Center of St. Louis at St. Luke's Hospital in St. Louis, Missouri, one of the most successful high tech programs in the world for couples with severe infertility problems. He has treated many thousands of infertile couples who travel to St. Louis daily from all over the world. His patients come from every state in the U.S.A., Europe, South America, the Middle East, Asia, and Africa. His patients include doctors, teachers, rock stars, politicians, astronauts, movie stars, scientists, truck drivers, lawyers, migrant fruit pickers, CEO's, princes and kings.

The author of three medical textbooks and more than 250 scientific papers on human fertility and reproduction, Dr. Silber is also a popular guest speaker and has appeared numerous times on *Oprah,* the *Today* show, *Good Morning America,* ABC's *World News Tonight, Nightline,* and many other national programs.

In addition, he is a professor and scientific collaborator at NYU in New York and at MIT in Cambridge, Massachusetts. He is widely sought as a lecturer at national and international medical meetings. Visit his Web site at www.infertile.com.

# About the Author